*f*P

ALSO BY MICHAEL F. ROIZEN AND MEHMET C. OZ

YOU: Having a Baby

YOU: Being Beautiful

YOU: Staying Young

YOU: On a Diet

YOU: The Smart Patient

YOU: The Owner's Manual

ALSO BY MICHAEL F. ROIZEN

The RealAge Workout:
Maximum Health, Minimum Work

The RealAge Makeover:
Take Years off Your Looks and Add Them to Your Life

Cooking the RealAge Way:
Turn Back Your Biological Clock with More Than 80 Delicious and Easy Recipes

The RealAge Diet: Make Yourself Younger with What You Eat

RealAge: Are You as Young as You Can Be?

ALSO BY MEHMET C. OZ

Healing from the Heart:
A Leading Surgeon Combines Eastern and Western Traditions
to Create the Medicine of the Future

YOU

Raising Your Child

MICHAEL F. ROIZEN, M.D.
AND MEHMET C. OZ, M.D.

with Ted Spiker, Ellen Rome, M.D., Craig Wynett, Lisa Oz,

Linda G. Kahn, and Nancy J. Roizen, M.D.

Illustrations by Gary Hallgren

FREE PRESS

NEW YORK LONDON TORONTO SYDNEY

Free Press
A Division of Simon & Schuster, Inc.
1230 Avenue of the Americas
New York, NY 10020

First Free Press hardcover edition October 2010

FREE PRESS and colophon are trademarks of Simon & Schuster, Inc.

For information about special discounts for bulk purchases, please contact
Simon & Schuster Special Sales at 1-866-506-1949 or business@simonandschuster.com.

The Simon & Schuster Speakers Bureau can bring authors to your live event.
For more information or to book an event contact the Simon & Schuster
Speakers Bureau at 1-866-248-3049 or visit our website at www.simonspeakers.com.

Designed by Mspace/Maura Fadden Rosenthal

Manufactured in the United States of America.

1   3   5   7   9   10   8   6   4   2

Library of Congress Cataloging-in-Publication Data
Roizen, Michael F.
You, raising your child : the owner's manual from first breath to first grade /
Michael F. Roizen and Mehmet C. Oz.
      p.   cm.
1. Child development—Popular works.   2. Child rearing—Popular works.   I. Oz, Mehmet, 1960–   II. Title.
RJ131.R62 2010
618.92—dc22
2010018092
ISBN 978-1-5011-1241-6
ISBN 978-1-4391-2783-4 (ebook)

NOTE TO READERS

CONTENTS

YOU

Raising Your Child

INTRODUCTION

Whether your child is an infant or a toddler, performing puppet shows at preschool or using your belly as a trampoline, we know how hard it can be to pry your eyes off your little one. Babies are as mesmerizing as they are miraculous, so it's easy to lose yourself in your adorable, sweet, gas-blasting bundle of beauty. When your infant graduates to being a little more mobile, perhaps you'll have a radar lock on him for other reasons, such as to prevent a monkey-bar mishap or to stop him from dunking your iPhone in his iCereal. So we appreciate that you've taken a moment to take a look elsewhere, and we suspect that one of the driving forces that has directed your attention to this book is that you have a big question: one that both excites you *and* scares the diaper decorations out of you.

How will my baby turn out?

Good question. How *will* your baby turn out?

As a parent or a parent-to-be, you've probably run through a couple thousand different life scenarios: Will he be healthy? Smart? Polite? Will she reach all of her milestones on time? Will she turn into a modern Mozart? Will he be able to throw a ball sixty yards? Will she be a good citizen? Will he grow up to be a CEO or have trouble holding a job? An everyday hero or a smack-talking punk? A selfless volunteer who wants to change a little bit of the world or the latest reality-show knucklehead? Will she grow up to find her soul mate, or, as someone else put it so nicely, will she have enough sense to know that if he likes her, he shoulda put a ring on it?

Some of these big-picture questions may not be easy to think about—especially during a time when you may be feeling such powerful feelings as love, joy, or even stress—but they are indeed the kinds of issues that will keep you up at night (more so than you already are).

Of course, it's convenient to credit (or blame) the genetic life force (aka DNA) for providing our children's biological and psychological blueprint for life. But more and more research indicates that the real life force that escorts children to their destiny has less to do with DNA and more to do with . . .

You.

Now, we don't mean "you" in the blue-eyes, big-feet genetic sense of the word, but in a much different way: how your behaviors, actions, principles, and all of the overt and subtle things you do as a parent shape the environment in which your child grows up.

That's right. This is a book about children's health, but it's as much about you as it is about your boy or girl.

In *YOU: Raising Your Child*, you'll get our best information and advice on all of the nuts-and-bolts issues that are important to handling the challenges of parenting. We'll teach you about allergies, infections, safety, nutrition, and the many things that you can do to help keep your child healthy.

But if this book were just an A-to-Z guide that listed everything from asthma to zoo animal obsession, then we'd close up shop and direct you to the nearest encyclopedic medical website. This book is more than a problem-solution guide. It's a book that will teach you how to be a smart parent.

What does that mean?

Many of us parent by instinct, and that approach works well much of the time. Smart parenting, in addition, is really about conscious decision making: selecting choices based on what we feel is best for our children in the short term and the long term. (Decision making starts from day one: Breast feed or bottle feed? Which vaccines and when? You'll see our take on the vaccine issue starting on page 392.) Many smart parents like to think of parenting as a "reverse engineering" process—that is, always keeping the end goal in sight. But we also realize that everybody has limited time and resources, so our book is also about balance, as we try to relieve some of the stress of parenting and also give you the essentials.

Ultimately, our goal is to teach you how to create the optimal environment for your child: an environment that's most conducive to your child thriving in all areas of life physically, emotionally, socially, and developmentally. Why? Because the latest research shows us that the environment—as defined not only by physical space but also by the behaviors of parents and other caregivers—is the number one determinant of your child's future in all of these realms.

In this book, which covers child health and development from birth to about age five, you're going to learn about cutting-edge research and a variety of developmental approaches. Among all of us on the authorship team, we've had fourteen children, and two of us are pediatricians—including one who's a full-time developmental pediatrician. So we've spent much of our personal and professional lives thinking and caring about the very same issues as you. A lot has changed since the days of Dr. Benjamin Spock—in terms of how the world works, the challenges of parenting that your parents didn't face, and what we've discovered about how a child's mind and body develop. You'll learn that kids are like dolphins (both *ping* their needs to their parents). You'll learn that some of the best parenting lessons are taught by children (they subtly send messages about where their skills, talents, and desires lie). You'll learn that kids actually learn *more* by doing *less* (cool brain section up ahead!). You'll learn that children are like mirrors (their brains are, actually), reflecting behavior that you, their caregivers, and other influential people in their lives model.★ And you'll learn that the most powerful messages you send your kids—from day one all the way up to day 6,574†—may involve absolutely no words at all.

We'll teach you about these amazing insights the best way we know how—through biology. Ultimately, all of these lessons do come down to biology, even the

---

★ That's actually one of the reasons why children raised in the same family can be so different; not only do you change the way you parent with subsequent children, but the environment changes, as well.

† That's eighteen years (including four days for leap years). Add another day if the child is born in 2007, 2011, or 2015.

ones that you wouldn't necessarily think would, like behavior. After all, we've always believed that explaining "why" can make the "what to do" much, much easier.

Along the way, we're going to ask you to join in a game of pretend, as you assume a metaphorical role as river guide (see Figure Intro.1). See, the way we think about child development—and smart parenting—is to imagine a child's journey through life as a boat ride down a long, often unpredictable river. You, as the guide, help control the direction and speed, while your youngster sits back and takes in everything around him (including watching you, so that he can eventually learn to paddle or steer on his own). This analogy, we hope, will help you understand parenting on several levels:

○ **Consider the boat that is your child's genetics.** Everyone is shaped a little bit differently, and that plays a role in how you can navigate the river, but it's hardly the only factor that determines the quality of your trip together.

○ **Your paddle really serves as your own behaviors, actions, and words.** It helps you steer the boat in terms of where you go and what your passenger sees. You can bring your boat to a standstill, you might crash into a rock and get stuck, you can choose which path (of many) the boat takes, you can go fast when needed and slow down when you need a break. You, for much of the time, are in control. But the biggest lesson of all when it comes to paddling is this: Sometimes you don't need to paddle at all to get where you want to go. In fact, there is such a thing as overpaddling—trying so hard to do right that you actually send your vessel in the wrong direction. Lots of times, you're better off going with the flow. Our mantra: Parent smart, not hard.

○ **The river represents the environment in which your child lives.** Sometimes there's rough water, and sometimes there's calm water. Sometimes you have a wide river with lots of choices of where to steer a boat and sometimes, in narrow sections, you just have to ride the rapids. The bottom line is that no matter how expert a guide you are, the environment has a bigger impact on you and your youngster's ride together than anything else. One of the great lessons we learn from traveling the river is that the easiest places to travel are the channels that are well worn and well traveled, and you'll encounter windows of opportunity in which to find those easy-to-navigate places. Your child will actually help direct you there.

⊃ **Your boat carries all the equipment you'll need.** You have maps to help you predict rough waters ahead ("I want to get a tattoo!" announces your daughter). And you have life vests, too, in case you run into some trouble. Both of them come in the various support systems that you already have and will develop en route, including your partner, friends, extended family, doctors, and even the internet, books, and other resources that can help you navigate a river that many before you already have voyaged successfully.

⊃ **The destination?** Well, those are all the traits, skills, attitudes, emotions, and behaviors that make up the person your son or daughter eventually becomes. As you can guess by now, your child's destination depends greatly on which path you take and how you lead the way—not by your words, but by your actions. But a big lesson we'll be exploring is that what you want for your child might not be right for her, so it's so important that you learn to read her signals and help her go where she naturally wants to go.

⊃ **Your ultimate goal as guide is to teach your passenger enough about the river so that she can eventually take the helm.** This handing-off process starts very early (think toilet training), and culminates when your passenger has attained all the skills necessary to be her own guide: how to make important decisions, how to be calm and confident in the face of adversity, and how to live a productive, satisfying, independent life. If all goes well, she'll be giving you a ride about two decades from now.

Since you're reading this, chances are that you've already embarked upon your river ride. Think of this book as one of your river maps, helping you plan the itinerary that will lead you and your child to your desired destination. Two qualities make for exceptional river guides: experience and knowledge. While you may or may not have the experience of parenting, we believe that this book can help you with the

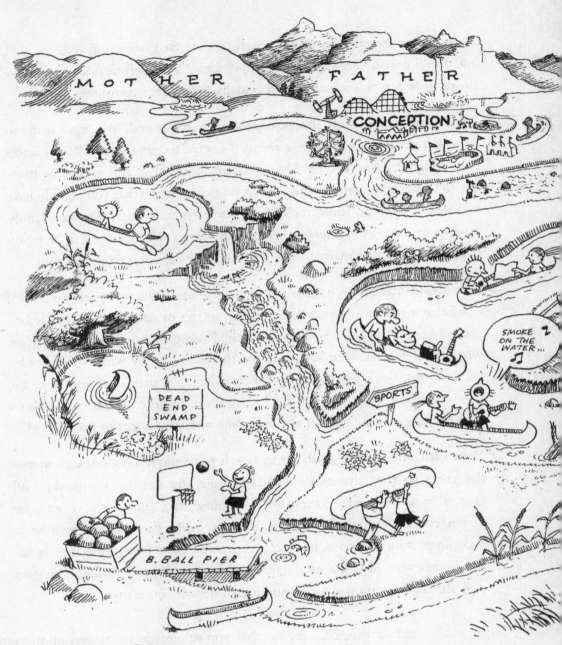

Figure Intro.1 **River of Dreams** As a parent, think of your role as river guide as you help steer your passenger down life's rapids, around rocks, and through gentle streams. These paths are not predestined; you have the ability to help your child find her strengths by creating an environment that allows her to thrive and enjoy all this journey has to offer.

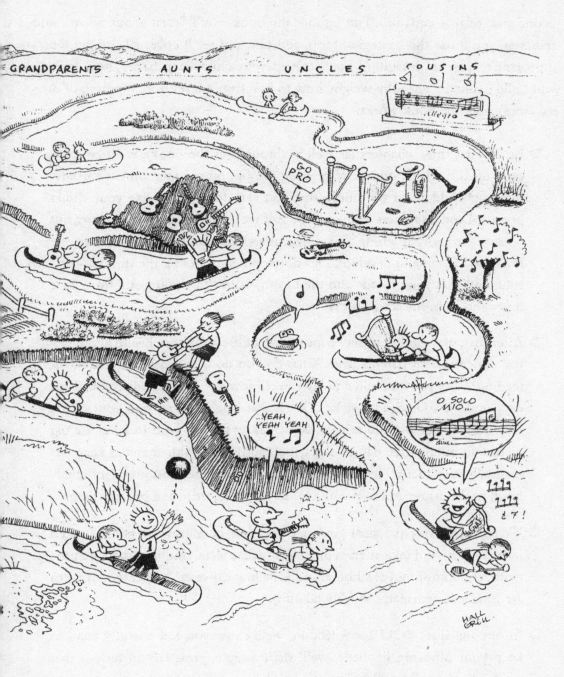

second part of that equation. Throughout the book, you'll learn about science and strategies, you'll use the strategies, tools, and tips, and we'll cover all the big topics important to parents, including how to help your child sleep better, how to help your child maintain a healthy weight, how to best treat a fever, and hundreds of others. Here's how the book works:

- In the first three chapters (as well as throughout the book), we'll concentrate on this whole notion of creating the optimum environment for raising your child—and the things that you can do to maximize your child's potential and happiness. It may seem as if we're dabbling in psychology, but what we're really teaching you is neurology: that is, the science of how the brain best learns and develops. This development relies on the stimuli (environment) that you provide and the healthy habits that you instill from your heart and from the start.

- After that, we're going to move into more of the hard-core health and medical concerns that parents have. What do you do if you have trouble breast feeding? Why is your child a picky eater? How do you treat allergies? What do you do if your child is sick? What is that bright red rash on your child's rear end? As doctors and as parents, we know that it's hard to keep the big picture in mind when day-to-day tribulations and health anxieties keep demanding your focus. This book takes you through the most prevalent childhood health issues and tells you how to diagnose, treat, and prevent them.

- We'll also provide practical guidance on some decisions and actions you'll have to make and take, such as picking a pediatrician, finding a day care program, childproofing your home, and installing car seats (80 percent of them are installed incorrectly, so it's vital info).

- In our signature YOU Tools section, we'll show you kid-friendly ways to keep your offspring in shape, we'll share simple, great-tasting recipes that your whole family will enjoy, and we'll summarize the various points of view about the hotly debated topic of vaccines. First-time parents will find our YOU Tool for newborns especially helpful; there we'll offer info on diapering, feeding, sleeping, bathing, and all the other mysteries of caring for an infant.

⊃ Our YOU Plan gives an overview of critical developmental milestones you can expect (but not obsess over, please), as well as some tips and tricks that will make the various stages from birth to age five a little bit easier. Think of it as the pocket version of our detailed map—good for a quick glance when you're in a hurry or need a refresher.

⊃ In our appendix, we'll cover issues that may be important to some of you, such as multiple births, nontraditional families, and a handful of specialized health concerns such as autism and attention deficit/hyperactivity disorder, or ADHD.

We know, we know. So exciting, so titillating, so promising that you can't wait to jump right in and devour dozens of pages on the fine art of applying cream to a diaper rash or teaching manners (not to mention the much more big-picture topics). But before you begin, we want to introduce you to a few high-altitude thoughts about parenting*—the recurrent themes that, while perhaps not front and center every day, should be on your radar screen as you undertake the greatest job in the world. Call them the YOU Parenting Principles, if you will:

Parenting = Complex

In life, there are some problems that have an easy solution:

Infection X + Medicine Y = Healthy U

When it comes to parenting, we'd like it to work that way, too. But parenting can be a little bit like intense detective work, in that there's not always a clear solution to whatever mystery you happen to encounter. See, in life, there are three differ-

---

* Did you know that parenting seems to lower your blood pressure? One of the many benefits, for sure.

ent kinds of problems: the simple (like baking a cake, where you follow a recipe), the complicated (like sending a rocket to the moon, where you use lots of teams to overcome the many challenges, but once you've succeeded, you know how to do it in the future), and the complex (like raising a child—it's always a moving target, with innumerable nuances and factors that make every situation different). Because parenting is complex, there isn't always a steadfast right or wrong way to do it; instead there may be stronger and weaker ways, but you also have to make decisions based on the unique qualities of your child. And that's what we're really after here—helping you learn about child development so you can understand the complexities and adjust for them along the way.

Parenting = Modeling

No two ways about it. You're a role model: a behavior model, an eating model, and an everything-else model. You'll learn in the first part of the book that the main way that children learn isn't through the words you use (the "do as I say"), but through your actions (the "do as I do"). We know this through the biology of mirror neurons, which we'll discuss in chapter 3. And it should serve as a guiding principle for you. For your child to be healthy, *you* need to be, too—not just in what you eat but also in areas such as your relationships with others and how you treat yourself. Kids learn more through what they observe than through what you tell them. Think of that next time you try to text while you're driving or lash out at someone with a series of bleepin' bleeps.

Parenting = Moving to the Middle

For lots of things in life, we're taught the superlative rules: Be the best, the greatest, the most amazing. Parenting shouldn't be about that. A lot of science shows that the two extremes of parenting are actually the most destructive to a child's development. While it's no surprise that having an absentee parent who gives a child no attention isn't healthy, the 180-degree turn is also bad. An adult who overparents—scheduling every waking moment or leashing your child to your body so he never gets to climb the playground equipment, for instance—can actually hinder development. (See why in chapter 1.) It's better to be somewhere in the middle, where you're giving your child enough attention but also knowing that exploration and independence are crucial to his learning. Here's the deep thought of the day: You can be the greatest parent in the world by not being the greatest parent in the world.

Parenting = A 3-D Experience

Doesn't matter if you don't sport glasses with red and blue lenses, the real trick to smart parenting is to provide a multisensory experience for your kid. You've heard that a child's brain is like a sponge, so you need to make the biggest mess you can. Spill everything: words, sounds, tastes, colors, shapes, smells, the world! As you do this, you'll find that your child will communicate (sometimes subtly) her preferences. Those clues will help you nudge her in the directions in which (1) she has the most interest, and (2) she has the most potential for success (very much related to her innate interest). Now, this doesn't mean that you overwhelm your child (see "Parenting = Moving to the Middle"), but it does mean that you are making an effort to satisfy all of your child's sensory needs.

Parenting = Challenging Genetics, Changing Genetics

One of the big notions that we'll be exploring in just a few pages is the new field of epigenetics. No doubt, you know about genetics. The union of Mom and Dad is what determines the genetic makeup of child. There's a lot to be said about how both physical and personality traits seem to come directly from parents. But cutting-edge information about pregnancy and child development demonstrates that we have the ability to change the way genes express themselves (or influence our traits), starting as early as in utero. Therefore, a child isn't necessarily tied to the actions of the DNA that she's born with. You can actually change how that works by adjusting what you expose your child to—you can turn genes on or off. So you play a crucial role in shaping the way that your child develops regarding everything from personality and behavior to his future health. Incredible indeed. You can change your child's life by changing the way his genes function. And you know what it all boils down to? You got it: the environment.

And that's really what *YOU: Raising Your Child* is all about. We're going to help you create the environment that allows your child to learn, to grow, and to be healthy and happy. This environment, as you now know, has as much to do with the river itself as the way you navigate it.

So grab your paddle and hop in.

After all, this ride *is* the ride of your life, and, believe us, your child is ready to go.

1

Let 'Em Grow, Let 'Em Grow, Let 'Em Grow

Establish the Best Environment Early On to Help Your Child Thrive in All Areas of Life

Even if you're new to parenting and haven't spent all that much time around children, you surely can think back to your own childhood and remember that there are as many kinds of kids as there are lotto-number combos. The princess-loving kids, the dinosaur-loving kids, the musical kids, the athletic kids, the kids who could dance in diapers the minute mom cranked the tunes, the kids who could read before they were even off the breast, the kids who could toot at a lion's-roar decibel level, the kids who were afraid of anything with four, eight, or one hundred legs. We could go on and on (more than we already have), and please don't take offense if we missed the kind of kid you were. (*Saved by the Bell* addict, were ya?)

We suspect that you get the point: One of the most wonderful things in all of life is that children are the crayons in the world's biggest box of Crayolas, so many different colors, and all beautiful in their own way.

That's part of the reason why we're here: to celebrate those differences and to help you nurture the unique qualities that make your child so fascinating.

That said, the reason you're reading this book, we imagine, is that there are certain aspects of parenting that you want to make sure you're doing the right way; the so-called normal way, the healthy way. Thankfully, you've come to the right place. Based on some common biology that most children share, we're going to talk about how you can create the ideal environment for all dimensions of your child's development.

By environment, we don't mean how you've prepared the nursery but how you've prepared yourself to meet the challenges and frustrations of parenthood. For nine months, a mother was the child's literal environment; now that he's breathing air, the parent is still the center of his universe (and we bet you thought it was the other way around). The toys you choose, the food you prepare, the music you play, as well as the emotions and attitudes you bring to your interactions with your child, influence how he is wired. We're not just talking metaphorically; we're talking about those two little twisty wires that inhabit every cell of the human body. Yep, you guessed it: DNA. So sit back and enjoy the *YOU* explanation of the most mysterious and wondrous process we can think of—how two single cells grow into your cute, smart, and mostly lovable little being.

Environmental Affairs: Nature or Nurture?

Above all the things that you will learn in this book, memorize this one: It's not the genes she was dealt that primarily control how your child will develop as much as it is how she manages the environment you create for her.

Translation: Child development is part nature and part nurture. But in a street fight, nurture whips nature upside its head, smacks it on its rear, and throws in a few yo-momma jokes for good measure.

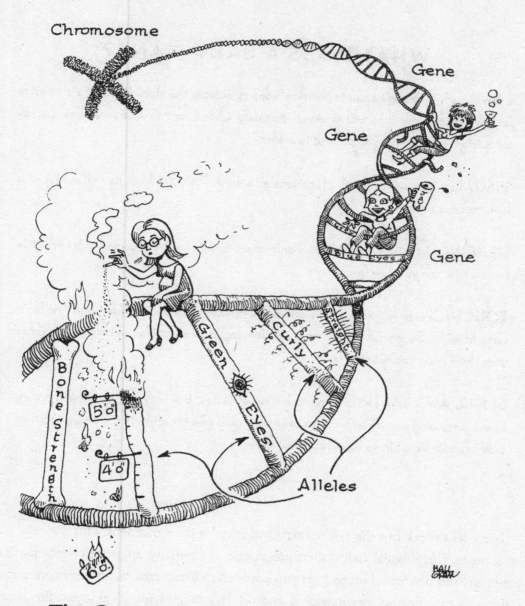

Figure 1.1 **The Gene Scene** It's easy to assume that your child is simply an adorable concoction of two sets of DNA. While true biologically, this doesn't mean that your child comes preprogrammed to be the person he will be. The field of epigenetics teaches us that the way genes function can actually change depending on actions you take, actions your child takes, and, ultimately, the environment in which your child grows up.

WHAT DOES A BABY WANT?

Even though they can't express their opinions right from the start, babies have already formed quite a few likes and dislikes—especially when it comes to having their senses stimulated. Here's what babies tend to prefer:

VISUAL: Infants will fixate on a face soon after birth. They like faces as well as toys with high-contrast patterns.

HEARING: Infants immediately recognize their mother's voice and tend to be sensitive to very high and very low frequencies.

TOUCH: Skin-to-skin contact stimulates the release of oxytocin, a hormone that facilitates bonding. So even if you're not breast feeding, it's a good idea to hold your child to your chest while you're bottle feeding.

SMELL AND TASTE: Infants prefer sweet tastes, but they can distinguish among sweet, bitter, and sour. (Fun fact: Two-day-old babies who breast-feed can distinguish their mother's milk from others based on smell alone.)

Now, let's break out the white coats and goggles for a moment. This concept has its roots in a biological field called epigenetics. Essentially, epigenetics tells us that genes have to be turned on to give you particular characteristics, and environmental influences can flip those switches on and off. In other words, it's not just the genes you pass on to your children that make them who they are, but the expression of those genes—and you have some mighty powerful control over that (see Figure 1.1). Early epigenetic research showed that some of a mom's actions and behaviors during pregnancy may cause epigenetic changes in a developing fetus; for example, smoking during pregnancy leads to changes that result in the way genes express themselves, resulting in such traits as small stature and even attention problems. More recent research tells us that epigenetic changes can happen all the time—not only in the womb but also after your baby is born—indeed, throughout life. Your environment steers your genes to operate in a certain way, predisposing you to certain illnesses, as well as to various behaviors, habits, and personality traits.

When we talk about the influence of the environment here, we're not just talking about exposure to smoke or other toxins. Something as intangible as a mother's parenting style can even affect how a child's DNA is expressed. This is not fluff or BS (bad science), but proven fact. Just one example from animal research: When baby rats receive less licking and grooming from their mothers than their siblings do, they mature to become more fearful and reactive to stress than their siblings who are raised with more licking and grooming. That isn't a genetic trait but, rather, an epigenetic one. Given the same DNA, less attention and more stress leads to a more fearful life for the individual.

Epigenetics isn't the only way that environment affects a youngster's development. Another means is what we call the "learning landscape." Not too long ago, it was believed that the mind developed independently of anything other than genetic signals; your ability to learn was simply a formula based on genes from Mom plus genes from Pop. It has become clear, however, that it's not just genes that dictate mental, emotional, and intellectual development. Instead the mind relies on the environment to give clues and signals about how it's supposed to develop and what it's supposed to learn. It's the landscape that you create around your child that influences how he or she learns.*

Think about it: Could you learn to swim, ice-skate, or ride a bike only from a book? Of course not; you need feedback from the environment, filtered through your body, to train your mind. A kid won't learn to play piano if he just knows the notes on paper. He has to feel and hear his environment to learn the skill.

In addition to providing a stimulating physical environment for learning, you can influence your child's learning by the emotional environment you create. If you sigh

---

* Researchers call this concept "embodied cognition"—that is, your ability to learn, memorize, and function is at least partially based on your physical interaction with the environment around you.

STRANGER THINGS HAVE HAPPENED

Right from the start, a baby knows the difference between family and strangers, and at about six to nine months, a child can actually develop fear of being touched or picked up by a stranger. "Stranger anxiety" doesn't happen in all babies, and it typically subsides by the time a child is about two years old.

heavily when your child asks you to toss a ball outside, you're less likely to raise the next Derek Jeter than if you leap from your La-Z-Boy recliner with enthusiasm. In the jungle, when Momma Monkey jumps away *fast* from a snake, that behavior is learned immediately by Baby Monkey, without the need for repetition. Here the emotional context created by the mother (stress, fear) signals to her baby that this info is of primo importance for survival, and the baby responds by locking it in posthaste.

So this new logic tells us that our minds and our environment are not independent—that we develop in a certain way, that we learn things in a certain way, that we become who we are in a certain way *because of the environment we're in.* This is especially important when it comes to kids because their minds are expanding at light speed as they gain the knowledge and skills they need to navigate the world around them.

Now, the point of this is not to dismiss the notion of genetics entirely. Without a doubt, children are born with a certain temperament. In fact, about 20 percent of kids are born with what's called a "high-reactive" temperament. That means they're likely to be startled by unfamiliar things, or they're very shy, or they tend to get scared of things like clowns or the dark. (As the children get older, this trait can develop into full-blown anxiety or depression.) These kids are certainly wired a bit differently. Their amygdalas—the almond-shaped region in the brain that deals with emotion—are overly active, even hyperactive (see Figure 1.2). So these children react emotionally to all kinds of triggers. This is not always a bad thing: Hypervigilance can also lead to being conscientious, punctual, and exerting great self-control. The environment in which a high-reactive child is raised can tip the balance one way or the other; for example, giving encouragement and support can make a shy child feel more comfortable and help bring him out of his shell, whereas dismissing his fears or pushing him beyond his comfort zone can make him want to retreat back into it. The bottom line is, even though there is some hard-core genetic wiring underlying the development of the mind, environment can influence genetic predisposition.

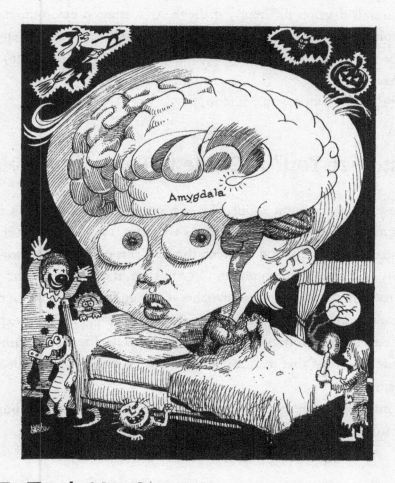

Figure 1.2 **To Teach His Own** One of the emotional centers of our brain, the amygdala, helps children learn by forming emotional attachments to information they process—whether good, bad, scary, or silly. That's an important lesson for all parents: If you want to teach your child and maintain his interest, you need to tickle the learning centers of his brain.

If you incorporate this concept of environmental influence into our river analogy, you will see how it easily makes sense. The way you might navigate a river depends to a certain degree on your boat (DNA) but even more so on whether it's a slow-moving stream or crazy rapids. You make different decisions and take different actions depending on what kind of environment you're in moment by moment, and that changes the kind of ride you have along the river of life.* Same holds true for kids: Their minds develop differently if they're in a stressed environment, a stimulating environment, a protective environment—any different kind of environment. Their minds also develop differently depending on how (or how often) that environment changes.

And that's exactly where you come in.

Who Are You? A Guide to Parenting Styles

Okay, so now you know a bit about why environment is such a key factor in how your child's mind develops over the years. As we again return to our river metaphor, it's easy to make the comparison between the elements of a river's environment and the elements of a child's environment. On the river, it's the rate of the rapids, the number of rocks in the way, the tree branches that'll guillotine you if you don't duck; in other words, as in life, it's a combination of the expected and the unexpected. For the child, it's everything from his home and his toys to his friends and family. They're all part of the landscape that determines how easy or difficult it will be for him to reach his destination.

But the most important element in determining how your child's boat will run the river of life is his river guide: you.

---

* If you allow us one more image to reinforce the point of environmental influence, listen to this: It used to be believed that in countries where people ride elephants, the guide's instructions controlled the direction of the elephant. But now it's theorized that it's the elephant who really dictates direction, and the guide's mind quickly rationalizes that decision. It's an example of matter controlling the mind, rather than mind controlling matter.

MIND YOUR OWN MIND

Odd as it may seem, one of the most significant features in your child's environment is *your* state of mind. Between 10 percent and 20 percent of mothers of newborns are affected by postpartum depression (not to mention the "baby blues," a milder form of depression that affects the majority of new moms), while one-third of moms with preschoolers also suffer from depression. As you might imagine, a depressed mom has a huge impact on a child's environment. Fewer than 20 percent of women with depression actually talk to their doc about it, but they should! It's also important for women to turn to friends and loved ones for emotional and social support. These networks will help you combat depression and the blues, which ultimately influence not just you but your entire family. When mothers are depressed, they may be physically present but neither emotionally nor psychologically available. Babies of depressed mothers may develop infantile depression and engage less with people and their environment. In the extreme, they may even fall off the growth curve. Children of chronically depressed moms may have difficulty forming close relationships throughout life. Also, children with depressed moms may be drowsy, passive, more temperamentally difficult, irritable, less able to tolerate separation, and more afraid or more anxious than children of nondepressed mothers. Because depressed moms don't talk as much to their babies, don't use "motherese," and are less responsive to their babies' cues, these children can experience language delays as well. The good news: Symptoms in children can be reversed if maternal depression is treated. Visit the website for Postpartum Support International (www.postpartum.net) for more info.

Until your child is old enough to hold a paddle and strong enough to navigate life's currents on his own, the job is yours. How you decide to manage the currents of childhood and parenthood is absolutely the number one environmental contributor to overall child development.

Our goal in this book is simple. We want to make it easy for you to set your course and go with the flow, rather than feel like you're paddling upstream. We're going to help you find the best paddle, and we'll help you choose the best route for

CRAZY CONFLICT

What happens when arguments get amped up a few decibel levels? It's not good—not only for the adults involved but also for the kids who are watching. So-called adverse childhood events (like witnessing abuse or domestic violence) have horrible long-term effects on children. While you may not want to rock the boat or paddle upstream because it seems too hard to get out of a bad situation, the consequences for your child are devastating if you stay in an abusive relationship. If you won't make a change for yourself, do it for your child's current and future health and happiness.

you: smooth sailing if that's your preference, or a safe white-water experience if you're more adventurous. In either case, the goal is to raise a child who is secure and skilled enough that you can eventually hand the paddle over to him to practice a few strokes here and there and, ultimately, to take total control for himself.

So where do we start? With a question that you need to answer now and reassess every so often during your parenting journey:

What kind of parent are you?

Yeah, yeah, yeah. You're loving, you're giving, you've made more sacrifices than a ninety-nine-year-old monk. We're with you, and we know that's the deep-down truth for the majority of parents in the world. Our question, though, is much more about your parenting *style*. What kind of environment are you creating for your child through your words, your actions, your approach to discipline, and your attentiveness?

There are two basic ways to think about parenting styles—one that reflects how you deal with authority, and one that reflects your overall parenting personality. So take a look at the following catalog of parenting descriptions to see what best describes you.

AUTHORITY Style

Zero Authority: *The Pudding Pop or Marshmallow Mommy*

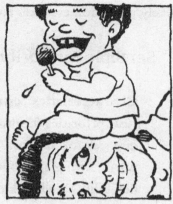

Puddin' Pop

Characteristics: soft, easy, sweet to the point of being unhealthy—i.e., a pushover.

This parental variety comes in all shapes and forms, but its most notable trait is the ability to say "Yes, sweetie" to offspring in any situation. As in: "Yes, you can go to bed whenever you like." "Yes, you may have cotton candy for dinner." "Yes, you may swing from the monkey bars with your teeth." More interested in being a friend than a parent, this type offers little guidance, often to the point of seeming to be disengaged or uncaring. These moms and dads have several predators: namely, their own offspring, as kids learn to manipulate parental units in all situations. Potential for destruction to relationship runs high.

Hyper Authority: *The Iron Maiden or Master*

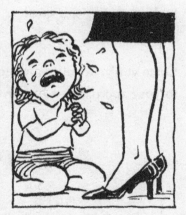

Iron Maiden

Characteristics: rigid, inflexible, superscary for everyone—i.e., a tyrant.

This fierce species comes with very sharp teeth and a loud growl to scare off any and all challengers in the quest for complete control. Parent will roar with a series of "No, not a chance!" responses, even to the most innocent of requests from offspring. Species rules the only way it knows how, having descended from equally controlling parents of its own. This beast creates a tension that can be felt not only throughout its own tribe but also throughout neighboring tribes as well. While the strong-arm approach can work to achieve short-term goals, long-term damage is likely, as tension escalates and offspring rebellion rates soar.

Sensible Authority: *The Flex-a-Family*

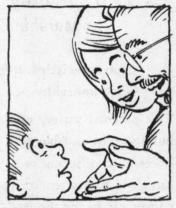

Characteristics: establishes ground rules with clear priorities (health, safety) and logical consequences for actions. Authority is exercised in a warm, loving environment, and is balanced with flexibility to allow kids to play and explore.

This species has a firm, foam-pillow-like quality to it: strong enough to provide support but soft enough to provide comfort. Parents work together and understand that raising the young requires a firm set of rules that teach offspring protective societal boundaries. But they also give offspring enough space to learn and grow on their own. Parents are not afraid to say no, but when they do, it's not about exerting control but about teaching why an action or behavior is unsafe or unacceptable. Success rates of raising a healthy, happy child are highest among this species.

Flex-a-Family

Once you've identified which species of parent you tend to resemble most in regards to your approach to authority, consider your overall parenting personality:

PARENTING Personality

The Hyper Parent

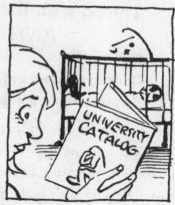

Hyper Parent

Characteristics: always on the go, go, go—moving, scheduling, social climbing—and doing everything for child, so that he never learns to do for himself.

The Hyper Parent views parenting as an extreme sport. Everything is controlled, and everything is the best (best pizza, best camp, best school, best neighborhood). Every minute is scheduled with not a minute spared for actually thinking or feeling or relaxing. Why waste time daydreaming when you could be working with flash cards? Gotta get your child involved in everything, and if he isn't the best, get a coach or a tutor who will make him the best. Make him shower in antibacterial gel. Do absolutely every single task by the book with no wiggle room at all. *Perfect* parenting, if you will.

The Absent Parent

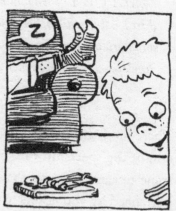

Absent Parent

Characteristics: solitary creature who camouflages self into the background or is too busy with own life to pay attention to the child.

Here the parent is as uninvolved as possible: plops the kid in front of the TV so the parent can take care of his or her own life. There's little or no social and emotional interaction. The thought process is clear: Let the kid fend for himself and learn the hard knocks as they come. "My parents didn't do one thing with me when I was a kid, and look at me, I turned out just fine."

The Go-with-the-Flow Parent (GWTFP)

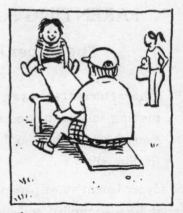

Go-with-the-Flow

Characteristics: adaptable, able to make decisions based on the specific situation at hand.

Life is unpredictable, kids are unpredictable. So the GWTFP remains flexible and adapts to any and all kinds of parenting situations and struggles. That means helping your child live in a balanced world that's neither too lax nor too tough. Life shouldn't be boot camp for a child, nor should it be a twenty-four-hour playground, either. It should be a little bit of both. The GWTFP knows how to balance appropriate stimulation with downtime and unstructured play. Providing free time is key to cultivating imagination and creativity (which teaches kids to think outside the box and to innovatively solve problems later in life). Unstructured play—at the beach, on the playground—also helps teach kids social skills as well as how to deal with the unexpected.

Note: A GWTFP should not be confused with a Marshmallow Mommy or Pudding Pop; there's a difference between laissez-faire and loving limits. And absentee parents can be darn totalitarian when they do show up. To produce the healthiest environment for your child's development, we recommend that you aim to be a GWTFP with a Flex-a-Family style.

• • •

There are big implications for parenting in any of the extreme environments: Each end of the spectrum can create tension for kids, albeit for different reasons. In fact, some research suggests that chronic stress (the same kind of stress that would be experienced by youngsters in any of these four familial situations) hinders the development of memory. Other studies suggest that the same kind of chronic stress in kids can be linked to obesity later in life. Still more science shows that a highly temperamental parent leads to all kinds of problems in kids, including anxiety, shyness, and behavioral problems. Not good, needless to say. This is also one of the reasons why nurturing your relationship with your spouse or significant other is so important to your child's health, as stress can come in the form of observing constant parental conflict.

Our goal as parents is to create the optimal learning environment for our children so that they develop competency and can eventually handle the world themselves. If your parenting style falls too far on the "easy" end of the spectrum, you don't give them the boundaries that they need to grow and to assimilate with their peers (not to mention assimilating with adults, too). And if your style falls too far on the tyrannical or hyper end, you're teaching your kids to live life scared, and that creates stress and anxiety levels that actually inhibit learning.

For some, finding that middle ground of parenting—the one in which you're strong yet flexible—will come naturally. But it's not always easy, and, at times, many have a hard time finding the middle. Sometimes it's because it's easier just to give in than to fight with your child or try to explain why-oh-why he can't have Guitar Hero when he turns two. And sometimes it's because having an iron fist can keep a child from even making such a request. And sometimes it's just easier after a long day to flip on the TV than read *The Cat in the Hat* for the eighty millionth time. The fact is that it actually takes a reasonable amount of work, discipline, and focus to live in that middle ground day after day, hour after hour, parenting challenge after parenting challenge.

Attention Attention: Finding the Middle Ground

If you're able to get yourself into the middle ground—a GWTFP and Flex-a-Family combo—the question arises: How the heck do you know when to flex and when to flow?

Your child's clues will actually tell you; your job is to pay attention. Like a bat flying through the darkness or a dolphin navigating murky depths, from birth, your child emits a constant stream of sonarlike pings—in the form of sounds, squirms, eye contact, and so forth—letting you know what he wants, craves, and needs. When you respond, he feels content and secure. Understanding your child's pings is instinctive: One of the first things that a mother learns is how to distinguish different types of crying—"I'm hungry," "I'm wet," "I'm tired," "I just want a little TLC"—and respond appropriately. This call-and-response is reinforced by Baby's actions (Baby cries, Mom picks up, Baby stops crying). Pings can be nonverbal, too: facial expressions or body language. (Think of the "I've gotta pee" dance.)

As your child grows, those pings communicate what kinds of things attract and intrigue her. Your job is to tune in, recognize, and respond to those signals so that you can, in turn, try to create the environment that she's longing (pinging) for.* How do you do that? By giving all sorts of positive feedback. For instance, when she oohs and ahhs, repeat the sounds back to her. Dole out smiles and hugs. When she shows from an early age that she's got Everest-exploring tendencies, build her a fort out of pillows. Resist the urge to squash the ant she's gazing at with such fascination. In addition to an encyclopedic knowledge of dinosaurs and Disney princesses, you'll be rewarded with a child who naturally loves to learn.

Your child's pings are her first attempt to grab the paddle and grind away. The danger is that if she gets no response from you (or a negative response), then you teach perhaps the worst lesson of all: not to try again. So what's your job? Tune into your baby's pings (sounds, squirms, eye contact)—and respond. What he wants from you most is your attention, so give it, especially when he reaches out to you or says a new word. If your child pings by showing an interest in, say, trains, then don't reject or override that signal and impose your own agenda—for instance, by replacing Thomas the Tank Engine with a baseball. Just go with the flow and see where those trains take you. That's because children are more apt to learn things that are interesting to them (same with adults, too); you'll read more about this in the next chapter.

* This is very similar to "signing" to your baby, a popular way that some parents use to communicate nonverbally. They teach their babies signs to help them express their needs before they develop the ability to talk, so they don't get frustrated. You don't need to take a class to use signs. Rather, learn to look and listen for your baby's pings and respond accordingly—you'll attain the same results.

The Motions of Emotions

While you may be anxious to get to the part where we explain the fastest way to get your child potty trained or reciting the alphabet, there's an important preamble to any kind of talk about encouraging your child's development. And that involves creating a foundation of good emotional health.

One of the ways we judge emotional strength is through a concept called "attachment." This emotional bond, which represents the sense children have that they can trust their caregivers, serves as the foundation for a healthy emotional life. Healthy attachment occurs naturally for many of us, especially if you had loving caregivers as a child, but some kids do suffer from what we call attachment disorder, in which they find it difficult to bond with their parents. Healthy attachment develops when a parent or caregiver is attentive and sensitive to a child's needs every day, as shown through prompt, consistent, and tender responses.

As a parent, you want to help create a child who can navigate herself down the river of life one day. Does that

FACTOID: In the early research on temperament, about 70 percent of the children studied fit three clusters of behaviors: 40 percent could be characterized as an "easy" child, who was positive, adaptable, and mild; 10 percent to 15 percent, a "difficult" child—negative, intense, and slow to adapt; and 15 percent were classified as "slow to warm up," indicating that they were negative, slow to adapt, and low activity. Over time, the difficult children accounted for a disproportionate number of behavioral problems, including ADHD, oppositional behavior, and other disruptive behaviors. They also exhibited general irritability and proneness to distress, and had difficulty controlling their negative responses.

What does this tell us? Well, many people think far more children are being diagnosed with ADHD these days than there used to be ("We didn't have that in our era," huffs Grandpop). But the truth is that we've always had it; it's just that it used to be called being a brat, and then it was called temperamental, and now it's called something else. We tell you this so you can realize that it's our language and classifications that have evolved—not necessarily an entire generation's behavior.

mean your job is to eradicate any and all disappointments, challenges, or obstacles? Of course not. It means that you need to teach your child to have the confidence and control to face and manage problems when they occur (which they inevitably will)—without overstressing, without panicking, without flinging a cup of milk across a restaurant when the waitress says they're out of macaroni and cheese.

We believe that you can provide your child with robust emotional health by focusing on what we call the Seven Strengths. Each is a particular characteristic that you can encourage in your youngster. As she grows, you can check in now and again to see how she's maintaining each and where she might benefit from a little boost.

1. **Happiness:** The parenting styles we talked about earlier directly correspond to levels of happiness in children. That's certainly pretty clear when it comes to the Iron Master/Maiden method of parenting. There's little happiness for a child who frets that he's going to get verbally assaulted if he happens to walk down the stairs a little loudly. But please don't make the mistake of thinking that happiness means that the child always gets his way and always gets rewarded for good behavior with a new Hot Wheels. Why? Because with that approach, you create an environment where desires are always gratified, which we know is not the case in life. True satisfaction comes from successfully meeting appropriate challenges in a nonpressurized setting—when a child feels confident that he will be loved for being himself, whether he's playing, working on a project, or simply exploring life. It's when a win is a real achievement that he has earned, not one that is engineered by his parents. While saying "no" may not always result in the most cheerful child, setting limits communicates to your child that you care about him, and there's a lot of happiness created (subconsciously, perhaps) when children know that their parents are there to protect them.

2. **Self-Confidence/Independence:** In the self-confidence spectrum, you see all kinds of kids. There are the ones who are bold, strong, and can strike up a ten-minute conversation with the UPS guy. And there are the ones who are so shy that they spend more time behind Mom's leg than on the jungle gym. We appreciate both kinds of kids. But it seems to us that the ideal is somewhere in

between. Think about it: If you were a passenger on a raft, you wouldn't want a river guide to be so bold and brave and reckless that he's being unsafe and taking you down a sixty-foot waterfall. But you also don't want a guide so unsure of himself that he doesn't allow you to experience any of the thrills of negotiating some rapids.

Kids, too, crave that sweet spot of having a guide (you) somewhere in between. In fact, they'll even be at a disadvantage (and in some case, even danger) if they're raised on either extreme. The ideal is to create an environment in which your child can develop confidence and independence—where he's forced to navigate a little bit of life on his own (with you watching), whether by interacting at the playground with kids he doesn't know or by letting go of the side of the pool and even trying the kiddie waterslide. While your impulse may be to keep him in a life vest until age eighteen, that doesn't grow a strong paddler with good decision-making skills in the long run. On the flip side, resist the urge to teach him to jump off the side of the pool if he's not yet comfortable putting his head underwater, as that can backfire, too. The best way to steer your child toward developing confidence (or rein him back, if necessary) is by putting him in age-appropriate situations and encouraging him to take a cue from Ferdinand Magellan and explore the world. Your job is to provide a map (or GPS) in case he gets lost.

3. **Resilience:** Go to any book or website of famous quotations, and surely you can find umpteen variations on this theme: "Show me a man who hasn't failed, and I'll show you a man who hasn't tried." Take any of them ("Get back in the saddle," "Try, try again," or "Failure breeds success"), and you have a perfect mantra for how to teach your kids resilience. It's okay to fail. Repeat: It's okay to fail. (At least at this stage; maybe *not* the message you want to preach when it comes to algebra class or when they move back home at age forty-three!) While you certainly are going to want your kids to try hard, to do their best, and to keep plugging at whatever task they're working on, you're doing your child a great disservice if you teach him that he has to hit the ball the first time off the tee, always color within the lines, or memorize multiplication tables by age three. The hard-driving, succeed-at-anything message often sent by the Hyper Par-

ent only sets up a child for future failures—not to mention rebellion. Because mistakes are inevitable, some children will, logically, figure that the best way to avoid them is not to try at all, lest they risk being imperfect (this explains bright children who underachieve).

What you want to do is flip the timeline: Let him experience failure now, when the stakes are low. Let your child try to solve problems. Don't rush in and put the puzzle together for him the minute he complains that it's too hard.* He may get only one or two pieces this time, but that will teach him to want to do better the next. Praise him for the effort, for the desire to learn and try out solutions, and for being brave when it took a lot for him to put himself out there. Dishing out praise that is *specific to effort and not about perfection* communicates to your child that you believe in him and think he is terrific no matter whether he succeeds or fails and that there is an adult in his life who is unconditionally devoted to him.

4. **Empathy and Compassion:** When you have a baby, there's no question: She's the most important thing in the world to you. And you send her that message every day with your love, with your attentiveness to her needs, with your warm snuggles and hug-me eyes. Absolutely, no question, you should do that as a parent. But at some point, you need to make sure that your child receives quite a different message: that she's not the only person in this world; that there are others who should be treated the same way, and that, really, her needs and wants are no more important than Sally's from down the street. Sounds a little harsh, we know, but this is another place where sensible authority comes in. You can love, care for, and protect your child all you want, but you also have to draw the line: to teach your child that it's not appropriate to hit other kids, to tease defenseless dogs, or to pull flowers off the neighbor's rosebush. The key to instilling compassion, of course, is communication. Soon enough, your child will pepper you with more questions than a public defender: Why? Why? Why? Why? The more "why" questions you answer—specifically about why other people matter—the

---

* Dr. and Dr. Roizen made *can't* a four-letter word never to be uttered by their children, or in their home.

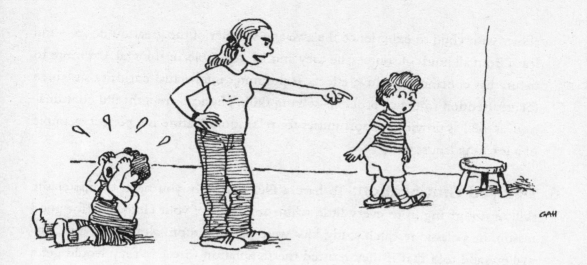

better. The earlier you teach your child to consider other people's feelings ("How would you feel if Izzy grabbed your tail or your doll?"), the better her chances of assimilating into a world that's a heck of a lot more diverse and unpredictable than your home environment.

5. **Playfulness:** When's the last time you let yourself really enjoy a game of hide-and-seek? It's hard to maintain a sense of playfulness when weighted down by adult responsibilities. There's always a phone call that needs to be returned, a mess that needs to be cleaned up, or a meal that needs to be prepared. But in the long run, do you think your child will remember that dinner was a little late one night or that after he found you hiding under a giant pile of dirty laundry, you tickled him until he couldn't breathe? Slow down and make time to play—at home as well as in parks.

Singing, dancing, and playing games with rhythm and music are fun ways to relax and let loose while stimulating your baby's brain. Exposure to music has actually been shown to increase the speed of learning and improve memory. For toddlers and older children, unstructured play with other children provides the opportunity to role-play, which reinforces their sense of empathy and compassion.

Kids who only play indoors are at risk of "nature deficit disorder": a lack of comfort and familiarity with the natural world. Getting outside and exploring allows your child to experience the awe and wonder of the great outdoors—and learn from all kinds of sources, be they animal, vegetable, or mineral. Exposure to nature has enormous positive effects: It promotes intellectual curiosity, sustained focus, attention to detail, problem-solving skills, physical strength, and coordination, as well as provides opportunities for relaxation. Nature is a perfect example of a learning landscape.

6. **Delayed Gratification:** To have a Flex-a-Family, you need to master the skill of not giving in to every little whim and want of your child. And for good reason. In a classic research study, kids were put in a room alone with a marshmallow and told that if they resisted the temptation to eat it, they would get a second marshmallow when the researcher returned. Decades later, those kids who could wait (as opposed to the ones who gulped it down immediately) ended up as higher achieving adults, with more satisfying careers and better earning potential. So how do you teach delayed gratification to a child who can't wait to eat the marshmallow? Some child experts advocate teaching them distraction techniques (how to take their mind off the "want" by thinking about or doing something else). Others suggest teaching them about setting long-term goals (saving up allowance to buy a special toy and then offering a special reward to teach how great saving is, such as giving them their money back after they've paid for the toy). The most important thing is not to give them everything they want the minute they want something. It all boils down to teaching your child how to be comfortable being a little uncomfortable.

7. **Spirituality:** Recent research suggests that one of the biggest influences on how a child develops emotionally is how grounded he is spiritually. In this context, spirituality doesn't refer to religion but to having a sense of one's place in the universe. For a child, this means how she fits into her immediate community—her family—as well as progressively larger communities she is exposed to (her neighborhood, her school, and so on). How can a parent help achieve this? Lots of ways, like creating family rituals around birthdays and holidays, participating in community events like parades, and volunteering as a family to help those less fortunate.

Now, the reason why instilling these strengths isn't as easy as it sounds is because we live in a world that's more complex than an organic-chemistry doctoral dissertation. There's a lot of stuff swirling around you, which can make mastering smart parenting difficult. But if you understand how to manage conflict and stress—and how to help your child do so too—it can make the job a whole lot easier.

Managing Conflict and Stress

Oh, life would be grand if every day were stress-free, conflict-free, and worry-free—if you could just kick back in your canoe and bask in the sunshine (fully UVA and UVB protected, of course). Alas, the period in your life when you are raising children is potentially the most stressful time you'll ever experience, what with kid stress, job stress, spouse/relationship stress, household stress, economic stress, extended-family stress, and so much more. And that's not even mentioning things like your own personality tendencies and that of your partner. Wouldn't it be great to be a kid again, when you played all day and didn't have to worry about money, about work, about anything except the fact that you wanted to stay up until eight-thirty and your parents made you go to bed at eight? Simple times. Or were they?

In an absolute sense, sure. Kids don't have your burdens. They don't have mortgages or in-laws. But children experience all kinds of stresses that simmer below the surface. The stress of encountering new people and situations. The stress of not being in control of their day. And the stress of knowing that they must rely on others for everything. They have few real choices. They can't switch siblings or parents or lives. They're in a perpetual state of learning, with the bar being raised on a daily basis. Geesh, talk about stress. Those stresses, unconscious for the most part, aren't always expressed verbally by kids. But they are there, and they do affect how kids behave.

Other forms of stress can be more apparent, and they differ depending on the child's age—whether it's the stress of jumping into a swimming pool for the first time, or walking into preschool, or eyeballing some four-legged beast that has teeth as big as a foot. Any of these can be very daunting for a kid.

The most potent form of childhood stress is tension between parents or the adults of the household. The problem is not the conflict per se—in fact, it's healthy for children to see that people disagree; otherwise they grow up with unrealistic notions about human interaction and avoid conflict, which can have its own negative consequences. Here's the real problem: While conflict is a part of any marriage or relationship, kids don't always see the resolution part of the equation.

Think about it: Mom and Dad fight about given topic. They throw a few barbs at each other, then give each other the silent treatment. Tension runs high, and the kid can feel that anxiety. Then a few more barbs (or dishes?) are thrown before the parents decide to take their argument private so that their youngster doesn't have to witness it anymore. Consequently, the kid never sees how two people can resolve their disagreements, make up, and move on.* Without witnessing the reconciliation process, the child remains in a state of anxiety worrying about the future of his parents' relationship.

It's neither realistic nor helpful to pretend that conflict doesn't exist. Nor is it healthy for a child to be exposed to constant fighting. (See page 442 on handling divorce.) Rather, a loving environment is one where hurts can be forgiven and differences of opinion can be resolved through mutual respect. It's your job to model that behavior.

Every day, zillions of factors go into what kind of environment you're creating for your child. Fortunately, if you fall off the flexible-parent wagon, you can always get back on and try again. While you're at it, admit your mistake to your child so he can learn from your experience that nobody is perfect. But when it comes right down to it, a strong factor in healthy child development is how you manage conflict and stress, and the behavior you model for your child.

Creating an environment that encourages healthy emotional development lays the foundation for healthy brain development as well. Before we start to explore the nuts and bolts of how the brain assimilates skills (such as motor skills and language skills) in the next chapter, use the tips below to help create an environment that's best for your child—not to mention for you.

---

* Though the kids don't need to see exactly how some couples make up.

YOU TIPS

Use All Senses. For optimal overall development, make sure to involve as many of your child's senses as possible in her experience of the world. While it may be easier just to rely on sight and hearing (showing an object and then saying the word aloud), don't hesitate to bring in touch, taste, and smell when you have the opportunity. All of that enhances the Learning Landscape. You can show an apple, say the word, and then let your child feel it and smell it (and taste it, depending on his age). A multisensory approach helps embed memories in the brain better than simply using one or two senses to make a point. Certainly you don't need to use every sense in every learning situation (nobody needs to taste mulch, after all); just look for opportunities to create as multidimensional an environment as possible.

Take It Outside. Getting kids to play outside has plenty of beneficial effects: It keeps a healthy mind in a healthy body and is an antiobesity agent (unless going outside means going to the neighborhood store for junk food). Playing in nature provides a valuable opportunity to learn from the birds and the bees, literally: to see how ants work together to move a stick far bigger than they are; to learn that the boy birds are the ones with bright plumage, not the girl birds; to see a chameleon camouflage itself to avoid detection (a great trick for hide-and-seek games later!). Kids who have experienced hands-on learning from nature do better on standardized tests, and for the wiggly kid on the ADHD side of the spectrum (see page 423), outside play can be the preferred means of getting those ya-ya's out. Howard Gardner, a proponent of the view that we have multiple intelligences, has proposed the notion of an eighth intelligence: being a naturalist, or having a sense of the natural environment. And going outside *with* your kids gives you the chance to practice smart parenting, or letting your child "ping" nature and have you express delight and joy in what he discovers (while also remedying your own potential nature deficit disorder).

Release Her Inner Olivia Newton-John. And let's get physical. A child's mind doesn't simply develop from passively processing what she is seeing and hearing. A lot happens when the child actively experiences her environment as well. Repeated physical actions—throwing a ball, climbing the ladder of a slide—lay down powerful muscle memories, and that's a huge way that both knowledge and intelligence are formed. It's a true mind-body connection, so rest assured that whenever your child is actively using her body, she's also exercising her mental muscles.

And Her Inner Columbus, While You're at It. In other words, let your child go out and explore. As parents, sometimes it can be hard to watch a kid roll in puddles, climb a tree, or stomp through mud after you just washed his shoes for the third time this week. But with a watchful eye, you should make an effort to let your child discover his world. Significant developmental benefits come to those who expose their minds to new experiences. In fact, it's this kind of spontaneous discovery that creates opportunities for learning. We're not saying that you should let your child run wild, especially in unsafe circumstances, but living in a bubble won't do much for helping his mind grow.

Teach Who Owns the Problem. Rather than telling your child no all the time, a smart tactic is to make him aware of the potential consequences of his actions so that he learns to make wise choices when you're not around to raise the alarm. Instead of shrieking at him every time he stands up on the chair, in a calm voice you can say, "I'd be disappointed if you fell because you'd get hurt, and we'd have to spend time in the emergency room rather than playing with your dolls or playing catch." While you sometimes need to be forceful with a "no," such as when danger is imminent, taking advantage of teachable moments early on can have a positive effect that will last a lifetime.

Just Watch. Throughout the book, we emphasize the importance of interacting with and stimulating your child. But that doesn't mean you have to play camp counselor all the time. In fact, you can learn a lot about what kind of stimulation she wants and what kind of emotions she has simply by sitting back and observing her behavior (she's pinging to you, remember?), her facial expressions, and the nuances of how she responds when exposed to certain things. Some of the greatest information about parenting doesn't come from this or any book; it comes from reading your child directly. By responding to her signals, you reinforce that she's getting attention, thereby creating a positive learning environment.

Go with the Flow. A mind is much better able to absorb things if it's engaged and interested. So the lesson for you is to follow your child's lead. If the ant hill is more interesting than the doll you just bought her, then go with the flow. If the box is more fun to play with than the toy inside, so be it. Open your own mind to learning something new, from your child's perspective. Enjoy play time with her; you'll be better for it, and so will she. Forcing a kid to sit inside and be drilled on his ABCs when he really wants to watch rain spouts drip is like paddling upstream.

Don't Neglect Downtime. Sometimes, in the wake of trying to be the perfect parent, we forget that children do not need to be stimulated *all the time*. In fact, having some time to themselves cultivates their imagination and creativity, helps them learn to think outside the box, teaches them to deal with the unexpected, and endows them with stronger social skills. In other words, think inside the sandbox. If your child is sitting playing by himself, don't jump in and try to push another toy or activity on him. Enjoy the downtime!

Control Your Own Stress. A child who watches a parent respond to stress by being anxious or fearful or angry will learn to do the same thing—and become hardwired to react that way in most stressful situations. Such reactions are emotional rather than logical, so it really pays to be in tune with your own signals so that you can control the messages you're sending your child about how to handle stress and conflict.

Learning Channels

The Biology of (Really) Early Education

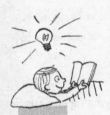

Forget YouTube. Forget *30 Rock*. Forget all things *Harry Potter*, vampires, or Dan Brown. The most entertaining thing in the world: children.

They ask the darnedest things: "Mom, can I have a pet armadillo and name it Army?"

They say the darnedest things: "All those clouds today must mean God is having a cigar."

They do the darnedest things: "Hmm, I can hide my peas in my glass of milk—and they'll never find them. *Ever! Mwah ha ha ha!*"

Makes you wonder what the heck goes on in those silly, brilliant brains of theirs, doesn't it?

Building on what we just described about creating an environment that promotes learning for your child, in this chapter we're going to talk about the nuts and bolts of cognitive development. We're going to take you inside a child's brain—how it develops structurally and how it works biochemically—and explain how all of that science helps kids learn and develop the skills they'll use throughout their entire lives. For those of you who measure milestones with accountantlike precision, this chapter will be right up your alley. But even if you're not the number-crunching type, you need to understand all of these intricate neurological systems and processes, because knowing how a child's brain works will not only help your little one be a smarter child but also help you be a smarter parent.

We think you'll be amazed by the brain's power and by the complexity and elegance of the mechanisms through which it works.

Building the Brain

It takes a bit of brain power to understand the ins and outs of the human brain. When you look at the biological infrastructure of the fattest organ in the body (yes, it's true: The human brain contains at least 60 percent fat★), then you can understand why it's so important to create a rich and rewarding environment for your child. We'll throw around a few words that may sound like they belong in a neuroscience textbook, but trust us: We'll make it understandable enough so you can dive into that squishy little cerebellum† of theirs and see all the cool things that are happening under the skull.

Let's start with the beginning of brain development, as in the *very* beginning. During the first thirty days of pregnancy, the fetus's central nervous system begins to take shape. A long, flat structure develops that forms a groove and rolls up into a tube. One end of the tube starts to swell—that's the brain. The rest turns into the spinal cord. By eight weeks into pregnancy, a large part of the brain is already formed. Now, the fetus is not doing long division just quite yet, but many parts of the brain are already in place: structures like the thalamus and the cerebral cortex, which are related to memory and learning. During the last few months of pregnancy, the brain

---

★ Fat itself is a type of tissue, not an organ, though visceral fat in the belly functions like an organ, causing inflammation. Here we are counting only healthy organs, not an abnormally fatty liver, which can be up to 90 percent fat, as opposed to a normal liver, which is 20 to 30 percent fat.
† As well as other parts of the brain.

BILINGUAL BABY

It's interesting to see how language works in bilingual families. If Mom speaks Spanish, say, and Dad speaks English, a child will answer his father in English and his mother in Spanish, even when those particular parents are speaking different languages than they normally do. Some bilingual kids mix the languages early on, and sometimes expressive language (what they say) is slightly delayed. But very quickly, those delays work themselves out, and when a child starts speaking in both languages, he will do so in full sentences that are contextually accurate and age appropriate.

grows and thickens and really begins kicking into action. (The spinal cord is actually responsible for the other kind of kicking you feel early on.)

Learning starts with the nerve cells of the brain: the neurons (see Figure 2.1). They carry information from one part of the brain to another, as well as back and forth between the brain and the rest of the body by way of the spinal cord and some specialized structures called cranial nerves. Those messages are what give us the ability to think, learn, feel, and move. Neurons are shaped like trees, with strong roots called dendrites and branches as well. Nerve cells receive info from their roots and send that info through the trunk of the tree (the axon) to the branches. Those branches pass along the information to the next neuron like a game of Telephone (or Whisper Down the Lane, if you prefer).

The branches of one neuron do not touch the roots of the next one. The message has to take a neurological leap of faith, if you will, by crossing the space between the two neurons, called the synapse. Its transportation mechanism? A chemical messenger called a neurotransmitter. As you'll see in a moment, the strength and complexity of the connections between neurons are the keys to learning and brain development.

The pace at which a baby's neural network is built is truly mind boggling: In utero, brains build 250,000 neurons a *minute* to result in about 100 *billion* by the time the baby is born. That's a heck of a lot of potential learning. Nevertheless, the brain can't afford to waste energy on learning everything there is to learn. To

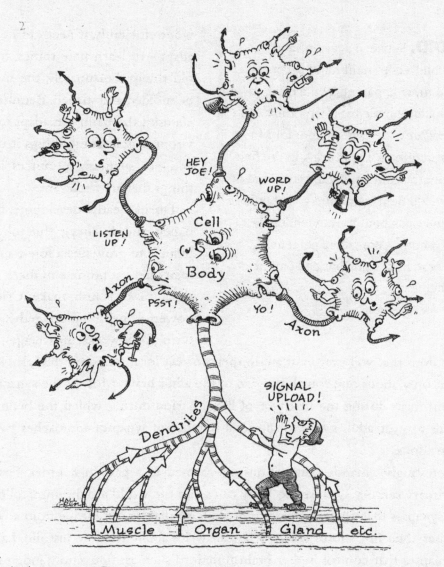

Figure 2.1 **Message Sent** The way we learn is through a process in which signals get transmitted from one neuron to another. When one neuron senses a change in our body's muscles, organs, or hormones, it interprets the signal and sends messages to surrounding neurons. All messages cross a space between neurons called the synapse. The more those connections are strengthened, through repeated exposure to a word, a subject, and so forth, the better the child is able to learn. When those connections aren't used, they go away—making it harder for us to learn new things as we age.

work efficiently, it needs to be able to adapt—to learn new things, to forget old things. Fortunately, the brain can be molded and shaped. Because of this *plasticity*, the brain can adapt to its environment, learning things it needs to and not spending resources learning things that are irrelevant.

During early development (pregnancy and infancy), the job of the brain is to grow like a forest and get as many trees as possible in there. Make it thick, make it lush, make it rich with powerful neurological redwoods. At term (forty weeks, on average), most of the neurons that will ever exist are in their correct locations, even though the baby's brain is only about one-fourth the size of the adult brain. Most of the synaptic connections form during the first year of life, a period during which the brain rapidly expands to near-adult size, and the total number of synapses approaches twice that seen in adults.

Interestingly, synaptic connections are formed in a particular order. First come the primary sensory synapses, so Baby can sense the world around him; followed by those synapses that control gross motor skills, so that he can escape from any threats he senses; then fine motor skills, so he can write about what he just did. Last come the synapses that control higher brain functions such as motivation, judgment, and reasoning, so that he learns what he may have done right and wrong in any given situation. These final pathways aren't fully functional until the late teens or even early twenties. Explains a lot, doesn't it?

Starting at about a year, as Baby is exposed to her new environment, the emphasis shifts from growth to pruning. Think of it as forest management: To encourage growth of the strongest, healthiest trees, deadwood and underbrush need to be cleared away. The brain does this by eliminating redundant and underused synaptic

COOL BRAIN FACTS
THAT WILL BLOW YOUR MIND

- The brain accounts for only 2 percent of the body's weight but uses 20 percent to 25 percent of the body's oxygen and energy supply.

- Messages travel between neurons at different speeds. Some seem like they're walking (one and a half feet per second), while others are fighter-jet fast (four hundred feet per second).

- In utero, the brain has no pain receptors, so it can feel no pain. Newborns feel pain with the same sensitivity as adults, but the sensation may be less localized (they don't know where the pain is coming from), and they may have a delayed response.

- While awake, the brain generates up to twenty-three watts of power, enough to light up a room.

- Simply opening your eyes activates 75 percent of your brain's energy.

- Children who learn two languages before the age of five have much denser gray matter as adults. They literally build bigger brains. *Muy bueno!*

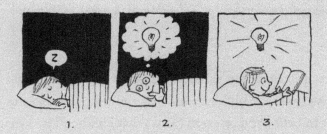

1.   2.   3.

connections. Baby doesn't need to know how to tap dance? Cut the rat-a-tat-tat connections. Baby hears both Spanish and English in the home? Strengthen the language connections. Baby gets put in a room all day to watch videos? Connections look kind of sparse. (Think Charlie Brown's scrawny Christmas tree.)

MAKING SENSE OF THE SENSES

We'd be remiss in talking about brain development if we didn't mention the fact that sensory development is a huge indicator of how well the brain is functioning. During the first few years of life, you should pay close attention to your child's vision and hearing. If things don't always add up, it may not just be a "sight" issue, but a brain development issue. You can read more about vision and hearing on pages 427–33, but for now, be aware that senses are more than just ways to interact with the world; they're cool little windows into the world of the brain as well.

About 10 percent of kids have problems integrating all of the senses—that is, perceiving info they receive from their senses and developing responses to it. These boys and girls may refuse to eat foods with certain textures or have aversions to baths or haircuts because they recoil from the sensation of water or a pair of scissors against their skin. They may be supersensitive to the sounds of fire alarms and vacuum cleaners or even feel disoriented while running and swinging (called gravitational insecurity). There are therapeutic techniques that can be used to help moderate these children's responses and get them used to the world around them. For instance, having a therapist or parent brush the body can help with tactile issues, while jumping up and down can help with gravitational issues. Your pediatrician or family doc can refer you to an appropriate occupational therapist or physical therapist if you feel that your child is struggling with sensory integration. Again, a key to regaining normal development is early intervention with an expert.

For the numbers folks out there, here's a quick recap: A child will have the maximum number of synapses she will ever have by the time she turns one. By age three, that number is cut in half. (And research shows that children lose synapses faster if the TV is constantly turned on.) This is why it's so crucial for a child to have appropriate stimulation from birth to age three so that she prunes neurons wisely.* (For many parents, making sure that their child has appropriate stimulation involves choosing a qual-

* There's even a national organization focused on that: Zero to Three (www.zerotothree.org); plus, it's the concept behind Early Head Start.

ity sitter or day care center, which we discuss on pages 323–28.)

Neurons are encased in a tough myelin sheath. This protective coating prevents the branches from tangling—and, thus, mixing up messages and disrupting connections—and insures that messages travel fast. Because myelin is made up of 80 percent fat and 20 percent protein, healthy fats are important for growing and maintaining a healthy brain. That's why we

recommend that moms-to-be take a DHA supplement during pregnancy. DHA, or docosahexaenoic acid, comprises over 97 percent of the omega-3 healthy fats in brains. It's also why we recommend breast milk (or infant formula fortified with DHA) until twelve months,* followed by whole milk (some brands are fortified with DHA) until at least age two. You should also try to incorporate healthy fats such as avocadoes, olive oil, and DHA-fortified milk into your child's diet from an early age.

The Biology of Education: How Kids Learn

By this point, you've already learned quite a few things about how children learn. In the last chapter, we talked about the learning landscape (how the environment and the mind make the best couple since Jay-Z and Beyoncé), and just a few moments ago, we shared info about the forest-management approach to neurons. Grow and prune, grow and prune. So where does that leave us?

* It appears that there's more fat in breast milk of women who breast-feed longer than those who do so for a shorter period—17 percent fat in women who nursed for more than 12 months compared to 5 percent in women who nursed for less than six, according to one study.

THE FIRST STEPS

When children begin to walk, generally between eight and eighteen months, they tend to have their feet wide apart and their hands up for maximum stability and balance. They also frequently walk with their feet and knees turned in or out. That's normal. Most kids eventually do develop a functional gait without special shoes or supports, but any concerns you have should be brought to your doc's attention, because occasionally children are bowlegged or have some other orthopedic issues early on. (See info on page 434.)

If you put the two together, you probably figured it out: The process of pruning those neurological connections is directly related to the environment to which a child is exposed. We prune connections that we don't use, as exemplified by the fact that we're not exposed to certain stimuli in our environment. (It's the old "use it or lose it" idea.) If a baby isn't spoken or read to, his brain might decide that he doesn't need those language neurons. The opposite is also true: We strengthen the connections that our brains deem important because of repeated exposure. That's why creating a routine is such an effective way to instill good habits in your child. More on this in the next chapter.

At a very primitive level, this method of shaping the brain developed out of a need to survive. The brain's main task, way back when, was to make decisions about survival, based on whatever information was available. See hungry beasts approaching the campground? Hightail it out of there. Next time you'll only need to hear a distant growl before you scoot. One of the really cool aspects of thought processing is that the human brain is an anticipatory system. We make decisions, we act, and we remember things that will help us with future decisions and actions. It was true for our caveman brethren, but it's also true for our wee ones: "If I cry in the middle of the night, Mom will come feed me. Isn't that awesome?! I think I'll do it again . . . and again . . . and again . . ."

To maximize your child's learning potential, we're going to let you in on a little secret that has to do with a concept called peak processing. While repeated exposure is critical to strengthening neural pathways, the timing of that exposure also comes into play. So when is a baby or child most likely to learn and retain information? Look at this chart to find out:

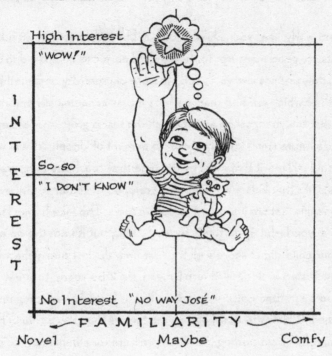

On the horizontal axis, we have "familiarity," ranging from novel to familiar. On the vertical axis, we have "preference," ranging from a child's exhibiting no interest to having very high interest. The perfect learning point (look at the star on the chart) happens when interest is at the absolute highest point, but familiarity is right in the middle.

In practical terms, let's see how this works: A child (or anyone, really) has to be interested to learn a subject. If she's bored, she's not going to process the information as well. But that information can't be too familiar, or else there's nothing to learn; what's more, it can't be too novel, because the child will have no context in which to understand the information. So the tricky part for a parent is to increase familiarity levels without going too far—because overexposure to anything can create boredom and frustration and thus decrease interest.

So go ahead and expose your child to soccer, violin, alphabet books, finger paints, and many different kinds of things (in moderation; you don't want to overstimulate

WILL YOUR CHILD BE GIFTED?

Starting at a very early age, your child will be subjected to lots of standardized tests. While these tests are good measures for how a child performs compared to other children of the same age, they are not always a good measure of creativity or something called task persistence (both of which are also markers for success academically and professionally). The problem is that the younger the age at which the test is given, the less accurate it is at predicting a child's future smarts. Only about 25 percent of kindergartners who are classified as gifted would still merit that label by the time they reach the third grade. The issue isn't with the tests, it's that kids are too underdeveloped at kindergarten level for tests to accurately assess skills that are important for future tasks. The take-home: Being classified as gifted can be a wonderful opportunity for some kids, but it's not the be-all and end-all. Just because your child didn't score well the first time doesn't mean she won't later, and just because she tested well early doesn't mean she'll be ready to meet the demands down the line. So be in tune not just to scores but to how she's keeping up with classes, homework (as she graduates to that), and all the factors that play a role in her education. And please be careful about putting too much pressure (or stimulation) on a child; rather, nurture her motivation. The pressure of being in an environment where the bar is set too high puts kids at a higher risk of problems than they would have had if they had just stayed the course of where they should naturally be academically.

No matter what level of intellect your child has, we recommend that you be careful in how you label him. Kids who are told they are smart often don't take risks because they're afraid to fail. Kids who are celebrated for being willing to try—regardless of their intellectual ability—continue growing even if they fail periodically, without taking it personally. We see this in research circles when we look at children who are asked to solve extremely hard puzzles. Some kids get frustrated and quit when they can't figure them out, while others enjoy the process and challenge and ask for another, even if they failed to complete the previous puzzle.

By labeling your child, you actually take away a little bit of his control—and, really, his destiny too. Another reason that it's as important for parents to praise a swing and a miss ("Good swing! Focus on the ball!") as it is to praise a home run.

his little brain). Your child will help guide you to what he likes and doesn't like. (Read his clues, or pings, as we discussed in chapter 1.) Then you can increase exposure to the things he likes, and perhaps reduce exposure to the things he doesn't. Think of yourself not just as the teacher but also as the student.

Because different parts of the brain are pruned and myelinated at different times, there are biological windows of opportunity when children are interested in and able to learn different skills. The exact timing differs from one child to the next. So, just as you wouldn't force a child to walk before she's ready, if your child doesn't show an interest in, say, ABCs at age two, put it on the back burner and try again in a couple of months. If, instead, you spend the next few months drilling him, when he does eventually show a preference, the material will be too familiar to fully engage his learning potential.

Sending Signals

In addition to having different interests, we all have different learning styles, and kids are no exception. Some prefer to learn visually, others prefer to learn aurally, and still others prefer to learn kinetically. Most learn through a combination of ways. But there's one form of learning that's universal: the learning that happens subconsciously. Kids take most of their cues from signals that you send them through your body language or the look in your eye. In fact, research shows that when communicating a message, the tone of voice is twenty times more important than the actual words of the message. And that's an important message for all of us to remember—whether we're parents of newborns or toddlers, not to mention tweens, teens, and beyond.

Nonverbal communication and the emotion it conveys account for more than 90 percent of what your child "hears" you say. The total impact of our parental messaging breaks down like this:

⊃ 7 percent verbal (words)

⊃ 38 percent vocal (volume, pitch, rhythm, and so on)

⊃ 55 percent body movements (mostly facial expressions)

IS YOUR BABY SMARTER
THAN A FIFTH-GRADER?

Without a doubt, there will be plenty of time to have your child take all kinds of tests: math tests, spelling tests, driving tests. But just for fun, why don't you see what kind of smarts that little bugaboo has now? Disclaimer: These tests are meant for fun and to give you an idea of how your child learns. If he does not pass or engage in these tests, it does not—repeat, not—mean that he's relegated to dunce-cap status. Nor does it predict future intellectual ability (as we explained on page 49).

FOR KIDS THREE MONTHS OLD

Put a finger in your baby's mouth and let her suck on it while you make eye contact and say "babababababababa" over and over. At first, your baby will suck a bit harder when you start saying "ba" repeatedly, but eventually her sucking will slow down. Now do the same thing, but at some point, say "pa" instead of "ba." You should notice the amount of sucking pick up when you switch from saying "babababababa" to saying "papapapapa." That change is a signal that your baby notices the difference between these sounds. Now, don't worry if your baby doesn't show a noticeable difference. It could mean that your finger is not properly calibrated to detect subtle changes in sucking interest. There are lots of things that affect what your baby does while you do this test. Babies have a hard time paying attention to anything, so it might just be that she needs to nap.

FOR KIDS ABOUT EIGHTEEN MONTHS TO TWO YEARS OLD

Find ten new toys of about the same size. They should be small enough for your child to pick up but, obviously, large enough that if she puts them in her mouth, she cannot swallow them. Five of them should be animals. The other five should be vehicles (cars, trucks, and planes). Watch the order in which your child plays with the toys. As she gains knowledge about types of categories, she will generally touch members of one category and then members of the other. When she gets older, she may alternate, touching an animal and then a vehicle, another animal and another vehicle.

FOR KIDS ABOUT TWO AND A HALF TO THREE YEARS OLD

Get some objects that are unfamiliar to your child. Two of them should be the same shape but different colors or textures. The others should be the same color or texture but *not* the same shape. Show the child the first object and say, "See this? This is a screwdriver." Then show the other two objects and ask, "Which one of these is also a screwdriver?" When the child reaches the point where she is learning words quickly, she should point to the object that has the same shape as the first object.

Words simply convey information. Emotion gives information meaning. That's why communicating emotion is at the heart of smart parenting. The ways you can convey positive emotion to a child include:

- ⊃ **Eye contact:** Parents who make eye contact with their children open the flow of communication and convey interest, concern, warmth, and credibility.

- ⊃ **Facial expressions:** Authentic expressions convey warmth, happiness, friendliness, and bonding. Don't forget: Smiling is contagious.

- ⊃ **Gestures:** A lively and animated parent captures attention and facilitates learning. Head nods, for instance, communicate positive reinforcement and indicate that you are listening.

- ⊃ **Posture and body orientation:** You communicate numerous messages by the way you walk, talk, stand, and sit. Standing erect, but not rigid, and leaning slightly forward communicates that you are approachable and receptive. Adults respond to this posture as well.

- ⊃ **Voice:** Parents (or talk show hosts) who drone on in a monotone are boring. Mix up your tone, rhythm, inflections, and volume to keep your child's interest.

CHILD DEVELOPMENT MILESTONES

Okay, we know that some of you are going to use the following chart to track every movement your baby makes. Please relax just a bit. This chart of average milestones is just that: an average. Some babies will hit them earlier, some later. But most will hit them just fine. As a parent, your instincts will kick in if some important milestone fails to occur for weeks on end, and your child shows signs that she's not developing as expected or establishing the building blocks that will help her reach future milestones. That's the point where you want to get an opinion from a professional. Developmental delays can certainly indicate problems, especially in the areas of language and motor skills. Some may resolve themselves naturally by the time a youngster enters preschool, but ongoing delays may warrant a discussion with your doc.

Think of this timeline as a TripTik pointing out great places to stop, look, and wonder as you ride the river. Here are the skills, traits, or habits a child will typically have developed by these dates:

Three Months

Social and Emotional
>   Social smile
>   Communication of feelings through face and body
>   Varied cries (hunger vs. pain)

Movement
>   Raises head and chest when lying on stomach
>   Stretches legs and kicks
>   Opens and closes hands
>   Brings hand to mouth
>   Shakes toys placed in hand

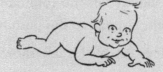

Senses

Watches faces and follows moving objects

Recognizes familiar things and people at a distance

Smiles at sound of voices

Begins to babble and echo sounds

Seven Months

Social and Emotional

Interested in mirror images

Responds to other people's emotions

Explores with hands and mouth

Struggles to reach for objects

Starts to have preference for a given person

Personality unfolding

Language

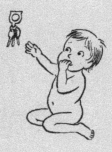

Looks when own name is spoken (generally eight to twelve months)

Responds to sound by making own sounds

Uses voice to show emotions

Babbles

Movement

Rolls front to back and back to front

Sits with support of hands at five months; without support of hands at six months

Reaches with hands and moves objects from hand to hand

One Year

Social and Emotional

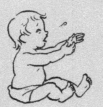

Shy with strangers (expression of this varies in intensity) and cries
    when parent leaves

Prefers regular caregivers to all others

Repeats sounds

Starts to imitate people during play

Learning

Explores objects by shaking, banging, and so on

Begins to use objects correctly, like holding cup to mouth

Begins to look at correct picture when object is named

Language

Responds to simple verbal requests and commands, including "no"

Changes tone when babbling

Says "Dada" and "Mama" specifically

Tries to imitate words

Points to desired object

Gross Motor

Crawls forward on all fours (though some kids skip crawling, which is
    not necessary for normal motor or cognitive development)

Sits up on his own

Pulls himself up to stand

Walks holding on to furniture

Stands without support for a
    moment

May walk a few steps without
    support

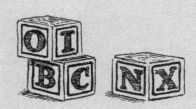

Fine Motor

Puts objects in container and takes them out (between twelve and fifteen months)

May stack two objects and/or bang two objects together

Pokes with fingers

Tries to make a mark on paper

Eighteen Months

Social and Emotional

Self-comfort (such as attachment to blanket)

Empathy, sharing, shame, guilt

Emerging independence

Social relatedness

Gross motor

Walks independently

Pushes and pulls large objects

Throws a ball while standing

Fine motor

Builds a tower out of a couple of cubes

Scribbles spontaneously

Language

Says ten to twenty words

Plays with dolls and cars

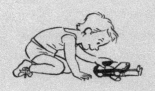

Two Years

Social and Emotional
Imitates others to please them
Excited about being with other children
Wants to be more independent
Shows defiance (may tell doll or imaginary friend "no")

Learning
Finds hidden objects
Sorts by shapes and colors
Plays make-believe games

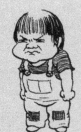

Language
Recognizes names of people and objects
Use phrases and two-word sentences
Follows instructions of several steps
Repeats words
Has vocabulary of fifty or more words

Gross Motor
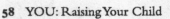
Jumps in place
Carries toys while walking
Begins to run
Stands on tiptoes
Kicks a ball
Climbs up and down from furniture

Fine Motor
Builds tower of blocks with a few blocks
Shows preference for one hand or another but handedness not
    completely established
Pours out contents of container

Three Years

Social and Emotional

Imitates playmates and adults

Can take turns in games

Expresses affection and wide range of emotions

Can separate from parents (fairly) easily

Learning and Language

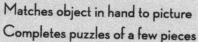

Matches object in hand to picture

Completes puzzles of a few pieces

Understands most sentences

Follows commands

Recognizes common objects

Uses three- to four-word sentences

Can say name and age and uses pronouns

Gross Motor

Climbs well

Walks up and down stairs

Kicks ball

Runs easily

Pedals tricycle

Fine Motor

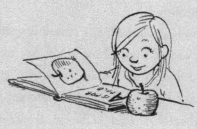

Can draw lines and circular
    shapes with pencil

Turns pages in book one at a time

Builds tower of more than a few blocks

WHAT EDUCATIONAL STYLE IS RIGHT FOR YOUR CHILD?

Soon enough, you'll be faced with some tough decisions about your child's formal education. You'll have to decide what kind of school you want to send your child to: public, private, charter, religious, home, or something else?

We're not here to give a stamp of approval to any particular kind (among the authorship team, we've had success with nearly all of the options). But we are especially interested in some of the lessons we can learn from the Montessori method of teaching. Developed in the early nineteen hundreds by Maria Montessori, the first woman to graduate from medical school in Italy, its approach to education is based on one pretty big principle: Kids learn according to their own pace, rhythm, and capabilities during periods when their brains are particularly receptive to learning. (She originally developed her methods to fit the educational needs of children with disabilities.)

Above all, Dr. Montessori believed that children weren't just little adults but that they had their own, unique developmental patterns. Therefore, they should be educated in a way that might be different than the way adults traditionally thought about education. She believed that children are dynamic, they learn about the world through their senses, they learn what interests them, they repeat activities, and, in many situations, they can teach themselves.

So how do the kids in these programs learn? Well, it's a very hands-on approach, as they use all kinds of materials that stimulate their senses. Children are encouraged to order things from smallest to largest, lightest to heaviest, palest to darkest. In one "work," the child orders blocks with different grades of sandpaper on them from smoothest to roughest. In another, different temperature water is added to small metal bottles, and the child orders them from coolest to warmest. The teacher acts more as an observer than an instructor (which is in line with what we've discussed about how smart parents watch for patterns and interest levels in their own children). The result is that students learn through discovery—often at times when they're by themselves.

Now, there are plenty of people who disagree with this method. Those who believe in more traditional approaches feel that Montessori children have fewer social skills because they work on their own at an individual pace and therefore may not transition well to a more traditional and less individualistic program. Some also take issue with the lack of imaginative play in many Montessori programs, which can vary from strict to modified. Indeed, Montessori may not be the best environment for a child who is extremely social or who can't sit still and focus independently on a task. The point is that you should consider all kinds of educational options when your child is ready to go to school. Don't just pick the same path that you went down. Despite the similarities that you may have with your child, each of us responds differently to different environments, so it's worth really taking the time to explore all of your options when it's time for your child to expand her educational horizons.

First and foremost, visit the school and see if you can imagine your child fitting right in. Look around. What's on the walls? If it's "No This" and "Don't Do That," it may be a stifling place for your child's brain. If you see evidence of creativity at play, it may be a great place for your child's brain. Are there just girl toys or boy toys? Is there a focus on right-brain activities (puzzles, spatial toys) as well as on left-brain activities (words, books, writing)? Do the teachers look grumpy? What about the other parents at drop-off and pickup? Do you see families that appeal to you, with children who might appeal to your child? We're talking future playdates and playmates here.

Got Skills? How Babies Develop

Before your child can develop into the virtuoso/MVP/CEO that you imagine she will become, she has to learn the basics. Based on what we've just discussed, there 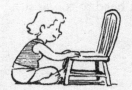 are a couple of essential things to remember about basic skill development. First, it seems that major milestones tend to happen in a logical, predictable progression. Example: Not too many children walk before they sit; that's because you need the trunk support you learn from sitting and rolling in order to walk.

Second, milestones happen in quite a varied range of time. Every child develops a little differently, and you shouldn't panic if yours doesn't hit every major milestone at the typical time or if your child develops a skill, loses it for a while, and then regains it months later. (See our developmental timeline on pages 54–59.) In many cases, the range for developing a certain skill can actually be several months long. On the other hand, if you notice a pattern of missed milestones, don't hesitate to seek professional help from a developmental pediatrician, as the earlier a youngster receives help, the greater the chance she'll get back on track.

There are three major categories of fundamental skills:

Language Skills: The suspense is unbearable; what will be Baby's first word? Mama? Dada? Squarepants? Though the first word will surely be one of the early milestones you'll enter into your child's baby book, it isn't nearly as important as all of the things that you can do to help him or her develop proper language skills. If you recall our previous discussions about environment and neurons, you have some sense of how language develops. As a child is repeatedly exposed to words, her neurons strengthen the connections needed to process the information. Meanwhile, the neural connections for sounds, words, or entire languages that the child isn't exposed to are pruned away. In essence, a child's brain says, "If I'm not exposed to the term *nuclear physics,* I have no need to spend all that energy remembering it." The opposite is also true: "If I hear *Mama* three dozen times a day,★ then, gee, that must be a pretty important word, so I'll remember it, store it, and use it." So the simple fact is that whatever words a baby ultimately utters first have probably been heard thousands of times before. The lesson: Talk to and read to your baby. A lot.

Gross Motor Skills: These skills involve the large muscle groups a child uses to move around. They include all the movements a child makes, from head to toe, as she

★ An hour?

learns to navigate the world and to use her own body. That means things like lifting her head, rolling over, sitting, crawling, pulling herself up, and walking. Environment plays a big role here, too. If a baby is sitting in front of a chair or table that's the right height for pulling herself up, she will. If not, she won't. Other factors, including maturation, opportunity, coordination, strength, and temperament, play roles in how soon a child will crawl, walk, or nail a perfect 10 on dismounting from a playground slide. But the real lesson here for many parents is not to panic if your child is a bit behind what's so-called normal when it comes to gross motor milestones.

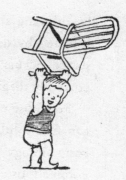

Fine Motor Skills: When a child gets a little older, we'll think of these skills in terms of things like holding a pencil or playing piano. For a baby, however, it's eye-hand coordination, which also includes Baby's ability to use hands and fingers for complex tasks such as picking up a Cheerio and bringing it to her mouth. The key to encouraging development of fine motor skills is providing a safe environment in which your child can explore the smaller things in life. (That means nothing sharp, nothing toxic, and nothing other than very digestible food so small that it can be swallowed. Use the toilet paper tube rule: If an object fits through one, it's too small for babies and toddlers to play with.) Simple materials such as wooden puzzles, Play-Doh, crayons, Legos (the big ones at first), and blocks are perfect tools for a baby to develop fine motor skills. And if you remember our chart on peak processing (page 49), that comes into play here in a big way. You've got to keep the stimulus novel enough so that your child stays interested, but also familiar enough to give her the time to practice and then master fine motor skills. One way is not to have all the toys out all the time; keep some in a closet and rotate every couple of weeks.

Abnormal Development: We know that many of you are highly interested in (and passionate about) the subject of brain development, especially as it relates to autism and various attention problems. In the media today, there's a lot of blame being thrown around, and there are still a lot of questions to be answered. You may be thinking about the subject as your child grows, wondering if he or she will be touched by developmental disorders that affect so many children. ADHD, for instance, occurs in 5 percent to 7 percent of children, while 1 in 110 youngsters are currently diagnosed with autism spectrum disorder.

For those of you who want more detail about autism and attention disorders, you can find a fuller discussion beginning on page 423. Here we'd like to address the basic biology behind these issues, because it all comes back to making those synaptic connections.

When those connections are at their peak, there are zillions of them—tree branch to tree root, neuron to neuron—far more than we need or can even handle long term. As we grow, those branches and connections get pruned down to only the essentials. In kids with attention problems, it appears as if those connections are getting pruned later. The result is that during childhood, there's excessive brain activity, making it difficult for these children to focus. Imagine branches getting tangled or power lines getting overzapped with energy. There's too much going on, and the system needs to slow down, but the brain is wired in such a way that it can't. Behavioral interventions and medications can help (see page 423).

For kids with autism (and that word represents a broad spectrum of similar disorders), the connections don't function properly. And that manifests itself in all kinds of issues, such as delayed or unusual language or impaired social development.

While you can't see inside your child's brain, you can see how it is functioning through his actions and behaviors. If something doesn't quite feel right, see if he has any of these characteristics. None of them signifies a specific diagnosis, but having any warrants further testing:

⊃ **Speech Delay:** The basic rules of thumb are that a child should be saying at least one word (however unclearly) by twelve months of age; at least twenty words by eighteen months; and putting two words together with a vocabulary of fifty words by twenty-four months. Another guideline is that a stranger should be able to understand 50 percent of what a two-year-old is saying, 75 percent of what a three-year-old is saying, and almost all of what a four-year-old is saying.

SEEING A SPECIALIST AND/OR A THERAPIST

If you and your doctor do determine that your child has some developmental issues, you may be referred to a medical specialist (pediatric neurologist or developmental-behavioral pediatrician) or psychological specialist to determine a diagnosis and a possible cause and the need for further evaluation. Or your doctor may simply refer you directly to a therapist to work on specific problems. Early intervention using experts trained in child therapy is important; seeing the right specialist can help your child get on track. Besides your doctor and interested individuals at your local hospital, a teacher may also have good recommendations. The three major kinds of specialists include:

PHYSICAL THERAPISTS: They evaluate the gross motor development skills such as walking by looking at physical capacities and limitations. Therapy includes not only play, but also exercise and behavioral training, as well as equipment or devices if necessary.

OCCUPATIONAL THERAPISTS: They look at fine motor skills and upper extremity use, as well as sensory processing function. They'll also use various equipment and training methods to help teach these developmental skills.

SPEECH THERAPISTS: They assess language skills and work on developing speech, vocabulary, understanding the meaning of words, and using sentences. (Hearing should also be assessed whenever there are speech issues.)

⊃ **Hearing Loss:** All children born in a hospital are screened for hearing at birth, but it is possible to develop hearing loss afterward or even for that screening to miss it. So if there is *any* question as to whether your child is hearing normally, he should be rechecked, and promptly. A hearing evaluation is also on the to-do list if there are concerns about speech delay, indistinct speech, and not turning when his name is spoken. It's not good enough that he hears; the question is whether he hears clearly enough to have the best opportunity to develop speech.

⊃ **Lack of Response:** Your twelve-month-old should look at the person calling his name; follow your finger when you point at something interesting; and maintain good eye contact.

⊃ **Lack of Cuddliness:** Don't attribute your babe's lack of affection to his father's genes. It's worth discussing with your pediatrician.

⊃ **Obsessions:** Your two-year-old shouldn't play with one thing obsessively to the exclusion of almost everything else (even if it is a typical interest, like dinosaurs) and shouldn't play obsessively with something that's not a typical plaything, such as flags or strings. Either can be a sign of an obsession disorder or autism spectrum disorder. Obsession really means getting stuck on a particular task, thing, or activity, ignoring everything else, potentially interfering with or inhibiting other learning experiences.

⊃ **Lack of Playing Skills:** Overall intellectual ability is very dependent on good language development. But visual-spatial skills (the ability to solve problems related to vision and spatial area matching) and problem-solving skills are big parts of intellect as well. So, see a pediatrician soon if your child is not engaged in play activities that involve manipulating things at a year (banging, throwing). By around eighteen months, he should be marking with a crayon, piling blocks, placing objects in containers and taking them out, using objects as tools, and problem solving: for example, figuring out how to get to something you do not want him to have.

⊃ **Decrease in (or Poor) Social Skills:** If your child speaks only in certain settings (home, for instance, but not at your Mommy and Me classes) or demonstrates a decrease or lack of development in social skills or interaction with others during the second year of life, it may be a sign of some developmental issues.

In most cases, it's not the individual signs but rather the combination that's telling. Basically, impairment in the social and communication areas of development can signal some kind of autism-related issue. Denial or delay in getting help only makes matters worse. Attention issues can exist on their own or in combination with other problems such as autism, obsessive behavior, and dyslexia (dyslexia is defined as when a child without other problems doesn't acquire academic skills and knowledge at the expected rate). The key to having a successful outcome is early intervention, to get your child on the best trajectory.

> **FACTOID:** Cerebral palsy, which affects about one in every five hundred newborns, is caused by some kind of brain damage that occurs most often in utero or, much less frequently, during birth. Characterized by motor delay, abnormal movement, or physical issues such as feeding problems or difficulty separating legs during a diaper change, cerebral palsy can't be cured, but therapy (again, the earlier the better) can help improve a child's skills and development.

No doubt, there are lots of essential points to consider when thinking about a child's early education. But this informal education—the education that happens before she steps one cute, little foot into school—is crucial toward developing a healthy and happy child. We hope you'll take a close look at our tips and strategies below, because they'll provide the knowledge and techniques you can use to create the ultimate learning environment for your child.

LET'S TALK ABOUT SEX

If you recently had a baby, the last thing you feel like talking about is sex. But we're not talking about your sexuality, we're talking about your child's sexual development. While most sex-related discussions will come when they're older than the age range addressed in this book, it is important to be aware that sexuality issues arise even with very young children. Some interesting things to note:

- Babies are sexual beings too; erections are perfectly normal and mean that the plumbing works. Don't worry if you don't see any, though; either way is normal.

- Toddlers become interested in noticing body differences as early as fifteen months.

- Kids have a sense of gender differences at eighteen months and become more aware of their appearance at this age, including their sexual organs.

- Around two years of age, they may start comparing their genitals to those of siblings, friends, cousins—and compare themselves to Mom and Dad.

- In the three- to five-year age group, you frequently see boys and girls playing dress up and assuming the role of the other gender. This kind of experimentation is perfectly normal and not to be discouraged.

The most common display of children's sexuality from infancy onward involves touching their genitals (especially boys—easier access). Instead of reprimanding him, use this as a teachable moment. Explain to your child that it's not polite to do that in public, in the same way that burping isn't. And you should explain to children of both sexes that the private parts are indeed private: They can touch them, and Mommy and Daddy can clean them, and a doctor can examine them when Mommy and Daddy are there. Everyone else is off-limits; if someone tries to touch their private parts, they need to tell you right away.

So what do you do with all this information? Well, for the most part, at this age, it's okay to just observe and make sure there's no abuse going on anywhere. It's perfectly normal for children to explore and wonder about bodily differences. You can do your part to cultivate a sense of normalcy about sex by answering your child's questions matter-of-factly and using the correct terms to describe their genitals. Accurate sexual knowledge is good. Research suggests that adolescents who have more knowledge about sex are less likely to contract sexually transmitted diseases and to become pregnant as teenagers.

Also, if you establish open communication about the subject at a young age, when your child does become sexually mature, he or she will feel comfortable coming to you for advice.

If your child is the one playing gynecologist at a tender age, it is well worth determining the source for this fascination. Could it be that he has been abused himself? Or is the babysitter hitting the porn channel after bedtime, with Junior sitting on the stairs watching? What shows are on the TV or radio when your son or daughter is at home or in the car? A healthy adult dose of Howard Stern may be unduly provocative for your school-age child.

The issue of sexuality is a complex one, especially as children get older. For now, the real strategy for parents is not to treat sexuality as a taboo but as one of many facets of a child's development, education, and exploration of the world.

YOU TIPS

Emphasize Play, Not Success. While it's true that kids follow the same basic learning patterns, it's also true that there are many nuances. Some kids learn better by hearing and seeing the information, while others learn by doing and practicing. No matter the method, what's really important is that you encourage your child to play with objects safely and explore the world around him. The point isn't to measure success or failure; it's to let him engage his intellectual curiosity. At this age (under five), that will create a stronger foundation for learning than drilling your youngster on any particular task.

Read It Loud and Proud. We can't say it often enough: Read aloud. Read aloud. Read aloud. Besides serving as wonderful one-on-one time, reading to your child will do amazing things for her future vocabulary. In fact, the vocab that a child has at the age of two is proportional to the number of words he's heard spoken to him before that time. Kids might not be able to respond verbally to you when they're little, but they're processing. Remember those neurons: With every sentence, you're building stronger language connections.

Say This, Not That. Sometimes it's easy to take the easy way out and say little or just use short phrases with kids, since they can't do much talking anyway. But everything you're saying helps their emotional development as well as their language development. Use these examples as guides for how to involve your child in your conversation:

Say "Do you think the doggie is hungry?"

Not "I'm going to feed the dog now."

Why: Questions initiate conversations and engage children with inflections in tone.

Say "Doesn't dirt look cool close up? Just try not to get any in your mouth, because it tastes yucky and can give you a tummy ache."

Not "If I have told you once, I've told you a thousand times not to eat dirt."

Why: Positive observations encourage curiosity; negative commands stifle it. Also, explaining the consequences of an action gives a child the knowledge she needs to make the correct choice on her own in the future.

Make Convo. The best way to talk to your child is by pretending that she *can* converse. Do you need a nap? It's been a long day hasn't it? These yams are pretty nasty looking, aren't they? Talk to her as if she were filling in the gaps. That will help her recognize language and word patterns that she'll need and use soon enough. Speak slowly and in short phrases, using gestures and facial expressions to reinforce the meaning of your words.

Drop the Background Noise. Having your favorite TV show host on in the background might be nice ("Say hi to Dr. Oz, bubby!"). But this kind of white noise makes it difficult for kids to distinguish between the sounds they need to know and the sounds they don't. So keep the TV off and make sure that the responsibility of filling the silence is fulfilled by the three-dimensional people in the room, not the two-dimensional ones. Even better, don't turn on the TV at all when your child is around, and don't even think about putting one in his room. Studies show that kids with TVs in their bedrooms tend to be more overweight and don't perform as well in school. Bottom line: TV can decrease brainpower.

Sign Up for Those Music Lessons.
And not because you're trying to create the next Bono. The advantages of music lessons go way beyond learning to play a little Mozart (or Metallica). Kids who study a musical instrument for three years do better than non-musical kids with skills not associated with music— such as verbal ability and, perhaps obviously, finger dexterity. Other research shows that music also improves overall memory. Fa la la la la, la la, la, la.

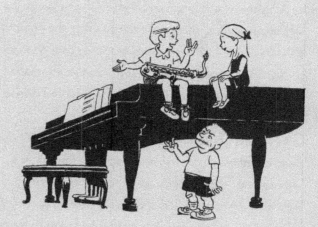

Do Art. One of the best ways to let your child's creative juices flow is to let her create all kinds of art, whether it's scribbling on a piece of paper or playing with paints and crayons. Besides allowing her to expand her imagination, this helps her develop those fine motor skills (holding a pencil or crayon, squeezing a bottle of glue). We suggest that you make art a regular part of your weekly routine, and try not to set too many rules (besides keeping the art on the paper, not the walls). The rug is going to be ruined by milk-soaked Rice Krispies anyway, so what's a little glue or paint to go with it? That way, your child will feel most free to express herself.

Show and Tell. Whenever you're out, be one of those pointer-outer parents. Point to things you see, hear, and smell; teach your child about the world. This applies wherever you are, whether it's in nature or at the mall. It's also really helpful to show your child how things change: Leaves change color, flowers bloom, batter turns into cookies, and so on.

Skip Disembodied Videos. There are a lot of baby videos on the market that purport to help turn your child into a genius. The problem is, though, that some research shows that kids who watch these videos may actually end up with a smaller vocabulary than those who don't watch them. What's wrong with them? While the videos may emphasize language-building skills, they use disembodied voices rather than visible speakers. Babies learn language not only through sounds but also by watching faces (kids on the autism spectrum tend to watch lips) and tracking how words begin and end. With just audio, the words sound more like gibberish than real language. And that's not even counting the point that a huge part of language development is the back-and-forth that happens during conversation, which is one of the reasons that even certain TV shows (the ones that encourage interaction, like *Dora the Explorer*) are better for brain development than some of these targeted videos.

Give Plenty of Tummy Time and Floor Time. When he's awake, that is. (Babies need to sleep on their sides or backs to decrease the risk of sudden infant death syndrome, or SIDS; see page 86.) The importance of tummy time is that it forces kids to work on the gross motor skills of lifting up the head and eventually rolling over. While you're at it, make sure that you reposition your baby regularly so that he learns to move his head in all different directions rather than, say, always looking to one side to see a favorite mobile, which can lead to a flat spot on one side of the head. To help correct such a spot, try moving the mobile to the other side for a bit and putting your baby in different spots in the crib, so he has to alternate where he's placing his head.* If the ground is free of (biting) dogs, cat dander, and dirt, then let your child explore the floor. That way, he can move around and learn to navigate all kinds of obstacles, like furniture and toys, which will also help him develop those gross motor skills. As he gets older, that should translate to time rolling a ball on the floor and doing all kinds of tumbling.

Make Junior a Genius. Okay, we're somewhat kidding here. The pushy-parent approach, more often than not, will backfire. Push a kid too hard, and he's going to find a way to push back one way or another. That said, it is interesting to note that the key element to attaining so-called genius status is practice. Extraordinarily accomplished kids tend to spend thousands of hours on a particular task. But those hours spent practicing aren't mandated by parents; they're done because the child wants to do them. So your job isn't to lock your child in his bedroom with his violin and a kitchen timer; it's to expose him to many things, so he can choose what he likes and be internally motivated to keep wanting to do it. Focus on all of his strengths rather than trying to improve every little one of his weaknesses.

Add DHA. Remember that the most important component of brain is fat, which helps improve the insulation of those brain cells to strengthen the communication of information from one neuron to the next. Here's one case when you should support the presence of fat: healthy fat. Research shows that children whose diets are supplemented with adequate levels of DHA perform better on cognitive tests and even have a higher IQ. Some grandmoms got us our healthy fats via cod liver oil, but these days, we can offer more palatable options: namely, supplements. Our recommended dose for kids (there's no hard data in youngsters up to four years): 30 milligrams a day for every year out of the womb up until age twenty (i.e. 60 mg at age two, 90 at age three, to 600 at age twenty). You can break up the pills and pour the liquid in healthy drinks.† For more nutritional info, see chapter 4.

---

* Another option is using a foam triangle wedge (available in baby stores) to help prop and hold the baby in various positions.
† We like to recommend you get nutrients in foods, but salmon and trout are the only fish in America that consistently have DHA. So we get them from where the fish do—algae, but from supplements.

Slow It Down. Your baby's noggin motor is churning right from the start. It's just that it's not churning at high speed, but a slow, steady setting. So especially in the first year of life, take things slow. It's great to expose your child to stimulation, but there's no need to create a circuslike atmosphere. Talk slowly and repeat your words. You're carving a channel in the brain, and the best way to make sure it's deep and wide is to take your time. "Motherese," or that singsong voice in which Mommy repeats what Baby says or describes what's going on at the dinner table, actually augments learning. It's okay to do singsong; just use real words that are pronounced correctly.

Routine Procedures

Help Your Kids Form Good Habits Right from the Start

If we had to define smart parenting in just a few words, we'd say it's all about instilling good habits and avoiding (or breaking) bad ones. We try to teach our kids that their positive habits will bring them health and happiness: Milk makes your bones strong, reading powers your brain, saying thanks earns you beaucoup brownie points. The not-so-great habits? They bring consequences that no child wants to endure: Hitting your friend over the head with a plastic bowling pin leads to time-out, not brushing your teeth leads to dentist drills, taking a whiz in the corner of the kitchen leads to mucho madness from Mama.

That's why we believe this chapter is so crucial, because it will give you the biological and psychological framework for establishing healthy habits and breaking unhealthy ones. While we'll detail guidelines for handling some of the major habits that kids form, such as sleeping through the night and toilet training, we believe that the overarching principles embedded within these specific illustrations will serve you well even after your child has mastered the art of the flush.

Habit formation is really about wiring the brain, and there are lots of reasons to lay down this neurological infrastructure early on. If you think back to our river comparison, you can imagine how much easier it is to navigate a river (or do anything, for that matter) once you've done it once, twice, a hundred times. Not only does repetition carve a deeper channel, as we described earlier, but also, in simple terms, the more often you run it, the easier it gets. So if you instill good habits early enough, the behavior becomes—and here's the crucial word—automatic. (Same holds true for bad habits, unfortunately.) Note that we say *you* here; it's your job to take the lead and show your child what's healthy and what's not. You've been down the river before and although your child's trip will be different from yours, you've got insider knowledge that can help set your child up for success.

The benefits of making good behaviors automatic are enormous. Biologically, living automatically is the body's lowest energy state, meaning that it's less stressful on the body not to have to work at everything. Habit reduces stress, allows us to pay attention to more important things, and, for a child, is a soothing influence. By promoting positive habits, not only will you take satisfaction in raising a well-mannered, well-groomed, and healthy child, but you'll also be able to spend more time bathing in the joys of parenting rather than battling the frustrations that can come with it.

Now, does that mean everything's going to be easy peasy lemon squeezy all the time? Of course not. It's going to take some time, effort, and savvy parenting to transition your child from the eating-sleeping-pooping machine that she is for much of her early life to the curious little kid who confronts challenges, explores the world, and uses a tissue. This chapter will give you the tools to help you pass your own good habits from one generation to the next.

Mirror Images: Show, Don't Tell

Children are true creatures of habit. Thumb in mouth. Finger in nose. Foot in sister's rib cage. Over and over and over. Sometimes, as parents, we believe that kids perpetuate bad habits simply because they either don't listen or because they have the sole intention of making our blood boil. While those may be reasons *some* of the

A HABIT GONE WILD?

With habits, as with many child health issues, there's a fine line between normal development and something that requires attention. While habits are normal, a tic might be a symptom of a health problem. So how do you tell them apart? For starters, a habit is more of a behavior or practice, while a tic is a repeated contraction of certain muscles and can't be voluntarily controlled much of the time. Most tics last for less than a year, but they affect up to 20 percent of kids—boys much more frequently than girls. Sometimes tics come in the form of muscle patterns (excessive blinking, for example), and sometimes they can be verbal (the child making a certain sound over and over). After the age of two or three, echolalia—when a child repeats sounds made by another person—can be a sign of autism, Tourette's syndrome, or another disorder. However, it's quite normal for kids to repeat babbles and words earlier on, when they're starting to put words together.

After you check out the tic with the pediatrician to make sure it's not something serious, you can let it work itself out. If it's caused by stress, then one strategy is to try to substitute a more innocuous behavior such as playing with a rubber band rather than pulling hair.

time, there are deeper psychological and biological reasons behind the formation of habits.

First, let's look at the psychological reasons why children form habits. Think about what happens when *you* are stressed. Some of you scream, some of you meditate, some of you turn to booze or fried cheese sticks. While some stress responses are healthy (meditation), many of them are not (fried anything). But the reason why we turn to our stress response is the same no matter what the particular response may be:

We're all seeking to gain some sort of control when we're in a situation that we don't control.

Think about the life of an infant. She has virtually no control 24-7. Can't talk, can't go to the fridge for a swig of Gatorade, can't turn the channel if you've plopped her in front of the same episode of *Barney* for the five hundredth time. Frustrating. So a child enacts her own stress response. Sometimes it comes in the form of a cry, but many times it comes in the form of a habit. In an infant, it may be thumb sucking or blanket stroking. As kids get older, they seek other ways to gain control (whining, tantrums) and soothe themselves (nail biting, hair twirling)—and those ways become habits.

Second, from a purely evolutionary perspective, back in the cave days, there was an advantage to a child forming habits—specifically, habits that would make him blend in with the rest of the tribe. If he could form habits that were parallel to the habits of fellow tribe members, then he wouldn't stand out, reinforcing that he was part of the team. Subconsciously, habits contributed to a child's assimilation into a community.

Last but not least, there's an important biological component to habit formation, and that comes in the form of something called mirror neurons. (See figure 3.1.) Simply, mirror neurons allow you to observe someone else performing an action (say, those fellow members of the tribe starting a fire), and that observation makes your brain want to perform the very same action. Yawning after someone else does is the classic example; it's not contagious in the viral kind of way, but it is in the neurological kind of way. Play peekaboo with your toddler, and he will do it right back. Working like tiny video cameras, mirror neurons are found all over the brain and help us assimilate all of the content we receive every day. That content comes in the form of actions as well as emotions, even allowing us to feel pain and empathy when those around us are suffering.

How do mirror neurons work? When you observe something, mirror neurons process that information in one part of your brain, then alert other parts of your brain that you should repeat the behavior that you just witnessed. This process is what causes children in the South to grow up speaking with drawls; it's what makes kids of hot-headed parents more aggressive.

The formation of habits depends largely on how these mirror neurons are firing. A common parental mantra—"Do as I say, not as I do"—just doesn't work because of mirror neurons. If you tell your child to eat vegetables while you're gobbling down cheese-smothered fries, what do you think he's going to want to eat? If you yell, scream, and throw pillows when you get angry, how do you suspect he's going to react when Tommy from next door breaks his truck? Exactly.

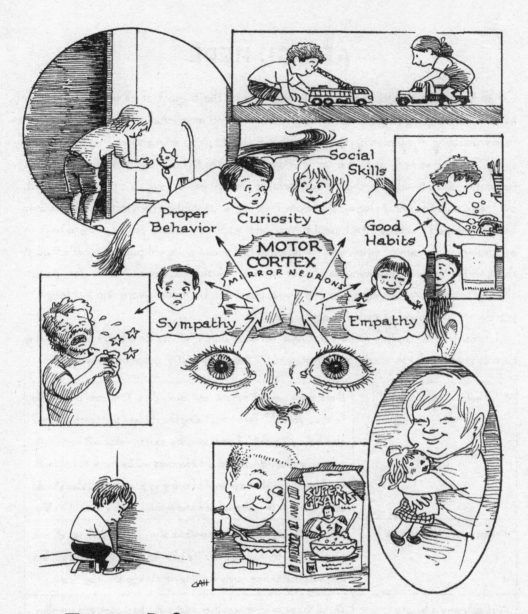

Figure 3.1 **Time to Reflect** As a parent, you are your child's greatest teacher, not through what you say, but through what you do. The component that makes that true: mirror neurons, which, as you might guess, help us learn through imitating the actions of others. In a child's development process, indeed it's true that nonverbal gestures, tone of voice, and actions all speak louder than words.

ATTACH HERE

Of all the things that children form habits around, the biggest of all is you. Yup, very early on, she's going to be attached to you literally and emotionally. Which is wonderful (and frustrating if you plan on seeing a movie without talking animals in a theater anytime soon). Starting as early as nine months and peaking at age two, many children experience separation anxiety—that is, they're comfortable with others as long as a parent is in sight, but the minute the parent leaves the room, it's a cry fest. On the one hand, this shows they have developed a secure attachment to you; on the other, it means you're going to have to endure some screaming when you try to leave the house solo, although in most cases, it stops within three or four minutes of your departure—trust us. Separation anxiety generally disappears between ages two and three, but it can be more severe and last longer if you do not use outside care on a regular basis.

Unresolved separation anxiety becomes an issue only when it's time to transition to day care or preschool. Here are some strategies for taking this often emotional step:

Well before the first day	Read books about school, and even do a little role playing by "playing school." Take turns being the student and teacher. It will also help your child if you describe exactly what will happen in school—and articulate that the teachers will be there to help with anything she might be scared of doing by herself. You also should make a visit or two, so she has some mental picture of what it's like.
When you're talking it up	Be alert to any worries or questions she may have. After all, it *is* a scary time for her. Tell her it's okay to feel sad or scared, but also emphasize how many exciting new things she'll be doing.
A couple weeks before	Do all the prep work together. Pick out a backpack and supplies, and get her to help you label things like jackets and lunch boxes. It's also not a bad idea to practice the school-day routine in terms of getting up, getting dressed, eating, and going. It'll help her reduce some stress—and get excited.

The night before	Let her pick out her clothes and lay them out so they're ready to go.
The first day	Let your child pick a toy or animal to put in her backpack; it can help comfort her early on.
Saying "See ya!"	Plan on staying for fifteen minutes or so on the first morning to help with the transition. You can look around the class, point out her name on the wall, all that fun stuff. Don't stay too long, and try to stay relaxed and loving (even if you, too, are sad!), because she'll pick up on your emotions. Have your special good-bye—maybe a hug and a special saying—and then go on your way. She may very well cry, but resist the urge to go back, because that will just teach her that you will rescue her every day. You can wait outside the classroom for a few minutes to be assured that, yes, she will stop crying and will go about her day.

The lesson here, of course, is that one of the best ways to establish healthy patterns in kids of any age is to lead by example. And isn't that what smart parenting is all about? We're teachers, we're leaders, and we've taken the responsibility as head boat guide to get our kids safely down the river.

Hard Habits to Make or Break?

Okay, it's time to dig in and learn the nitty-gritty about some of the biggest habit-related challenges that all parents face such as getting your child to sleep through the night, transition from diapers to toilet, turn off the TV/computer/DS Lite, and stop the high-pitched screaming in the middle of your cousin's wedding. We approach

WHAT GOES BUMP IN THE NIGHT

Dad yelling when his Giants win isn't the only thing that can startle your child out of a sleep. Here are some other things that may, too:

NIGHTMARES: They may start in infancy but won't be remembered or articulated until between two and five years old. Nightmares occur during stage 2 (REM) sleep, and they're the ones in which the kid wakes up, screaming in fear, and remembers both the dream and the comforting. It may take a little while for the child to fall back asleep.

NIGHT TERRORS: These happen in a much deeper stage of sleep (stage 4). Typically, a child will wake up frightened, confused, sweating, and disoriented. He'll go back to sleep quickly and will have no memory of it the next morning. Unlike the parents! These are usually more common in boys than in girls (the opposite is true for nightmares) and affect less than 4 percent of kids.

SLEEPWALKING: This doesn't usually happen until about age five. Children who sleepwalk generally have no memory of getting up, walking around, or even eating. Though it's rare that this would be a repeated problem, it also reinforces the need to have safety latches and locks on doors, cabinets, and windows, plus gates on stairs.

these topics with two goals in mind—one, to give you the tools to handle these specific situations, and two, to have you think a little more broadly about each subject and consider ways that you can use the underlying principles to address any other habits you might want your child to make or break.

Sleeping: Especially when you're in a sleep-deprived state yourself, trying to get your baby into a sleep routine can be more difficult than a one-thousand-box Sudoku puzzle. But it's worth every ounce of effort (promise!). And it's never too early to start. From the get-go, do everything you can to help your child internalize the fact that there is a nighttime routine in which she will go to bed and fall asleep. (Eventually this will also include staying asleep and staying in bed.) Even when she's waking for middle-of-the-night feedings, there are still things you can do to begin to influence whether she's a good sleeper or not. We can't emphasize enough how important good sleep is to a child's overall health. Sleep supplies the brain with energy; it also helps the brain grow and assists with wiring the circuitry for learning. Along with proper nutrition, it is the most important thing that a child needs for her development. Poor sleep (or "junk sleep," as some sleep experts call it, equating it to junk food) can impair brain development and is sometimes to blame for poor performance, inattention, bad moods, exhaustion, behavior issues, even obesity. (A child's mood can be a barometer of whether or not he's getting sufficient sleep. If your child is generally happy, then he's probably getting enough.)

Although each child is different, here are some ballpark numbers to aim for:

> One to four weeks old: fifteen to sixteen hours a day
> One to twelve months old: fourteen to fifteen hours a day
> One to three years old: twelve to fourteen hours a day
> Three to six years old: ten to twelve hours a day

Here's the kicker: Signs of sleep deprivation are nearly invisible in babies and young kids, so it's virtually impossible for parents to see if sleep deprivation is causing any damage. The harm actually becomes visible around the age of two, when a child who's been tired for two years becomes defiant, noncompliant, and ready to color the inside of Grandma's house with his Crayola 64.

So follow these strategies for instilling good sleep hygiene in your child; it'll benefit all of you.

⊃ Early on, your baby will be in a constant sleep-eat cycle, but that doesn't mean you can't begin teaching him about the difference between night and day: that there's hustle and bustle during the day and quiet during the night. (You're not really influencing his circadian rhythms; they're inborn.) During daytime naps, go about your business. The household noise will help teach your child to sleep through some noise and not be startled at the slightest disturbance.

⊃ Nighttime for babies is any time after seven or eight o'clock. Before bed-time, provide as little stimulation as possible. No music, no mobiles, no bright lights, no excessive talking. You want to teach your child that night-time is boring, so a good choice is to sleep. If you do otherwise, he'll grow to depend on stimulation and associate bedtime with entertainment. This is especially important during nighttime feedings, to help him fall back asleep. Blackout shades or curtains help set the scene, especially in the summer-time, when the sun rises early and sets late. An example of reducing stimu-lation would be changing from the standard daytime pattern of (1) feed, (2) change, (3) play, and (4) sleep to (1) change, (2) feed, and (3) sleep, under dim lights with no "props"—that is, no music, no rocking your child to sleep, no using a bouncy seat to get her to sleep and then switching to the crib, and so on.

⊃ You can induce sleep by giving your child a warm bath, reading him a story, and even adopting a simple gesture, like stroking a finger from the forehead down to the top of the nose. Some kids get so good at this conditioned re-sponse that it takes only two or three strokes before their eyes start getting heavy.

⊃ If you can teach your child to soothe himself with a rag doll or a small blanket in the crib (start this after six months, when he is less at risk for SIDS—see page 86), he'll be able to fall back asleep on his own rather than relying on you for rocking, nursing, or finding the lost pacifier. If you rock your baby to sleep, guess what? He'll come to expect that. Don't run into Baby's room every time you hear a cry or whimper; babies make a lot of noise when they sleep. First, assess the sound. If it's a cry, is it an "I just woke up from a dream and am feeling disoriented!" cry or a "Get in here and feed me and, while you're at it, check out the present I left you in my diaper!" cry? If it doesn't sound urgent to you, wait a few minutes to see if she can figure out how to put herself back to sleep. If you rush to her side, you'll be depriving her of the opportunity to practice self-soothing techniques. Not only that, but she'll learn that fussing or crying is a sure way to get you

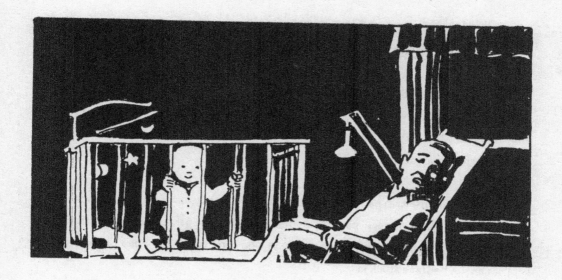

into her room and to pay attention to her—a bad habit you don't want to reinforce. And if you feel guilty about letting her fuss a little bit (let's face it, who doesn't?), ask yourself this: If you ignore her for a few minutes at night, does she still smile at you in the morning? Of course she does. She's forgotten. It's harder on you than it is on her; remember that. And also remember that the habit of self-soothing is a coping skill that will be hugely beneficial to her down the line.

⊃ If she is hungry in the middle of the night and you are the primary caregiver, have your partner give her a bottle, so that she doesn't rely solely on your comfort to fall back asleep. This will give you a break as well as give your partner a chance to bond with her as well. If she's still waking up after fifteen to eighteen months, try giving her water in a sippy cup or bottle; it is less rewarding than milk, and she won't like it as much and may eventually stop asking for it. You can make the transition to water by gradually diluting the milk over time. This strategy also helps prevent ear infections and milk rot, or lots of cavities from her going to sleep with teeth bathed in milk from that last bottle.

REDUCE THE RISK OF SIDS

SIDS (sudden infant death syndrome) mostly affects children under six months, peaking between the ages of two and four months. There's new evidence to suggest that the risk may be associated with a decrease in certain brain chemicals, but every parent needs to know how to reduce the risks of SIDS:

- ⊃ Make sure the crib has a firm mattress that fits tightly and is free of suffocation hazards, like bumpers, pillows, stuffed animals, sheepskins, and comforters—anything soft that a baby (especially one who can't yet lift her head or roll over) can get her face stuck in.

- ⊃ Keep the room cool, as heat may contribute to SIDS.

- ⊃ Put Baby to sleep on her back and don't put her in bed with you; she'll be at increased risk of someone rolling on her and suffocating her. If you choose to sleep in the same room, keep her in a crib.

- ⊃ Don't smoke or expose Baby to secondhand smoke.

- ⊃ Interestingly, use of a pacifier when falling asleep decreases the chances of SIDS.

⊃ For an older baby who is definitely not hungry and is waking up only out of habit, there are many different approaches, ranging from the "Let 'em cry till they're blue in the face" technique to the "She looked so sad, I just brought her into our bed" pitfall. We recommend a middle ground in which you reassure her that you haven't abandoned her but also let her know that she needs to put herself back to sleep.

One technique is to let her cry for several minutes to give her a chance to self-soothe. If that doesn't have the desired effect, peek in and gently pat her hand or her rear end. Resist the temptation to talk to her, pick her up, rock her, or engage her in any way. Then leave the room. If she continues to cry, wait a little longer before going in the next time. If your baby really is capable of sleeping through the night, this technique should take only a couple of nights to succeed (sometimes as little as one night; rarely as long as two weeks). If you can't stand the thought of leaving your baby crying alone in her room, an alternative is to park yourself in a chair in her room and sit there silently in the dark. She'll cry for your attention, but if you resist giving it to her, she'll eventually get bored and go back to sleep.

➲ Try not to be the only one who ever puts your child to sleep. Get grandparents and babysitters in on the action early. That teaches your child not to be dependent on one person for the nighttime routine. If you're nursing, occasionally pump a bottle and let someone else give it to Baby at bedtime. Over the first few weeks and months, it may seem warm and wonderful to put your child to sleep yourself every night, but down the line, you may want to, say, go out on a date (what a concept!), and if your child can't be put down by anyone else, you can forget about it.

➲ Never take the child into your bed unless you plan on doing it permanently. That's an extremely hard habit to break. If you do choose to cosleep (that is, having your child in the bed with you, either for convenience, for keeping a closer eye on the baby, or for family bonding), that's fine. But it's important to note that cosleeping does increase the risk of SIDS and infant death, most often through suffocation.★ Make sure that the place of sleep, whether a bassinet or a bed, contains no soft things that can cover the baby's mouth and interfere with breathing, such as a comforter or pillows. Though there are some strong advocates for cosleeping, we recommend separate sleeping quarters. If nothing else, it'll improve the chances of keeping your romantic life in good shape.

★ And, of course, never sleep in the same bed if you've been drinking or taking recreational drugs.

➲ Make napping a habit early on. The best times for naps are typically at nine in the morning and two in the afternoon, when a baby's circadian rhythms will make him the sleepiest. Don't try to outmuscle sleep by forcing a nap that conforms to your schedule or by keeping him awake during the day. Depriving him of a nap does *not* mean he'll be more likely to fall asleep at night. Unlike teenagers, young children will not sleep later in the morning if they've gone to bed later at night or skipped a nap during the day, so the hours they miss end up increasing their total sleep deficit. Of course, not all kids are exactly alike, so pay attention to your child's natural rhythms and your own household schedule, and make adjustments.

➲ Some kids nap until they're four or five; others give it up before age two. Most transition from two naps a day to one between twelve and fifteen months. Watch your child's cues for when to reduce the naps to once a day. When she is taking two fifteen-minute naps a day, it may be time to go down to one a day, which, hopefully, will last longer. Make sure that you're home in the early afternoon and you put your child in the ready-to-nap position in the same way, making everything calm and nonstimulating. If you run around and do errands during your child's natural nap time (after lunch), he'll learn to nap in the car seat or stroller. This can be a curse: Every time you want him to nap, you'll have to take a drive or stroll for an hour—a real pain in bad weather. Instead of feeling pinned down by having to be home for a couple of hours in the early afternoon, think of it as an opportunity to catch up on phone calls, housework, or paperwork, or even to just put your own feet up.

➲ A child who has been sleeping through the night may begin to wake up in the middle of the night if he's having a growth spurt, he's developing a new skill (crawling or walking), he's teething (more on page 99), he's anxious (for example, about starting preschool), or his routine has changed in some way. Just practice the same techniques you used to teach him to sleep through the night in the first place: Keep things calm and quiet, and either allow him the opportunity to self-soothe or camp out in his room for a few nights until the phase passes.

BED-WETTING

Though common, bed-wetting (medical term: enuresis) tends to go away for most kids by age four or five. Of kids who wet the bed longer than that (boys more often than girls), as many as 10 percent may do so all the way through adolescence, especially if a family member was also a bed-wetter. If your child has always been a bed-wetter but is approaching the age of overnights, there are some simple strategies you can use. First, check with your doctor to make sure your child does not have a bladder infection or some other cause. Second, don't lose your cool! Punishing the bed-wetter does *not* help. Third, with an older child, matter-of-factly have him help strip the bed and change the sheets, dividing and conquering the labor, without making a big deal of it. And for sleepovers, there are great medications such as the antidiuretic desmopressin (DDAVP), which reduces urine production by the kidneys. DDAVP comes in pill form as well as nasal spray. These meds are expensive, so most families don't use them nightly, unless the laundry bill outweighs the pill cost. Other strategies:

⊃ No fluids after dinner, or only sips until seven o'clock.

⊃ Get him up to tinkle before you hit the hay. Even if he is already asleep, stand him by the potty, aim, and let it flow. You may have to help him aim, depending on how soundly he sleeps.

⊃ Try a Potty Pager or other wireless silent alarm, which, upon sensing moisture, wakes up the sleeping child by vibrating. These devices work great and usually come with a money-back guarantee. (Sorry, you don't get the bonus ginsu knives.)

⊃ Reward with cool underwear when he stays dry so many nights in a row.

Toilet Training: At a certain point, either kid or Mom has had it with the diapers. That means it's time to transition to toileting. Generally, there are three approaches to toilet training: One is initiated by the parents, often in the first few months of life. This is unusual. Some cultures, for example, start training babies as early as six weeks old, by holding the child over a potty seat when it's time and saying "*psshhhhhhh.*" The second is initiated by the child, usually around age two. The third is more socially driven, meaning that the, say, three-year-old wants to do what everybody else is doing, or the mom knows that Junior won't get into preschool unless he ditches the pants with the Pampers. This is not the ideal situation, because the added deadline pressure makes it much more difficult to, uh, perform.

Our recommendation: You'll have the most success if you start training as soon as your child gives you the clues that he is ready, such as:

⊃ He wakes up dry (showing he has some bladder control).

⊃ He can (and will!) follow instructions.

⊃ He imitates other family members' actions.

⊃ He gives you signs that he needs to go. (The tinkle-tinkle-squirm dance is pretty common, as is clutching the crotch.)

⊃ He says he doesn't like the way it feels to be wet or soiled. (Superabsorbent disposable diapers don't help here, because children don't feel the wetness. For this reason, kids who wear cloth diapers often train much earlier.)

⊃ His pooping schedule is predictable (for instance, every afternoon after his nap).

⊃ His poops are well formed and not mushy.

Here are the steps to take:

⊃ Buy a child's potty (one with traction for the floor), so she can sit comfortably rather than having to balance her small body over the big hole, even with the small potty seat that goes on top of the toilet. Most kids feel better having their feet on the floor rather than dangling. Plus, it's less scary than to be so high up. If you're going to use the real toilet, place a stool under her feet.

➲ Read books about using the potty (*Everyone Poops* and *Once upon a Potty* are all-time favorites) and watch videos to get in the mood. (We recommend *It's Potty Time.*)

➲ Talk to your child about why we use the potty and what the signals are: When she feels like she has to go, it's time to sit on the potty. Emphasize that she'll be now going to the bathroom the way Mommy and Daddy do. By now, she should have seen lots of family members going to the toilet.

➲ You can conduct a dry run-through (emphasize dry) by showing her how to sit on the potty with her clothes on. Then show her how to pull her pants down and sit. With boys, you can teach them to pull their pants down, lift the seat, and aim for one particular spot in the bowl while standing. Using a Cheerio or a piece of toilet paper can improve little boy aim immensely. But sometimes it's easier to teach boys to pee sitting down first.

➲ You may have the most luck by escorting your child to the toilet every twenty or thirty minutes and have him try going. That's because many kids don't recognize they have to go until it's too late. And if you're trying at

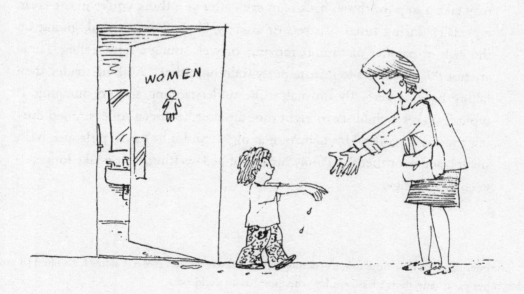

regular intervals, chances are you'll hit jackpot at some point—a perfect chance to use positive reinforcement. It's a labor-intensive system, but a very quick one, especially if the child exhibits the signs of readiness listed above. Many parents using this method report that their children are trained within a week or two.

⊃ Instill routines. Always encourage your youngster to use the toilet before bed, before going in the car, after dinner, and so on. Of course, you can't fully control the times that their bowels and bladders need emptying, but you can nudge them along. Another routine to start right away: Get your child into the habit of washing his hands afterward.

⊃ Positive reinforcement works much better than scolding. (Sadly, lapses in potty training are one of the leading causes of child abuse.) Many parents will offer an M&M or a Cheerio after some piddle lands in the potty. Though we'd prefer that you pick a nonsugary reward, we are on board with using the reward system here.

⊃ Understand that this is an evolving process. Just because your daughter went a week without any accidents doesn't mean she's potty trained forever. She may take a step (or three) backward even after you think you're in the clear, especially during times of stress or anxiety, like starting school, giving up the crib or pacifier or thumb, moving, or welcoming a new sibling. These are not the best times to initiate potty training, either.* Making strides, then falling back, is perfectly normal, so be understanding and encouraging. It typically takes a child six to eight months after he's been toilet trained during the day to control his urination at night. And if he's a deep sleeper, has a small bladder, or there's a family history of bed-wetting, it may take longer—even years longer.

* Summer can be a nice time to start training because fewer clothes make it easier for a child to pull down her pants (and there's less laundry when she has an accident).

UNCONTROLLABLE CRYING

If your infant or young child is wailing like an over-dramatic soap star, stop and consider that there could be a very quick fix. Some of the more common reasons for a big old tear session: an eyelash (or some other foreign substance) in the eye; she's wet; his testicle is caught in an awkward position in the diaper or car seat; a hair is wrapped around a digit (or even the penis). The lesson: Do a quick total-body once-over to see if you can find the culprit. Another tactic that has worked for some of us: a kiss, then a drop of gas-relief medicine like Mylicon. And then another kiss.

Tantrums: It doesn't take an expert in Pavlovian psychology to know that children can use tantrums to get what they want: Kid wants candy in supermarket, Mom says no, Kid whines, Mom says no, Kid screams and hurls himself into neighboring carts, Mom says, Oh, okay, just this time. Next time Kid wants something, he immediately goes into cart-hurling mode.

No question that tantrums (especially the public ones) can be some of the most frustrating times we have as parents. Choose your battles. If your kid is known to throw a whopping tantrum if he doesn't get extra milk in his cereal, what does it hurt to give him some extra milk? Obviously, you don't want to give in too much or all the time, but it's important to let kids "win" sometimes. The easiest thing is to give in; to do anything to stop the insanity. Intellectually, we know that's not good, because it reinforces bad behavior. Practically speaking, it's much harder to stand your ground. Harder, but not impossible. These strategies should help:

⊃ Certainly, some parts of a child's temperament and personality are intrinsic, but much of our kids' behavior comes from modeling. Youngsters who see their parents lash out (at each other, at kids, at the Bears) are much more likely to lash out when they're angry. So the first step is to try to stay calm and cool, even when disciplining your children. His mirror neurons will kick in, and over the long run, you'll likely have far fewer public displays of destruction.

⟳ We believe that the best way to handle temper tantrums is through prevention. Learn to predict the times when your child may be more likely to toss his milk at the people at the next table. That way, you can either avoid public situations or perform a timely intervention. The truth is that tantrums are surprisingly predictable; they often happen when kids are overtired, overstimulated, or hungry. (Same holds true for adults, right?) These explosive moments are typically preceded by a sullen or quiet period; the proverbial calm before the storm. Then when he tries to do something he can't do or is denied something, it's not long before a little whining morphs into a category 5 hurricane. If you do your best to keep your child well fed, relaxed, and well rested (quiet time can be as effective as naps), fewer of those storms will make landfall.

⟳ You shouldn't let a child's habit of throwing tantrums deter you from saying "no." Kids need boundaries for many reasons, and they need to know "no." However, you may find that it's more effective to avoid using the N word directly. Changing the way you tell your child that you're denying him something can be a good way to diffuse a volatile situation. Maybe you explain briefly why today's not the day he gets to jump puddles. Maybe you start with a positive: "I love chocolate chips, too, but we're having dinner in an hour." Or maybe you deflect the reason for saying no off of them and on to you: for example, explaining to your four-year-old how sad you would be if he fell off the porch while trying to mount the railing (like the big guy he saw at the park) and hurt himself. Remember, who owns the problem? "I would be disappointed if you chose to do that, because we would need to spend time in the hospital and miss the fun here."

⊃ Make sure all caregivers in your child's life know your ground rules regarding behavior and discipline. Consistency helps kids establish good habits. Inconsistency creates confusion and a side order of tantrums (more on this in our YOU Tips). It might be worth a family conference with grandparents, aunts, and uncles to make sure you're all on the same page; that's much healthier than having a fight with Grandma and Grandpa after they let your little princess watch back-to-back Disney videos when you have a no-TV policy (see page 97). And when you need to call in the heavy artillery with the grandparents, bring them with you to the pediatrician's office, and make sure you tell the pediatrician at the start of the visit that you want to hear more about strategies for instilling good habits rather than perpetuating bad ones. You can even email or call the pediatrician before the visit to set the agenda.

⊃ If you're in a place where you can ignore a tantrum comfortably (say, your own home, as opposed to church), then go ahead and ignore it. No response from you eventually means he won't lash out to get one. For a child, drama without an audience is like a glass without wine—there's nothing to it. But beware: If you're going to ignore it, you have to stick to that. If he learns that your ignoring it for thirty minutes eventually leads to a great display from you, he will work even harder to overcome the ignoring phase to get that delayed reward. Whatever the cause of the tantrum, figure out what works to pull your child out of it and stick with that. Sometimes kids just want to be heard. If a two-year-old is saying, "I want my tricycle," it may be enough just to reinforce to him that you hear and understand him. "Yes, I understand, you want your tricycle. Yes, you want your tricycle." Speak back to him in his manner.

⊃ With some children, tantrums can lead to hyperventilation. There may be crying involved, or not. These spells can be frightening, because children can lose consciousness. If this happens, lay the child down on the floor so he doesn't fall. Exposure to intense stimuli (like a cold cloth on the face) in the first fifteen seconds or so can help snap him out of it. Medications aren't recommended, and you should try to handle these tantrums the same way you'd handle others (see above).

CHILD ABUSE: A PRIMER

While we're discussing issues of discipline, it makes sense to talk about the extreme end. It's not a pretty topic. In fact, it's one of our least favorite, and we wish we didn't have to address it at all. But the fact is that many kids are affected by various forms of child abuse: According to official reports, abuse affects sixteen out of every one thousand children under the age of three. The actual rate may be as much as ten times higher. Child maltreatment includes neglect (60 percent of reported cases), which is defined as lack of parental care resulting in actual or potential harm to a child; physical abuse (20 percent); sexual abuse (10 percent); and psychological abuse (7 percent). Scary stats, no doubt. Even parents who intellectually understand the dangers of abuse and say that they would never ever abuse their kids become abusive under certain circumstances. Some of the causes include unrealistic expectations of a child (for instance, thinking that a five-year-old should "know better" than to wet the bed), inconsistency in child rearing (having many different people care for the child can lead to inconsistent rules), parental exhaustion (shaking a baby who won't sleep), and being in a household where there's already domestic or substance abuse. Parents who are stressed themselves—emotionally, physically, psychologically, financially—are at greater risk of abusing their children. So if you feel your own life slipping out of control, seek help before you do anything to your child that you might regret.

In addition to monitoring your own reactions, you need to be on the lookout for signs that other people may be mistreating your child, and nowhere is that more important than in the area of sexual abuse. Male offenders are more common than females, and the majority of perps are people known to the child, such as relatives, significant others, and authority figures. (See our take on male babysitters on page 328.) The key to prevention: supervision, supervision, supervision. Also, be attuned to your child. If she comes home from somewhere and is acting strangely or shows resistance to going to someone's house, trust her and try to provide a safe space for her to talk about her feelings. And if you suspect sexual abuse, see your pediatrician immediately. Not tomorrow, now.

Now, there are going to be some children who have behavioral and anger issues that exceed the typical tantrum. In that case, the safety of your child and others should be your priority. A simple time-out will (see page 104) be inadequate here, and you may need to seek professional help. No kid feels good about himself after he's just kicked, screamed, and writhed on the floor and still didn't get his way. So when a child eventually does pull himself out of a tantrum, it's a good time to use positive reinforcement. "You did a good job calming yourself down."

Finally, we encourage you to be understanding. Sometimes kids kick and scream because they're overwhelmed, tired, need to release tension (often after being picked up from preschool or day care), or are having trouble dealing with something they can't articulate. They're not trying to outmuscle you or win a power game; a tantrum may simply be the only means available to them for expressing pent-up emotion. Sometimes they just need to "talk" things out. A hug, with some close talking and reassurance, can help too.

TV/Entertainment: We don't believe that TV is bad per se (heck, we're on the tube ourselves), but for kids, spending too much time in front of the TV (or later, playing video/digital games) isn't all that healthy. For one, while they're watching, they aren't engaged in healthy activities, like socializing, reading, exploring, creative play, and running around outside. Plus, kids tend to model behavior they see on TV that you don't necessarily agree with. And that's not even mentioning the violence, sex, and fast-food commercials (On average, kids see fifteen food commercials a day!) they'll be exposed to. The average kid watches about three hours a day, but that number gets much higher as they get older. Not surprisingly, excessive TV watching is associated with childhood obesity. So follow these strategies for limiting their time in front of the TV, no matter how much they love the dude with the square pants.

➲ After they turn two, you should limit them to one to two hours a day of screen time (under two, they don't need to be watching much at all, if any; as they get older, screen time includes time spent on computers and video games, as well), according to the American Academy of Pediatrics and researchers looking closely at baby brain development. And prescreen what they're watching to make sure it's a quality choice. Shows that encourage active participation (like calling out answers or dancing along) rather than passive viewing are best. If you want them to emulate bratty behavior, then make sure they watch the average sitcom. Funny, yes. But monkey see, monkey do applies here.

⊃ No TV in your youngster's room. TVs in the bedroom are associated with a higher incidence of childhood obesity, sleep problems, and behavior problems. In general, eating in front of the TV in *any* room of the house should be kept to a minimum, because it leads to mindless snacking and lots of extra calories (see page 137).

⊃ Videos and DVDs may be a better choice for kids than TV, because you can vet the content beforehand. Some of our recommendations: Rabbit Ears Productions' series of classic children's stories for preschoolers, *Veggie Tales, Sesame Street, Blue's Clues,* and other shows that encourage interaction. Videos are also a plus because they don't expose Junior to fast-food commercials; of course, you can always record a show and fast-forward through the commercials. A nonprofit organization called Parents' Choice Foundation regularly reviews videos, programming, magazines, and books for children on its website at www.parents-choice.org.

⊃ Limit the time you have the TV on in the background. That's a habit your child is going to copy—not to mention the fact that you probably don't want your child learning language skills from TV people. TV can be a distraction, preventing your child from tuning into *your* language. Also, beware of the adult content on shows you may have on for yourself (soaps, news, *The Dr. Oz Show,* and so on), because children will absorb and repeat what they see.

While there are plenty of nonscreen options for entertaining your child in healthy ways (playgrounds, games), the number one alternative is reading. It's one of the best ways to interact with your child in a peaceful, cuddling environment, plus it gives her the intellectual foundation for academic success and does wonders to improve the neural circuitry that's being formed in these early, critical years. See more in our YOU Tips.

Hygiene: For a while, it's just you, your baby, a bathtub, and some baby wipes. But it takes more than that to teach kids good hygiene habits that will improve and maintain their health as they grow up. Follow these guidelines for making sure that you're keeping things squeaky clean.

Tooth Care:

⊃ When your child starts cutting teeth at about six months, you can help soothe some of the pain in her mouth with a teething ring. (A frozen bagel or wash cloth works equally well.) For severe discomfort, a dose of the anti-inflammatory pain reliever children's ibuprofen may be necessary. We don't recommend using topical products (ones you apply to the skin and other tissue) containing the local anesthetic benzocaine (for example, Orajel) because of the potential side effect methemoglobinemia, a rare life-threatening condition that impedes red blood cells' ability to deliver oxygen to the body. Children with this disorder (about 1 in 250) can literally turn blue (cyanosis) due to oxygen deficiency.

⊃ No bottles in bed, no bottle propping. If your child falls asleep with a bottle in his mouth, it increases the likelihood that his teeth will rot from sitting in pools of lactose, the natural sugar found in milk.

⊃ Don't start kids on soda or candy. If they're not exposed to these cavity creators, they won't crave them. Same goes for juice, especially in a bottle while sleeping, In fact, juice is double forbidden and double bad because it bathes the teeth in sugar and with the exception of orange juice, contains empty calories. Instead encourage eating whole fruit and drinking water as they get older.

ARE CAVITIES CATCHING?

All cavities are symptoms of a bacterial infection called dental caries, which is the most common disease of childhood. Nearly half of all children have cavities before they enter kindergarten, and most of that is because of transmission of bacteria from mother to child (although sometimes from nanny to child) through activities such as cleaning a pacifier that fell on the floor in your own mouth, wiping your child's face with your saliva, tasting food off of your child's spoon, or prechewing food (common among some Caribbean cultures).

Having your child's cavities filled does absolutely nothing to cure the disease. Unless you also take steps to eliminate the infection, your child will more than likely be back in the dentist's chair within two years. Those steps include fluoride treatments, use of an antibacterial rinse, regular flossing, brushing with fluoride toothpaste, and avoiding sugary foods. Bacteria need sugar to live, and the rising amount of sugar in children's diets has led to an increase in the number of cavities dentists are seeing in the under-five set; cavities are caused by the frequent eating (or drinking) of sugar, not the total amount consumed. When we eat sugars, bacteria ferment them into acids that erode teeth.

In addition to the long-term effects of tooth decay—the single best predictor of cavities throughout life is cavities in childhood—the immediate effects on your child can be wide ranging. Early childhood cavities can interfere with speech development and affect mood, learning, and nutrition. The best way to avoid dental caries is to take your child to the dentist every six months beginning at age one.

⊃ Give your child fluoride supplements if you use well water. (Check with your dentist or pediatrician first.) Also, if you have fluoridated tap water, it's better for a kid to drink that than bottled spring water; just use a Brita pitcher or faucet filter after pouring off the first two glasses of the day if you're concerned about purity. And have your well water tested for pesticide and other contaminants that have a stronger effect in small people with developing brains.

⊃ Pay attention to baby teeth. Just because they're going to fall out doesn't mean you should ignore them. If baby teeth get infected, the risk is that the adult teeth may not grow in properly when the time comes.

⊃ By age one, brush your child's teeth once a day, even if it's with a clean finger and minimal toothpaste. You can use a damp washcloth to wipe teeth starting as soon as they appear (as early as four months), then graduate to a toothbrush when there are enough teeth to brush. By the time your child reaches two, you should be brushing him twice a day.

⊃ Use fluoride toothpaste (after age 3); some natural toothpastes don't have it. Only use a pea-sized amount and teach your child to spit, not swallow. Beware of yummy-flavored children's toothpaste that kids may want to snack on, as fluoride is poisonous in large amounts. Keep toothpaste out of the reach of children and always supervise brushing.

⊃ Use a soft nylon-bristle brush. Have your child brush for about two minutes, making sure to hit every tooth, top and bottom, inside and out. You can play games (like hide-and-seek of the teeth, or counting to ten) to help kids stay engaged and to make it a fun and habit-forming experience. They should do it once and you once. Musical toothbrushes can keep kids brushing for the whole length of the song.

⊃ Ideally, the first dentist visit should happen around age one—certainly no later than two—and every six months after that. In the beginning, the dentist will check for normal tooth development and oral health. As your child gets older, your dentist may recommend applying fluoride varnishes or treatments or sealants, or taking X-rays.

⊃ Don't be afraid to get a second opinion on your child's teeth. It's not uncommon for dentists to misdiagnose cavities, and some pediatric dentists even argue that small cavities don't need to be filled at all; that cavities essentially heal themselves by circulating calcium and other minerals in and out of the tooth. Many dentists are switching to a model that promotes the remineralization of teeth through procedures like fluoride varnishes. Filling cavities does not stop tooth decay, which is caused by bacteria that live in the mouth (see box, page 100).

Hand Washing: Hand washing should be a habit that you model when you come in from outside, change a diaper, go to the toilet, and prepare and eat food. When children start going to the toilet, they should begin to wash and dry their hands by themselves. A stepping stool helps ensure easy access.

Bathing: While it's going to be quite some time before your child is able to bathe herself, it's important to start a good bath routine early, so that it becomes a happy habit. You'll give sponge baths until the umbilical cord falls off, but after that, you bathe Baby in a small tub or sink. We don't recommend the kitchen sink; it's not the cleanest to mix food remnants with private parts.

Use warm water (test it first) and a mild baby shampoo. Gently sponge the body and hair, and make it a playful time, so that your little one associates bath time with fun. (Tupperware and measuring cups make for great bath toys.) We recommend making it a habit before bed several times a week, but not too soon after a meal. And never ever turn your back on your baby: no answering the phone, no running to get a towel, no siblings in charge of watching the baby, no nothing except all eyes on her.

Thumb Sucking: Some babies learn to suck their thumbs when they're in the womb. Why? Not because they're bored and there's no Placenta Library to check out books to pass the time. It's because it's soothing and calming, and even after they're born, it's a natural reflex. Other kids don't find their thumb until six months and some never pick up the habit. The reason for concern down the line is that it can interfere with teeth and mouth development. Most kids stop by six months or so, and that's fine. If it continues beyond age two, mention it to the child's dentist.

We recommend using a behavior modification sticker system to reward for however many hours a child can go without doing it (give a sticker as positive reinforcement). Giving toddlers gentle physical reminders (like taking the thumb out) can help. If positive reinforcement doesn't work, some parents have had success with putting mittens on their child's hands or applying bad-tasting nail polish to the thumbs to discourage the sucking. You can also use similar techniques if your toddler turns into a nail biter.

. . .

We can't emphasize enough that it's much easier to establish good habits early than break bad habits later, so we encourage you to think about how your family will address these issues before they become problems. Below we also offer some more practical advice that will help you devise systems that will pay dividends when it comes to the health of your child—and the sanity of your family.

YOU TIPS

Be the Leader. It can be hard to control your anger when your child insists on wiping boogers on the babysitter's purse. And we understand that parenting can be challenging; after all, they did name it the terrible twos. But if you take one message away from this book, it's that your child will emulate your behaviors. So behave yourself. It can be the greatest gift you ever give your kid.*

Call a T.O. The perfect time-out works like this: Teach your child that if he does something that you tell him not to, you will give him a warning and a slow count to three. That counting gives him a chance to stop what he's doing and correct the behavior. If you reach three, then he's going to the time-out place in your home. Many of us will give a warning at one. If the misbehavior doesn't stop, we'll say clearly, "I asked you not to put your sister's doll in the dishwasher. That is two." At three, the time-out starts.

Make the time-out place a chair where there are no stimuli; the idea is to make it a boring place where kids don't want to be. You keep him there for the number of minutes equal to his age (four minutes for a four-year-old and so on).† After your child serves his time, you explain why what he did was harmful and not acceptable and ask if he understands. But don't make it a lecture; just state the facts. You make punishment a habit that children don't like, and they'll change the habit that got them there in the first place.

By the time the child is three or four, she may ask if her behavior is good or bad and may even give herself a time-out. This signifies that she knows right from wrong, still needs to test limits, but is mature enough to take ownership of her behavior. Just like imaginary play, time-outs can help youngsters figure out their boundaries.

Wrap Him Up. Boys and girls respond differently to anger, stress, and discipline. Girls, who tend to have more advanced language skills, will use their words, whereas boys may feel like

---

* Though she may believe it's that wicked-cool cell phone you give her a few years down the road.
† No, don't put a six-month-old in time-out for thirty seconds, smarty pants.

hitting someone or something. One of the strategies that we have found effective (and by *we*, we mean Dr. Oz) is this: When a boy is reacting emotionally or physically, go ahead and wrestle a bit with him (playfully, not WWE-like). This gives him a chance to vent physically without actually hitting anything, and it also helps diffuse the situation. (Good-natured wrestling should be supervised by a mature adult—hello, Mom!) When kids don't have language to vent frustration, roughhousing can help. (The periodic broken lamp is less expensive than psychiatry bills later on in life!) Plus, think of all the subconscious cues going on: Yes, you may be restraining him, but the physicality also means that you're hugging and comforting him at the same time. It's a strong statement to a kid: It shows that you're engaged with his emotions but also establishing your role as the parent and the authority. Note: If your daughter sounds more like the boy in the description above and needs a good wrestle rather than just a hug, this is not a cause for alarm. The above is a generalization, and individual temperaments vary tremendously.

Recruit and Educate. So you've got it all down. Time-out strategy, going-to-bed routine, saving the pudding for last. Works like a charm—until you leave your precious petunia with grandparents who think it's perfectly fine for her to stay up until ten and draw on pillows with Sharpies, and who buy a toy for Junior every time they walk into the store. One of the toughest parts about parenting is training the *other* caregivers in your child's life to follow your routines (especially since you may feel guilty admonishing someone who's nice enough to help you out and give you some time off). Plus, it's a long list of people, including relatives, nannies, babysitters, older siblings, day care workers, and anybody else who can break an instilled habit with just a few bad minutes of icing-covered animal crackers. That's why it's worth your time to talk frankly with those close to you not just about *what* you do but also *why* you do it. Even prepare a "mommy sheet" to give to all caregivers (with emergency numbers, too). At the same time, don't fret if the grandparents spoil the kids once in a while. Creating conflict only highlights the event in the child's memory. Let it slide by like a small stone in the river that your parenting boat brushes by. And find a different time when nerves and tempers are calm to address discipline style points with them.

Mind the Manners. It's never too early to start getting your child in the habit of saying please, thank you, and excuse me. Even before he starts talking, your repetition of the words at the right times helps build the language patterns and habits of using good manners. But please have reasonable expectations of what toddlers can do. For example, you won't likely get a two-year-old to sit through a four-course meal at a fancy adult restaurant. But it is okay to teach your toddler that he can sit with the family at the dinner table for ten minutes or so. Gradually increase the time as he gets older. To up the odds of success, make sure that the food is ready to be served—don't waste your ten sacred minutes on meal prep—and keep your child engaged with lots of talk and interaction* so that being at the table is associated with fun. If you absolutely can't resist having your toddler accompany you to a restaurant, be considerate of the other patrons and bring books, small toys, and coloring supplies to keep him occupied.

Start the Reading Habit. To combat the effects of TV, turn to books. Here's what we recommend.

- ⊃ Start with picture books and read them every day, even if it's just for five minutes. Make it a habit your child will grow to love and expect. Board books are great: Kids can't rip the pages. Cloth books are also good for babies: They can chew them, and you can leave them in the crib. There are also neat waterproof books for the tub; in some, the pictures change color when they're wet.

- ⊃ You can change books or stick with the same one over and over if that's what your child likes. Follow her lead. It doesn't matter if the story is the same; what matters is the interaction and the process.

- ⊃ Rhyming books, such as Dr. Seuss, are great for language development. After a while, you can leave off the last word of a line, and your child will be able to fill it in.

---

* Preferably, interaction that does not involve tossing spaghetti like a rodeo lasso.

⊃ Pick up a book yourself. While he's playing, take some time to read rather than flipping on the TV. Modeling, modeling, modeling!

Laugh Away. Laugh with your child, but never at your child. Being able to laugh with someone at a situation can be a powerful coping tool. Example: Junior is trying to pitch his best tantrum, but instead you tickle him until he can't help but laugh. Or make your silliest face. Or try balancing a spoon on your nose. The tickling can serve the same purpose as wrestling. Wrapped in a hug, he receives the message "I love you and we laugh together." It doesn't always work, but it's worth a try from time to time.

Distraction Action. One of the telltale characteristics of a tantrum is that a child in the midst of one gets caught in a behavior loop that no amount of logic or cajoling can break. Once he gets sucked into this vortex, there's often little you can do except ride it out. But if you can learn to identify the signs of an impending meltdown, you can try to distract your child before he gets sucked into the black hole. First, feed him a healthy snack if there's a chance he's losing it because of low blood sugar. If that doesn't work, break into a silly song, start a game of chase, or try the tickle technique (above).

Get On the Go. Leave it to traveling to throw even the best habits off track. Some tips for keeping things as smooth as possible when you're on the road:

⊃ To help with time-zone shifts, put your child to bed at the new location's bedtime and adjust his meal schedule too. (For infants, feed on demand.) Get outside as much as possible because the daylight can help the body adapt to the new time.

⊃ Don't give antihistamines to make him drowsy; it can actually decrease his chances of adjusting to the new time.

⊃ Carry antibacterial hand sanitizer and practice good hygiene all the time to minimize the spread of germs. Perhaps the only thing more challenging than traveling with a child might be traveling with a sick child.

⊃ Have two binkies/blankets/snuggle items when you travel. If one hits the deck, all hell does not break loose. You simply pull out the second identical item for immediate comfort mode.

4

Good Taste

Instill Proper Nutritional and Activity Habits for Baby and Beyond

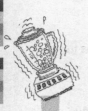

n the beginning, parents find themselves using a lot of four-letter words: Baby. Cute. Mama. Dada. Uh-oh. But the four-letter word that may prove to be the most crucial is this one: fuel.

Fuel in the form of breast milk or formula early on (and foods and drinks soon thereafter) lays the foundation for your child's overall health and development. The fueling process starts out simply enough: You've basically got a choice between natural milk and the artificial kind. But as your baby gets older, the world becomes a little more complex. You have to deal with all of the higher-calorie milk variations (milk shakes, milk chocolate, Milk Duds, Milky Ways), and you also have to help your child navigate the unhealthy temptations that he's going to encounter every day and at every meal.

We've spent the last two chapters discussing all the crazy-cool things happening inside children's tiny skulls; now we're going to move a few inches lower to dissect all the things that go into their mouths and dribble onto their bibs.

Proper nutrition influences brain development, behavior, and attention span, and it plays a major role in whether your child is at increased risk of obesity, asthma, heart disease, impotence, cancer, blindness, memory loss, and other later-in-life health problems.

If you return to our river journey analogy, you can think of nutrition as part of the paddle that you use to guide your raft. (Remember from our introduction that the paddle represents all of the individual choices you will make as a parent and, later, your child will make on her own.) When it comes to nutrition, your goal is to build such a strong paddle that your child will be able navigate the river easily and tirelessly throughout her entire life.

Just think about how foods affect your own energy levels: If you don't eat enough of the right foods, you feel so sluggish that it's as if you haven't even put a paddle in the water. And some foods (think sugar) make you want to paddle like a maniac for about fifteen minutes and then let you down so quickly that you peter out immediately thereafter. The effects are even more dramatic for your child. Healthy nutrition gives him the energy, stamina, and strength to navigate the river optimally and consistently so that he can deal with obstacles along the way.

The tough part is finding the best ways to help your child avoid treading water in the River of Trix or getting caught up in the Currents of Cookie Dough. It's not easy, we know, to resist the come-hither power of the glorious fruit-flavored drink box, the fast-food mascots, and the umpteen sugar- and fat-laden options along the way.

The good news is that fried-food addiction is not inevitable, because most taste is a learned sense. That's right. If you lay down the groundwork for proper nutrition now, you can teach your kids to *want* to eat right—to prefer water over pop, to like real fruits over berry-flavored candy, and to order a side of broccoli rather than a side of fries, even when they don't have you along to steer them in the right direction.

In this chapter, we're going to guide you through a child's early nutritional development. We'll start by discussing the benefits of breast milk and how to manage some of the challenges you may face if you do decide to nurse rather than bottle-feed, then move into some of the strategies you can use when your child transitions to solid foods. After a brief interlude in which we explore the biology of blubber, we'll spend a little time discussing physical activity. The ultimate payoff of learning about these subjects: Your child will be well on her way to developing a healthy brain, a healthy body, and a healthy life. Don't know about you, but we'll take that over a corn dog any day.

Breast and Beyond: The Early Meals

When your child is born, there's no question as to where Baby's first meal is coming from. There's no "Let's go to the baby-food court," no ordering up some kid-sized lo mein noodles or ministeak to the maternity ward, no hoping for a baby-friendly helping of Grandma's secret meat loaf. You've got two choices: You either feed her with the milk that comes from your breast or, if that's not an option because of physical reasons or adoption, the formula that comes from a can (or powder you add to water). We're going to spend the majority of this section taking you through the beauty and biology of breast milk—nature's perfect baby food. More about formula in just a few pages.

We firmly believe that breast feeding is the best way to nourish your child. Your body knows exactly what your baby needs and puts together the best possible cocktail in the form of breast milk, which contains protein, healthy fat, sugar, vitamins, and minerals, and some protective immune fighters. Breast milk will help your child grow and enjoy good health. What might be most amazing is that the composition actually alters as your baby grows, adapting to her changing needs. And yes, there's clear evidence that breast milk helps protect against infection, allergies, asthma, and many other conditions. If that's not enough of a reason to breast-feed, consider that you give your baby—and lose from your waist—500 calories a day when nursing!

Here's how breast milk is formed (see Figure 4.1): When you're pregnant, the hormones estrogen and prolactin cause the milk glands and ducts in your breasts to increase in size. The glands are where the milk is produced, and the ducts are the tubes that carry the milk from the glands to the nipples. Your nipple is actually built

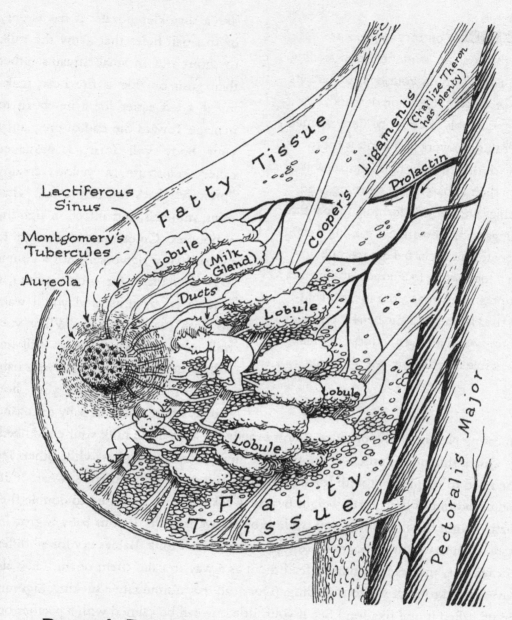

Labels in figure:

Lactiferous Sinus

Montgomery's Tubercules

Aureola

Fatty Tissue

Lobule

(Milk Gland)

Ducts

Lobule

Lobule

Lobule

Cooper's Ligaments

(Charlize Theron has plenty)

Prolactin

Pectoralis Major

Fatty Tissue

Figure 4.1 **Breast Is Best** Mom's hormones stimulate her body to produce milk. Nature's perfect meal, breast milk gives a baby all of the nutrients she needs early in life. If you breast-feed after the baby is six months old, you will need to supplement with extra protein to meet his growing needs.

like a sprinkler nozzle: It has twenty or so small holes that allow the milk to squirt out in small streams rather than gush out like a fire hose, making it a tad easier for a newborn to manage. Toward the end of pregnancy, your body will form a substance called colostrum, a yellow, creamy "premilk" that's full of proteins, vitamins, minerals, and infection-fighting antibodies. Colostrum is enough to nourish your newborn until a couple days after birth; for most women, it is replaced by milk, and you'll wake up with swollen breasts. When your milk comes in, your breasts will initially produce far more than your baby needs or can handle. As your hormones adjust and your baby establishes an eating pattern, you'll produce almost exactly the amount of milk your child needs.

Quick side note: Some women produce enough for quintuplets, while others feel the need to supplement with formula. All babies lose weight in the first week of life, then rebound to their birth weight by two weeks. They're supposed to double their birth weight by six months, and triple it by twelve months. If your baby is growing faster than that, you do *not* need to supplement breast milk. Babies cry for all different reasons, and it's tempting to feed them as a way to calm them down. They also have a need to suck without feeding. (Docs call that nonnutritive sucking; Sigmund Freud called it oral fixation.) See if your little one can be calmed with a pacifier or a thumb; if so, then you know he's not really hungry.

Now, the most important thing to remember about breast feeding is that not only are you passing along all the nutrients your child needs but also some others that he may not need or want courtesy of the foods and drinks that you're consuming. So before we even get into the nuts and bolts of proper feeding techniques, it's essential to get your own nutritional house in order first.

For optimum nutrition, keep taking your prenatal vitamin and make sure to get enough of the following nutrients, deemed especially beneficial for improving your baby's health, as they also buttress the quality of your breast milk:

FACTOID: How do kids develop a love of tomatoes and garbanzo beans? You. As fetuses, they develop a sense of taste through the foods that you eat, the flavors of which get passed to the amniotic fluid. Strong tastes like garlic and spicy foods are especially potent. Breast milk can also transmit flavors that influence your baby's developing sense of taste.

◯ **Protein:** two or three servings a day of organically fed poultry (skinless), seafood (non-bottom-feeders and small fish; think wild—including canned—salmon, trout, mahimahi, sea bass, flounder), eggs, low-fat dairy, and soy. Fish protein is super healthy, but you should limit seafood to about two or three servings a week to avoid potential overconsumption of mercury and other trace elements. Salmon and trout are great sources of the omega-3 fatty acids EPA and DHA, as well.

◯ **Calcium:** 1,300 mg a day from supplements and low-fat dairy products, calcium-fortified orange juice, soy milk, tofu, broccoli, spinach, sardines, beans, sesame seeds, oranges. Consume no more than 600 mg in any two-hour period, because that's the maximum your body can absorb at a time, either from food or from a supplement. If you choose pills, we recommend that you take a supplement containing calcium citrate, vitamin D_3, and magnesium at least twice a day. The magnesium (one-third the dose of the calcium) is needed to prevent constipation or bloating from the calcium. Note: Do not take calcium supplements if you have kidney dysfunction.

◯ **Iron:** 20 mg a day from poultry, seafood, dried beans and fruit, egg yolks. Your multivitamin often includes more than that, and that's okay while you are pregnant, breast feeding, or menstruating.

⊃ **DHA:** 600 mg a day. An algae source, available in most drugstores, is ideal, since it avoids any toxin concerns and is very palatable in pill form.

⊃ **Vitamin C:** 800 mg a day from citrus fruits, red peppers, broccoli.

Above all, aim to have a healthy, balanced diet and drink plenty of fluids. It's best to eat five or six smaller meals throughout the day rather than have three larger ones. We also recommend that you avoid spicy or gas-inducing foods, as well as caffeinated beverages and alcohol. If you do drink alcohol when nursing, do not breast-feed for at least four hours after your last drink, or longer if you're still feeling the effects.

If you become engorged (when your breasts are so big and swollen with milk they feel like they're going to explode) while still under the influence, use a breast pump to remove some of the milk and dispose of it. There's no need to pump and dump otherwise: Once the alcohol is out of your bloodstream, it's out of your breast milk; it doesn't accumulate.

FACTOID: If your baby is nursing after six months of age, he needs extra protein because breast milk no longer provides all the nutrients he needs. That can come in the forms of puréed meat, tofu, cheese, and rice and beans.

The good news is that while you can't see what's in your breast milk or measure how much is coming out, you can get a pretty good idea whether it's doing the job. If your baby is gaining weight appropriately and soiling diapers often, then you're most likely giving him enough of the foods he needs. If he's not gaining weight, then you will need to talk to your doc about possible feeding problems.

While breast feeding often works very smoothly for both mom and baby, the real trick, if you choose to nurse, is sticking with it in the face of some challenges. So consider these steps to help the process go as smoothly as possible:

The Hold: Holding your baby to your breast isn't like hauling a bag of groceries. It requires a much more delicate approach. Besides making sure that he gains easy access, you need to support his head and back during the feeding. Above all, relax. Anxiety or stiffness on your part will only make your baby fussy and uncooperative.

The best way to make sure that your baby is feeding well and comfortably is to employ one of these four positions:

⊃ the cradle hold (the classic position)

⊃ the cross-cradle hold (gives more control over his head)

⊃ the football hold (good for nursing twins)

⊃ the side-lying hold (especially good for women who have had Caesarean sections because it takes any pressure off the incision, as well as for night-time feedings)

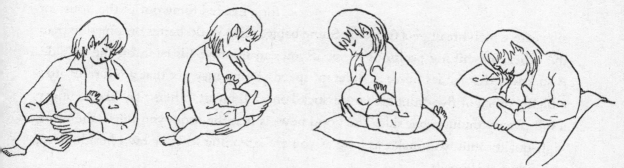

Cradle Hold   Cross-cradle Hold   Football Hold   Side-Lying

The Latch: When you hold your baby's mouth to your breast, you should hear a transition from short, quick sucks to long, slow, deep gulps, during which you can hear swallowing and see his jaw moving up and down. When that transition occurs, you will often feel a tingly sensation in your breasts. This is the "letdown reflex," and it means that your milk is flowing freely to your baby. Apart from a sharp pain deep in your breast when your baby first latches on (it usually goes away within the first few weeks), breast feeding should not be painful. If it is, check to make sure that your baby is properly latched on: His mouth should be wide open, covering most of the areola. If he's not latched on, gently put your finger inside his mouth, breaking the suction, and try again.

Most babies feed from both breasts at each feeding (burping in between; more below). The milk with the best nutrients, or the highest amount of brain-strengthening fat, comes from the breast that has been nursed for a while. So if your baby prefers a long sojourn on one side and only a quick visit on the other, that's fine; you can either pump the "off side" and save for a needed foray out of the house or alternate which breast gets first dibs. Some babies seem to do better on one side than the other; try shifting positions to see if you can improve his latch on the off side. Also know that babies nurse at different speeds: Some may get that good milk after a highly efficient five-minute "power suck" on each breast; others may like to linger a full twenty minutes per side. The good news is that the more you nurse, the more high-quality milk you make, as long as you are attending to your own health, sleep, and nutritional needs.

If your child is having a hard time latching on, it could be caused by a number of reasons. He may not be fully awake and stimulated. You can help keep him alert by removing his clothes, which will wake him up in a hurry. He also may have trouble if you have inverted nipples (that's when not enough of the nipple is exposed for your baby to latch on to). You can use plastic devices found in pharmacies that fit into your bra to help stretch the skin around the areola, which causes the nipple to poke out. If you do have inverted nipples, it's best to start using these devices in the third trimester—though nature often works itself out, so this may not be necessary. Also, you'll want to be on the lookout for white spots that may develop on your baby's tongue. That's called thrush, a type of yeast infection that may hinder him from eating well. Thrush is easily treated with nystatin liquid. The prescription antifungal medication is administered as a 1.25 milliliter squirt onto the tongue (or tongue and cheeks if you see white plaques there too) four times a day.

The Burp: You should burp your baby before moving him from one breast to the other, and then after he finishes. Hold him so that his head is over your shoulder, and rub or pat his back gently in an upward motion. The key to a successful burp: Provide a little counterpressure under his stomach with your collarbone. The gentle pushing against his belly, not the back pat, is what really does it—although patting does dislodge bubbles. You can also do the rub-up strategy: Place a thumb on his belly and the rest of your hand on his back, and gently rub both upward, as if you're coaxing the gas bubbles up with your hand motion. This can be done over the shoulder, with Baby sitting on your lap with one hand as head and trunk support, or with him lying over your knees.

• • •

There are many health benefits to breast milk, which is why health care professionals advocate for it so strenuously, but that doesn't mean it's your only option for first feedings. Some women have jobs that prevent them from nursing or pumping as frequently as they need to; some women are on medications or have medical conditions that don't mix well with breast feeding; some mothers of multiples find the process too overwhelming; and some babies have medical conditions that require close monitoring of fluid intake. You also should not breast-feed if you have a serious infection, smoke, or are doing illicit drugs.

Our recommendations for formula: Choose one made from cow's milk rather than soy protein, because cow's milk is most similar to human milk. And read the label to find one with the highest concentration of vegetarian DHA. How much formula to give? Generally, add 2 to 3 ounces to your baby's age in months per feeding. So a one-month-old would get 3 to 4 ounces per feeding, a two-month old would get 4 to 5 ounces, and so on. When he hits about 32 ounces during a twenty-four-hour period, it's probably time to try a little solid food. This is not an absolute rule; some babies grow great on less than that, and every now and then there's the kid who seems to need more. The tricky part is that they may feed slower by breast than by bottle, and if bottle feeding, they may drink fast and more than they need. You'll know that when you see it, or, rather, wear it: Overfed kids tend to be really spitty babies. It's nature's way of saying, "Give me less, or else!"

And don't panic if your one-month-old wants only 2½ ounces at a time. As long as he's gaining and growing, you're doing great, even if he didn't happen to read the baby textbook telling him how many ounces he should weigh at what age. He should be doubling his birth weight by around six months, and tripling it by a year. If he is far below that curve, it's worth touching base with your pediatrician to see what else might be going on. If he's far ahead of that curve, stop giving him a bottle every time he makes a sound; he's likely getting far more than he needs.

From Liquid to Solid: Transitioning to the Hard Stuff

If it hasn't happened already, there will come a time when your baby is going to need to kick the bottle. Not entirely, at first. But his mind, fingers, eyes, and stomach will be craving more variety in his meals. This transition phase can be tough for parents.

OPERATION ORGANIC

Because more and more studies show that it's best to avoid early exposure to some of the toxins found in pesticides, it makes sense to eat organic when you can. Because it can be expensive, we know that it's not always possible to do so all the time, but it does make sense to pick some foods and make them your priority, like perhaps milk and some of the foods that tend to have the highest pesticide content (for example, peaches, apples, lettuce, potatoes, and strawberries). So it's a good time to take advantage of green markets and organic farm stands, or even grow your own (and get your child involved!). It's also smart to research your produce at your local market to see where it's coming from, since not all countries have the same pesticide-control standards. You can find other hints about organic food at RealAge (www.realage.com).

When is it okay to start solid foods? How much food can he have? Is there anything he can't have? Is it really necessary for spaghetti sauce to end up in his ear every . . . single . . . time?

After your baby is a few months old, you'll start hearing it from neighbors, in-laws, the mailman: When are you going to let that poor little dear have a piece of potato? While there isn't one set of rules that applies to every child, we can give you general guidelines for moving from an all-liquid diet to one that includes solid food. Anecdotally, it seems that it can help babies sleep through the night, and it can also bring more fun interactions between child and parent.

At about four to six months of age, when your baby can sit up in a high chair, start by mixing 1 to 2 tablespoons of baby cereal with 1 or 2 ounces of breast milk or formula in a small dish. *Don't* put it in a bottle. Feed that concoction to your baby twice a day, using a spoon and a "here comes the witty bitty airpwane" voice if you like. It'll be pretty watery, but that will help with the transition, and after a few days, you can increase to 2 to 4 tablespoons of cereal, while keeping the liquid at just an ounce or two; that will make for much thicker feeds.

For the best chance of success, feed your baby when she's calm and alert. Don't wait until she's out of her mind with hunger, but also don't try feeding her right after you've nursed or given her a bottle. If she's a little bit hungry, she'll be most receptive.

If you start too early, your baby will tell you—not in the funny E★Trade commercial kind of way but via a reflex called the tongue thrust. That's when your baby sticks out her tongue and spits out the cereal. Though parents think it's just because she doesn't like cereal, it's actually a reflex that goes away when the baby is about four months old and is related to the way she uses her tongue to strip milk from a nipple. If that's what happens when you give it a try, just wait about a week and try the cereal again.

As far as which cereal to try first, it depends on what's coming out the other end. If Junior is a Loose Pooper (sounds like a *Seinfeld* character, eh?), start with oatmeal or rice baby cereals, which are more constipating. If she's plugged up, then start with barley baby cereal, which makes stools looser. Whichever you choose, try it at least four days in a row, unless she gets a rash on her bottom, vomits profusely each time you try it, or has another dramatic reaction. If she does, she may have a food allergy, and you should stop giving her that food immediately. (For more on food allergies, see chapter 7.) After those first four days, you can add another food. Keep following this pattern, trying each new food for four days before adding another one. (For advice on making your own baby food, see page 135.) Your early options include:

⊃ Another kind of cereal

⊃ Puréed vegetables such as green beans, carrots, peas, squash, and sweet potatoes. Make sure to alternate green and orange ones; too many orange foods can make your kid look orange—that's called carotenemia.

⊃ Baby fruits, like applesauce, bananas, pears, apricots, and peaches. Don't mix these with the cereal, because once she has cereal with fruit, she won't want to eat it plain ever again!

This will take you to five to six months of age, a time when the typical daily schedule should look like this, with bottles or breast milk upon waking, between meals, and before bed:

> Breakfast: cereal and fruit
>
> Lunch: veggies and fruit
>
> Dinner: cereal and veggies

As your child eats more, she may want slightly less formula or breast milk; just let her self-regulate. If she only wants a few bites of something one day, she'll make up for it the next. And if she acts like she absolutely doesn't like one particular food that you are determined she eat, just keep trying it, because for most kids, reexposure breeds familiarity, which usually gets them liking it. It can take at least ten exposures to develop familiarity—and liking. In fact, many kids will forget they didn't like it, making this a great trick for older kids with picky eating habits.

At six months, you can add either baby meats or meats puréed in a blender. Meats can include beef, lamb, ham, and then turkey. Save chicken for at least nine months of age, since it can be the most allergenic.

Hard-boiled egg yolk can be an entertaining food—especially outdoors, since it can be made into a three-foot-wide radius of mess for great, tactile, exploratory baby-feeding fun. The egg white has to wait until your child is twelve months, as it too is highly allergenic before that.

Now your schedule will look something like this:

> Breakfast: cereal and fruit
>
> Lunch: cereal, meat, and veggies
>
> Dinner: Meat, veggies, and fruit

You can mix it up; just make sure your child gets two of each group a day. Once she transitions from puréed baby food to regular solid food, typically around her first birthday, you'll want to make sure that she gets three balanced meals a day (think protein and veggies) and snacks (fruits and starches), too. You want to be careful that the snacks aren't more appealing—and less healthful—than the meals, or else your child will learn to load up on snacks and scrimp on dinner. Make breakfast and lunch bigger meals than dinner, and you'll be guiding right for life. Also, rethink your notions about rewarding with food. You don't have to reward a good behavior with a dessert-type snack every time she does something right. Simple praise, rather than food, can be a reward.

Though you don't need to calculate nutritionals at every meal, try to think about overall nutritional balance. A good ballpark figure is for kids to have about 20 percent to 25 percent of a day's calories from protein (important for muscle building), 20 percent to 25 percent from healthy fat, and 50 percent to 60 percent from healthy carbs: whole-grain starches, fruits, and veggies.

Another note about nutrients: Children need 800 milligrams of calcium, and toddlers, 500 to 600 milligrams daily. Since 60 percent of bone mass is accumulated by puberty, around age thirteen, you want to make sure that kids get enough early on to build a strong skeletal foundation.

Here's a sample of how a perfect day would look for a toddler:

Breakfast: 100 percent whole-grain cereal, whole fruit, milk

Snack 1: fruit or 100 percent whole-grain crackers, water

Lunch: ½ sandwich (cut up when children are little), applesauce, carrots, milk

Snack 2: yogurt

Dinner: protein (beans from a burrito, tofu, fish, eggs, lean beef, lean pork, or skinless chicken), starch (100 percent whole wheat pasta, couscous, brown rice), green veggie, fruit, milk or water

THE BLAME GAME

If you look at all the statistics we listed on pages 125–27, you can see that childhood obesity has increased faster than the national deficit. And you may be asking yourself why this happened. It's not one reason; it's a whole bunch of them. Kids have more access to junk food. Manufacturers are combining more addictive ingredients—saturated fat, simple sugars and salt—in prepared treats like Cinnabons that cause kids to want to eat more calories. Schools are eliminating or decreasing time spent in recess and phys ed. Kids spend more time in front of the TV, so they're not only sitting more, but they're also exposed to lots of ads for junky foods. Today there's less of a sense of community, so kids spend less time outside and don't walk to school. That's just scratching the surface. We could go on and on about all the things that make it difficult for kids to maintain a healthy size. But in the end, the choice is up to you: You can either engage in the blame game and come up with all the reasons why it's easier for your kid to eat ice cream and entertain herself with her PlayStation Portable, or you can be a leader and make the changes that will improve your child's life now and in the future.

Keep in mind that not every bite needs to be eaten at each meal. Children self-regulate far better than their parents, and if your child eats less at one meal or in one day, it will tend to balance out with what he eats over the next day, or few days. As long as he is continuing along his expected growth curve (see pages 449–50), and not crossing into percentiles that are too high or too low, then let him self-regulate rather than force-feeding him. Toddlers who are chronically overfed will eat more than they need to later on—a preventable problem if you read their cues better when they're young.

While it seems that this feeding schedule should be easy enough to follow, we know that it's not. That's because there are picky eaters (see box on page 124); there are also eaters who are obsessed with sweets. And that's not even considering the fact that kids get pummeled with confusing messages from marketers (advertising sugary cereals with fruity names), which children don't have the context or knowledge to interpret. Candy is found right at the supermarket checkout counter, and fried nuggets come in the shape of dinosaurs. (What's in *those* bad boys is what's *really* scary.) So it can be a challenge. And while you don't want to make your child neurotic about eating—a sure recipe for a future eating disorder—you also want to teach him the difference between nutritious ingredients that promote good health and non-nutritious ingredients that can bring about disability and disease.

DON'T MAKE SUCH A FUSS

We've all seen kids who decide that the only thing worth eating is a chicken nugget. Or a bowl of pasta. And that's it. Oh, the picky eater, the child who asserts that he likes only a few things and refuses to let his tongue touch anything else. The real issue, of course, is not one of taste but one of control. To avoid future food wars, try these strategies to avoid raising a picky eater:

➲ Provide lots of choices, and don't be afraid to parallel cook. If Junior never eats fish, then have a different protein available and encourage eating fish when there is positive peer pressure to try it. For instance, when Junior's best buddy, whose parent has told you he eats fish like a champ, is coming over, plan to have fish for that meal. Observation of peers and older siblings or cousins can be a powerful motivator.

➲ Food repetition is okay, as long as there's balance overall, or a multivitamin makes up the difference. Children may go for days, weeks, or months wanting only peanut butter and jelly, or whatever the latest taste preference may be. While it may drive you nuts, look on the bright side: You've got an easy meal that goes down without a fuss. Choose organic fresh peanut butter made from only ground peanuts, available at most health food stores; the emulsifiers in commercial peanut butters stimulate latent allergic tendencies (see chapter 7).

⊃ Keep exposing her to new healthy foods; some may stick. Try food games like: "How many raisins can stick to a celery stalk filled with cream cheese ?"

⊃ When you feel a battle coming on, take a step back. Will your son be scarred for life if he does not eat two more carrots?

⊃ Add a daily multivitamin. This provides an insurance policy against an imperfect diet. But read the label: Some brands recommend a half vitamin for children under two and a whole tablet for those two and older, while other brands recommend one vitamin for under age two and two tablets for those over two.

⊃ For kids with autism, texture can be a challenge. These children may only eat one texture (only puréed foods) or color of foods. Some of this group inhabit the extreme end of the picky eating spectrum that is unacceptable nutritionally, where even a multivitamin won't be enough, since they are missing out entirely on other food groups (often protein or fat). To help, find one of the foods that they tolerate—something crunchy, for instance—and mix in enriched foods (like enriched cereal) that can help them get the nutrients they need. Starting with puréed foods and working with an occupational therapist who specializes in feeding can help too.

The Weight War: Reducing the Risk of Childhood Obesity

Here we're going to help you devise an eating plan that goes on the offensive by providing your child with the nutritional firepower to feed and develop her brain, build her immune system, and help all of her internal systems run at peak performance. But we also want to help you run defense: that is, to protect against the evil forces that contribute to childhood (and eventually adult) obesity. Together these two strategies will score you big points, not only for the health of your child but also for the well-being of your entire family.

Obesity is the most obvious chronic disease among kids, and yet the majority of cases are preventable. The responsibility starts with you. While adults have a lot of problems they can blame their obesity on—bad boss (stress), bad marriage (more stress), bad luck, bad genes (leading to issues with their thyroid gland)—children very rarely have a genetic or medical condition that contributes to obesity. The main cause of childhood obesity is simply harmful eating habits (promoted by marshmallow parents). The strategies we outline below will help you instill healthful behaviors.

In case you were thinking that a chunky child isn't a serious problem, just consider these facts:

⊃ There was a 54 percent increase in obesity in children under the age of thirteen from the 1980s to the 1990s. Currently, 20 percent of children between six and nineteen are obese, while in some cities and among some racial and ethnic groups, the figure is more than 30 percent.

⊃ Childhood obesity dramatically increases the chances of being obese in adulthood. For example, there's a 41 percent chance of being an obese adult if you're obese at age seven, a 75 percent chance if you're obese at twelve, and a 90 percent chance if you're obese as an adolescent.

⊃ The medical consequences of childhood obesity are staggering. It hugely increases the risk of developing hypertension, type 2 diabetes (it used to be called adult-onset diabetes but now occurs even in kids as young as nine!), coronary artery disease, joint problems, stroke, and certain cancers as well as many other conditions. And did we mention that being overweight correlates with lower academic achievement? That's probably not the life you want for your child.

⊃ The first year is especially important: Infants with greater body fat and rapid weight gain have an increased lifetime risk of cardiovascular disease and diabetes. Toddlerhood is also key: Those who are chronically over-fed and not allowed to self-regulate will start picking portion sizes that are more than they need. Singing the praises of the "clean plate club" does not help.

> **FACTOID:** It's not sugar that makes kids hyperactive. When it comes to foods, it's more likely stimulants such as caffeine that may be doing a number on your kid's energy levels, taking him from a docile dude to one who looks awfully similar to a two-foot tornado. Plus, caffeine may interfere with sleep, resulting in an overtired kid who is bouncing off the walls. Kids with attention deficit/hyperactivity disorder (ADHD) have the opposite reaction: Stimulants calm them down and help them to focus. Don't forget that chocolate has a lot of caffeine.

⊃ As you can imagine, or perhaps you even remember firsthand, the psychological consequences of obesity can be just as damaging as the physical consequences. Overweight kids have a harder time interacting with peers, they're chosen less often as preferred playmates, they have lower self-esteem, they get bullied and teased, and they have to deal with negative stereotypes and discrimination throughout life.

⊃ Having one obese parent gives a child a 40 percent chance of becoming an obese adult; if both Mom and Dad are obese, the odds double to 80 percent. Taking care of yourself sends the message to your kids that it's important to eat healthfully. They emulate what you do, not what you say.

Luckily, you can avoid these potential threats by teaching your child how to eat healthfully from the start. If you already missed the boat, be assured that this isn't an irreversible process. If your child is headed down the overweight path, you can redirect him. But don't delay: Biologically, the best time to make changes that will stick is before he turns six. After that, he's eating lunch, maybe even breakfast, at school, and we all know about school lunches.

The Biology of Blubber: How Food Becomes Fat

Before we teach you some family-friendly strategies for raising a child of a healthy weight and size, we're going to teach you about the biology of why we eat and what happens to food in our bodies.

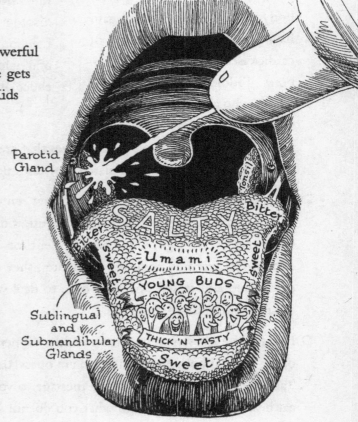

Taste: One of the most powerful muscles in the body, the tongue gets a lot of action in childhood. Kids play with their tongues, stick out their tongues, even tickle their tongues. In the eating process, the tongue, along with the nose, gives youngsters information they need to determine whether they want to eat a certain food. That information is governed by the five elements of taste:* sweet, sour, salty, bitter, and umami (which recognizes the inherent deliciousness in fatty foods like cheese and bacon). While there is some

* Babies have ten thousand taste buds at birth; that number drops to about three thousand by the time they reach eighty years old.

genetic component to what we think tastes good and what we think tastes like landfill, you can actually program taste buds to like certain foods; simply exposing kids to a certain food about ten times increases the likelihood that they'll like the food. On the flip side, *not* exposing children to certain foods (think sugary foods or foods with saturated fats) means that their tongues will not learn to like them in the first place.

Appetite: People tend to think that appetite is controlled by the stomach: that the amount of food a kid has in his belly determines whether or not he's hungry. But the reality is that appetite is controlled more by what chemicals are present in the brain and how big you make your stomach (see Figure 4.2). If you enlarge the stomach through regular overeating, it will send "empty" signals even when it has enough food in it. There are two main hormones that transmit these messages from the stomach to the brain. One is a gremlin called ghrelin. When ghrelin levels are up, your child is going to feel like devouring a six-pack of Happy Meals. The other chemical, leptin (love leptin!), sends the opposite signal. When leptin levels are up, your kid feels satisfied. In many ways, the real battle over appetite and cravings comes down to this chemical battle. The bottom line: If your child eats healthy foods—those high in protein, healthy fats, and fiber—you will increase his leptin levels, and that will keep him satisfied. If your child eats harmful foods with fat-promoting substances like trans fats, sugar, and high-fructose corn syrup, or if you enlarge his stomach so that reasonable portion sizes don't fill him up, his ghrelin levels will go through the roof. And his stomach will soon follow.

Fat Storage: You've heard it before, but we'll say it again: Food is energy. When you eat food, your body breaks it down and, through the digestive process, provides nutrients to the liver. Your blood transports these nutrients to all of the places that blood travels: your knees, brain, lungs—everywhere. Whether they're protein, carbohydrates, or fat, all nutrients get turned into the chemical glucose to power all the organs, muscles, and systems in the body. Without food, the body doesn't work. But the food that's not used? All that extra glucose is eventually stored as fat. Contrary to popular belief, eating fat isn't what makes you fat. Eating more calories than you expend—no matter what form—is what makes you fat. Now, in the first few years of life, children actually have a low number of fat cells (it's called low adiposity, in

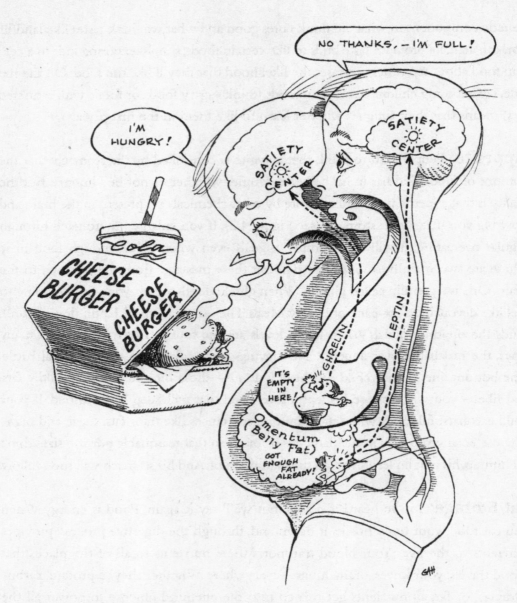

Figure 4.2 **Food Fight** Even if a child is active, his body (and mind) is in a constant tug-of-war over hunger and satiety—two sensations controlled by hormones. While leptin curbs hunger, the gremlin called ghrelin can make a child hungry. Marketing messages may make temptations stronger, so the key to fighting childhood obesity lies in creating an environment that encourages healthy eating, to increase leptin and shut down ghrelin.

case you're wondering). But starting at age four to six years, that number of cells begins to increase (docs call it adiposity rebound), and the cells accumulated during this period will forever want to be fed. That's thought to be one of the reasons why overweight children are at such high risk of becoming overweight adults.

Fat Burning: Truth is, when it comes to managing body size, the same formula applies to children as to adults. The big battles are won and lost in the kitchen, at the supermarket, and when dining out.* But the small battles, primarily around physical activity, can also make a big difference, especially over an entire childhood. A child who sits in front of video games and only works out his opponens pollicis muscles† is going to be in far worse shape than the kid who plays tag, jumps all over the playground, creates a jungle gym out of couch pillows, and is enrolled in the local gymnastics class. That's because physical activity increases muscle, which increases metabolism—that is, the rate at which calories are burned and used for energy—and not just when the child is active. Just as movement or activity increases metabolism, the opposite is also true: The more a child sits, the slower his metabolism, thus increasing the rate at which he stores fat. No two ways about it: You have to instill in your child not only that she must move, play, and explore the world with her body but that it's fun to do so as well. Better yet, get off the couch and join her. (See our exercise plan on page 376.)

· · ·

Even if you've always known how important nutrition and activity are to a child's health, we hope that this chapter has given you some perspective and biological insight into *why* it's important. Sometimes, as parents, we may choose certain things simply because they're easier (and we're exhausted). Just keep in mind that it's a lot easier to prevent weight problems and poor nutrition early on than to deal with the consequences later. In addition to our recipes and exercise suggestions in the YOU Tools section starting on page 309, use the following tips to get your child on the right track from the start—or get him back on track if, by chance, he's drifted off course.

* See *YOU: On a Diet* for a plan full of eating strategies that can be used by the entire family.
† They're muscles in the thumb.

WATER, WATER EVERYWHERE

They'll bathe in it, they'll drink it, and in a few years, they're going to be filling balloons with it. But how do you insure that your water is safe? The scary thing is that water is not guaranteed to be safe, even expensive bottled water. So here is our four-step plan:

1. If you are on a public water supply: Look at your municipal water company's annual report, called a CCR, or Consumer Confidence Report. It is usually mailed in July, but you can request it from your water company at any time. Check the report for six potential contaminants:

   ⊃ Lead

   ⊃ Nitrates (from fertilizers)

   ⊃ Nitrites

   ⊃ Germs and bacteria (usually from animal or human waste)

   ⊃ Chlorination disinfection by-products such as chloroform and a group of four chemicals called trihalomethanes

   ⊃ Dangerous other substances such as arsenic, cyanide, mercury, benzene, and trichloroethylene

   Those of you with well water (not covered by the CCR) will want to have it tested for all six pollutants.

2. If these levels are below the federal limit and therefore considered safe, get a test kit that will pick up four contaminants. Water from your town might be okay, but water in your house might pick up contaminants like lead from your pipes, or bacteria that can grow on carbon filters. The standard test kit costs about $20 and is relatively easy to read.

3. Public water supplies will usually contain trace levels of chlorine by-products such as trihalomethanes and chloroform. These can easily be filtered out with a granular activated carbon (GAC) filter. If other contaminants are present, like arsenic or lead, you may need a more sophisticated reverse osmosis water filter. Get professional consultation before your baby's birth or as soon afterward as possible. Five types of filters, described below, are available at a cost of less than $200 each. Whichever kind you choose, remember to change filters regularly and keep them clean.

⊃ Carafe filters (Brita, as well as others): These are good for drinking water, unless lead is an issue.

⊃ Faucet-mounted water filters: These usually don't have a lot of filtering capacity and generally are not recommended.

⊃ Above-sink filters with separate housing that taps off the faucet: These are often the most economical and convenient in terms of being long lasting and effective.

⊃ Under-sink filters or whole-house filters: These can come in multiple stages and can have greater filtering capacity needed for special hard water, sulfur, or contamination issues. A whole-house filter is also excellent if you want to keep the bath water free of contaminants. This is the most expensive option and usually requires a plumber to install.

⊃ Shower or bathtub filters: These have limited capacity and need to be replaced more often but are helpful in cutting down on exposures when bathing your baby.

4. No matter what, always run water for a few moments and let it go down the drain before you drink from your tap, or even use water to bathe or cook. This gets rid of a lot of toxins and bacteria stored in your pipes; in fact, it may be the most important step to having clean water, either at home or when you're out.

YOU TIPS

Take a Deep Breath. It's often hard to breast-feed if you're stressed, distracted, or nursing on the go. If you don't get a proper latch, your baby will not get enough to eat and will be hungry again in no time. Try to set aside quiet time for nursing. Sit in a comfortable chair with good back and arm support, and set yourself up with everything you need ahead of time: a glass of water, a book or magazine, soothing music, and the telephone within reach. After you and your newborn have gotten the hang of breast feeding, your body will respond automatically to the baby's stimulation of your nipples, and you'll be able to multitask if you like.

Know How to Pump. There will come a time when you're going to want to have a little extra milk on hand: like, when it's Dad's turn to feed, or you'd like to go out for a night, or you're going back to work. Planning ahead for these events or transitions by pumping extra bottles of milk will help reduce the stress. You also may want to "pump and dump" if you consume spicy foods or a glass of wine. If you're pumping only occasionally, a hand pump will do. If you're going to be pumping regularly, it's worthwhile to rent a powerful hospital-grade pump. And if you plan to have more than one kid, it may be more cost effective to just go ahead and buy the thing. The best time to pump an extra bottle is shortly after your baby's first feeding of the day, as most women have plentiful milk in the morning.

Even though the actual pumping is initially an uncomfortable experience—no way around that—know these guidelines: You can store breast milk at room temperature for four to eight hours; in an insulated cooler for a day; in the fridge for a week; and in the freezer for three to six months. (Remember to mark the date you pumped it.) We recommend that you use glass storage bottles, especially when freezing, because plastic ones may leach the endocrine disruptor bisphenol A (BPA). In fact, make sure that all of your bottles, including water bottles, are free of this chemical used in the production of plastics. Also, always wash your hands before touching your baby's mouth or feeding him (the bisphenol A from receipt paper is much higher than that even in the worst baby bottles). Do not store milk in plastic bottle-insert bags, as they are porous and will increase the chance of your milk going rancid.

Make Your Own Baby Food. If you want to make your own food, you can purée it in a blender, then freeze the extra in ice cube trays and defrost a cube or two at a time. If you microwave baby food, always stir it with a clean finger to make sure it is not unevenly hot or scalding. (The same goes for any food that you nuke.) Let the baby-food industry make beets, turnips, carrots, collard greens, and spinach, because these veggies may contain large amounts of chemicals called nitrates when grown in some parts of the country and can cause anemia—a deficiency of red blood cells—in your wee one. Overexposure to nitrates can even turn your baby blue. Baby-food companies screen their produce for nitrates; if you want to be mega-sure, buy organic versions of these products. If you feel compelled to make them yourself, then serve the vegetables fresh and don't store them, as storage can increase the nitrates.

Reduce Toxins. Don't microwave foods in plastic to avoid absorbing bisphenol A and other plastic residue into the baby's food. BPA is an endocrine blocker that may have long-term effects on hormones and metabolism. And avoid cosmetics and deodorants that contain phthalates. These toxic chemicals, used to soften vinyl, are easily absorbed and passed to your infant through breast milk.

Eat Together. In this era of soccer games, dance recitals, Mom's working late, sister's facing a deadline for her Pluto project, and brother's putting together a PowerPoint presentation, it's easy to fall into the trap: Eat quick, eat in front of the TV, eat junk. Big mistake. Of all the things you can do to influence the health of your child, perhaps the most important is to make family dinner a priority. Research shows that having family dinner more than twice a week can positively influence a child's waist, eating behavior, school achievement, and overall psychological development. It's also a great opportunity to model table manners. The more family dinners, the better; see if you can go for more than five a week. You can also try family breakfast or other meals that suit everyone's schedule.

Play Red Light, Green Light. Kids love this game on the playground, but you can also play it in the kitchen to teach young kids about healthy foods. Make a short list of green-light "go" foods such as vegetables, fruit, and nonfried fish; red-light "stop" foods such as soda; and yellow-light "treat" foods such as 100 percent whole-grain, 100 percent omega-3 chia muffins or Lifestyle 180 Bars. (See kid-friendly Lifestyle 180 recipes starting on page 329.) It makes it fun for kids and teaches them principles that will last. Other cool games that work well with some kids:

⊃ Find the best cereal in the store, based on what you learn from labels.

⊃ Have a kids cooking day, on which you pick one healthy meal that your kids can assist with.

⊃ Toss out the junk at a friend's house (with said friend's approval).

Create a Mantra. Kids can be motivated to change their behavior if you introduce a fun system that gets their little imaginative and competitive minds churning. One we love: The "5 to Go!" system developed by the Cleveland Clinic. Here's how this one works:

⊃ 5 servings of fruits and veggies a day.

⊃ 4 servings of nonfat dairy a day, for calcium and vitamin D_3.

⊃ 3 compliments (give and get, to create a positive environment that goes both ways).

⊃ 2 or fewer hours of screen time.

⊃ 1 hour or more of play/exercise.

⊃ 0 sweetened beverages, other than reduced-fat milk (children under age two need full-fat milk).

You can also come up with your own set of five messages or a daily checklist of five things you need to eat or do, then four things, then three, two, and one. Throughout the day, you can play the game of tracking how each kid has done, making it a daily competition.

Start Early. A basic biological fact: Kids will not crave foods they're not familiar with. As soon as your kid starts eating solid foods, really concentrate on the YOU strategies: no added sugar or syrups, fewer than 4 grams of saturated fat per meal, no trans fat, and only 100 percent whole-grain foods. If your kid doesn't taste high-sugar foods such as candy, cereals, and soda, she won't grow to like them (and won't "Please, Mama?" for them all day long). We also recommend that you teach your child to look at nutrition labels as soon as she can read. But please don't make it an obsession; some think that obsessing too much can instill eating-disordered behavior in children.

Talk Smart. One of the ways that you can reinforce the notion of eating healthy foods is by talking about the healthy foods your child should be eating, rather than dwelling on all the unhealthy ones she should avoid. You know what they say about temptation, especially when it comes to the forbidden Froot Loops.

Don't Use It as a Carrot—Even If It Is a Carrot. You should avoid using food as either a punishment or reward, because it sends mixed signals to a child. "Do something good, and I get a doughnut!" Might seem nice at the time, but what message does that send? Good behavior is rewarded with bad food; a notion that hurts kids in the long run.

Don't Avoid Healthy Fat. We've seen it happen: Parents have success on a low-fat diet, so they decide that their kids need to follow it too. Not a great strategy. Kids need healthy fat for brain development.

Establish a Healthy Household. It's much easier to maintain a healthy routine when you establish principles and practices that make healthy living automatic. Some easy ones that you can instill include packing healthy lunches rather than relying on less healthy in-school options (we YOU docs are trying to help schools serve healthier choices); and making at least one family activity a week something that involves physical activity, such as a hike or bowling night instead of a movie and popcorn.

No Watch, No Eat. After a long, hard day, it's tempting just to gather around the tube with your plates to watch the evening—er, reality show. But it's not a good idea. Kids (and adults, too) eat much more on average in front of the TV than when they're sitting at the table. Why? They lose awareness of the sacredness of food, and the act becomes mindless—a sure recipe for overeating. When you concentrate on eating, you can pay better attention to your body's signals that you're full. Not only that, but kids take about 150 fewer steps for every hour of TV they watch, so it's a double whammy: Eat more and burn less!

Play, Play, Play. Buy some balls, go outside, run, run, run. We've gotten very far away from the days when kids would play for hours outdoors, and we need to get some of that back. There are many creative ways that you can get your kids moving without having them feel as though they're doing a workout. Routine walks or hikes in the woods are a great physical activity for both parents and kids and also provide good one-on-one time. For those of you who want a little more structured routine for your children, try our kid-friendly workout on page 376; it will get their bodies moving and their minds engaged.

Park the Stroller. Walking is one of the easiest and best exercises around. Simply getting rid of your stroller—we recommend at age three—will increase not only your child's activity level but also her engagement with her surroundings. We know, it's a lot easier to run errands when you don't have to run after your child at the same time. But the extra effort is well worth it.

Be Assertive. You don't have to be chained to your kitchen and a slow-cooker to feed your kids good foods, but you do need to speak up when you eat out. Order off the menu if you need to. Remember, if a chef can put lettuce and tomato on the side of a burger, then, my goodness, you've got the start of a salad going.

Stop Forcing the Clean Plate. We share your concern about starving children around the world, but their plight is not improved by forcing your children to give their plates a good tongue bath. If they've had proper nutrition throughout the day, it's okay to let their hunger determine whether or not they finish their meals. Or, it might even be better to just start with smaller portions; cut the meat in half or, when dining out, order smaller meals.

Use Peer Pressure. Lots of times peer pressure can be a really bad thing, but you can also flip it so that it works in your favor. Kids model other kids' behavior (you read about mirror neurons in our last chapter), so encourage your child to hang out with his friend whose parents have the same healthy habits that you strive for. Once your child sees that Ethan thinks carrot sticks are a yummy snack, he'll want them too.

Take Care of Yourself. You can preach all you want about broccoli and grilled chicken, but if your idea of dinner is a cheese ball with a side order of prime rib fat, then your children are going to want no part of the good stuff. You need to show them the right way. As we've said before, children won't treat themselves the way that you treat them but, rather, the way that you treat yourself.

Consider a Change Up. Some parents have success feeding their children their main meal at lunch rather than dinner. Oftentimes, kids are so tired at night that feeding becomes more of a battle than it needs to be. It's a good strategy nutritionally, as it insures that they get at least one balanced meal for the day.

Add Water. If you do serve fruit juice (calcium-fortified, we recommend), cut it with an equal amount of water or twice the amount of water so that your child doesn't consume as many empty calories and doesn't get used to the intense sweetness.

5

Gross Anatomy?

The GI System Provides Some Crazy Clues About Your Child's Health

Remember a time when you got together with your friends and a mug/glass/bottle of your favorite beverage, and you'd talk and talk and talk? About what was happening in your relationships, about what was happening at work, about what was happening in the world. These days, if you're lucky enough to escape the craziness that has enveloped your household, you still may find time to meet up with your friends. But the topics of convo have changed quite a bit. No longer do you banter about shoe sales, *Dancing with the Stars,* office politics, or your husband's mad habit of cracking his knuckles while you're dead asleep.

Now discussion centers around poop. Baby poop.

How much poop, how little poop, consistency of poop, color of poop, who pooped, who didn't poop, and the time it took you two hours to clean the poop-from-hell off of the crib slats, the walls, and all seven legs of Junior's Whoozit.

If you've been a parent for even a day, you surely know how endlessly fascinating the workings of a baby's GI system can be. Our collective obsession with the process of elimination has nothing to do with how easy it is to make a lot of crappy jokes about the subject. (See?) It's because our instincts as parents are dead-on: We know that understanding the state of a baby's GI system doesn't simply help us save money on bleach; we know that it's in the GI system where we often see signs of trouble. When things are going in and out in ways that are different from what we expect, our alert level rises. As well it should.

GI health is essential for a child's overall health and behavior. That's not just because there could be acute problems, the primary subject of this chapter. But there's collateral damage to consider too. Digestive disruptions can make children irritable, anxious, sleep deprived, and even affect their ability to focus and learn. We adults act the way our guts feel, and kids are no different. Even subtle discomfort can lead to less-than-happy kids.

In this chapter, we're going to take you through the inner workings of a child's digestive system from top to bottom, and we're going to talk about all the things that you might have to deal with along the way—including what comes out the top and the bottom. But this chapter isn't only about learning how to handle issues like constipation, diarrhea, appendicitis, and the like. It's about how to optimize your child's digestive system and, in the process, optimize her health.

Food Moves:
The Biology of the Digestive System

There's a good chance that, like most folks, you basically think of GI issues in terms of two types of problems: the aforementioned "out the top" and "out the bottom." We prefer to think of GI problems in terms of two other categories: ones that are mechanical and ones that are related to absorption. The mechanical issues have to do with how the child's GI system is built; perhaps there's a kink somewhere along the digestive route that keeps the system from working properly. Absorption issues, as you might imagine, have to do with the child's ability to absorb nutrients. The struc-

CONNECT THE TUBES

As early as in utero, docs check to make sure all the components of the GI system, from the mouth to the anus, are connected. If the esophagus is not connected to the stomach, for instance, the child will vomit. While this problem is fairly uncommon, an ultrasound in utero can catch it; since the tube is blocked, these babies have extra amniotic fluid because they haven't been able to swallow it, and there will be no evidence of what's called a gastric bubble, because air can't pass through the esophagus to the stomach. If undiagnosed, the child will have trouble feeding (choking, sputtering, and so on). If the large intestine is not connected to the anus, the child cannot defecate, which is why Baby has to poop before going home from the hospital. In either case, surgery can connect the tubes properly.

tures may be intact, but something is preventing the body from getting the nutrients it needs.

The tough part is that it's hard to know if the system was built to spec or not. It's not as if you can do a quick eye check and know that a part of the intestines is folded the wrong way or that a nutrient in a particular food isn't agreeing with your child. So what you need to do is look for the big sign that things are progressing normally or not: growth rate. If your child is growing at a consistently normal rate (see our growth charts in the appendix), then it's more likely that she's getting most if not all of the nutrients that she needs and that her GI system is working pretty well. The good news is that most GI issues—both mechanical and absorption related—can be fixed or are outgrown.

Before we take you through the symptoms of and solutions to specific gastrointestinal problems, it makes sense to learn a bit about that tract and also about how a child's digestive system differs from that of an adult. After all, kids aren't just mini-adults. They have their own biological and anatomical characteristics that make them even more special than the little munchkins already are.

So on this quick tour of the body's sewer system, let's take it from the top.

Unless you (or your child, if he's feeding himself) have really bad aim, the diges-

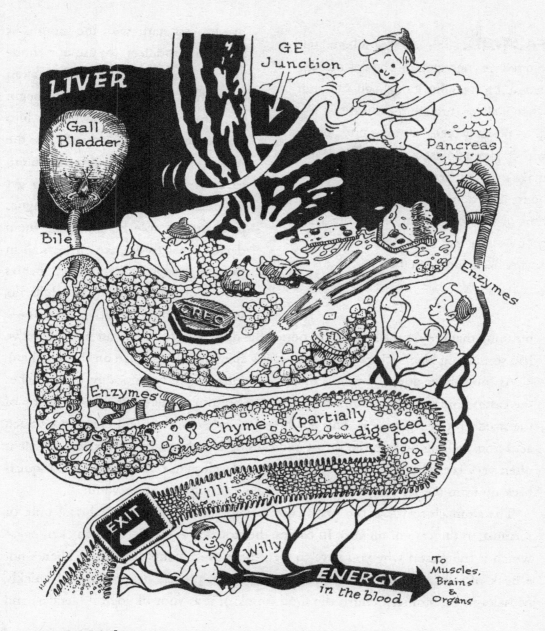

Figure 5.1 **GI Whoa** It's inevitable: Every parent is going to have to deal with some level of gastrointestinal distress at one point or another. The digestive process, one of the many amazing bodily journeys, typically works just fine. But the occasional bugs or genetic disposition to cranky bowels can sometimes make for an anatomical (and literal) mess.

FACTOID: Some say that mineral oil can relieve constipation. The downside is that it has no nutritional benefits, and when it slides through the intestines, it quite possibly takes vitamins out along with it. If you do use it to help your child, make sure that you administer it two hours after a meal to give the body more time to absorb important nutrients. The good news is that mineral oil comes in flavors like lemon and mint.

tive process starts with the mouth. As adults and toddlers, we use our choppers to grind our food so that it can be digested. Enzymes in saliva begin to break down carbohydrates into simple sugars. Babies naturally use the sucking reflex they developed in utero to latch onto breast or bottle to get the nutrients they need. Their tongues play a major role here, helping them decide what to eat, as you learned in the last chapter. Remember, babies have more taste buds than adults do, so they're more sensitive to tastes—meaning that they're really going to notice the difference in, say, breast milk, if you've had something bland (chicken) or something spicy (poblano sauce on that chicken).

As food slides down, it moves into the esophagus pretty smoothly, then reaches the gastroesophageal junction, which joins the bottom of the esophagus to the top of the stomach (see figure 5.1). This is where a muscle contracts and prevents stomach acid from spilling up into the throat and causing heartburn. In infants, this muscle is often very lax, which is why they're prone to developing reflux, where food squirts back up from the stomach into the esophagus, causing spit-up or vomit.

The stomach serves as the first major storage facility of food (or breast milk or formula, in the case of infants). In babies, the stomach is the size of a chicken egg,★ which is the reason why you have to feed them every couple of hours. There's not a heck of a lot of room in there, so the digestion process happens pretty quickly. Muscles in the stomach churn the food (think of it as your biological blender) and

★ At days one and two, it's about the size of a marble; at day three, about the size of a ping-pong ball; and by day ten, the size of an egg. An adult stomach is about the size of a fist or grapefruit. But you can stretch your stomach to over-football size. We wrote a book on why and how not to do that: *YOU: On a Diet.*

mix it with gastric juices and chemicals that break down the big bits into small particles. These particles are eventually absorbed (mostly in the intestines) into the blood to be used as our building blocks or as energy to power organs, muscles, and tissues all throughout your body.

Once food leaves the stomach, it moves to the small intestine—that brainy-looking tube of an organ. In

fact, the small intestine doesn't just look like a brain, it works like a brain, too. The small intestine produces about 90 percent of your body's serotonin, the chemical that, when found in the brain, gives you that happy, click-your-heels-together feeling. That's one reason why your gut influences the way you feel so much; if your gut isn't happy, neither are you. In a child, the small intestine would stretch about nine feet if it weren't wrapped around like a switchback hiking trail. While there's a difference in size between adults and kids (adults' small intestines average about twenty-six feet), the length is proportional to body size. In children, the small intestine is about three and a half times their height.

In the small intestine, food mixes with bile, a green liquid that breaks down fat in the same way that soap removes grease. Bile is made by the liver and stored in the gallbladder. Meanwhile, various enzymes continue to break down carbohydrates into simple sugars and proteins into amino acids. Then the magic takes place. Throughout the membranes lining the small intestine are blood vessels that absorb the nutrients from broken-down food and deliver them to the liver and then into tissues and organs throughout the body. Chemicals that the body doesn't need all that much, such as some excess vitamins, water, salt, and fats, are not absorbed and are passed along to a reservoir located between the small and large intestines called the cecum (pronounced *sea*-come).

Once this waste goes to the large intestine (the colon), much of the liquid gets drained out so the body can use the fluid—leaving the solid mass that we all know.

Feces travel down the colon and into the rectum before they're diaper deposited for you to dispose of. The reason why infants tend to have bowel movements after every feeding is because in a baby's colon, there's not a lot of room to store waste, so it's got to rocket-ship it out of there. That processing time increases as the body grows.

The typical transit time from stomach to anus varies and is measured in minutes and hours rather than in days. But that system doesn't always work as smoothly as it should: Sometimes it works too fast (diarrhea) and sometimes it works too slow (constipation). Later in this chapter, we'll explain why these problems occur, as well as what you can do about them.

The Rules of Stool: The Primer on Poop

When it comes to adult bowel movements, there are two kinds of people in the world—the ones who look and the ones who don't. (We recommend that you do look—to use your own poop as a proxy for your health. A nice S shape means that systems are running pretty smoothly. Pellets mean they're not.) But when it comes to a child's poop, you have no choice but to look. And smell. And, many times, *hear*, come to think of it. This primer will give you an idea of what you should be on the lookout for as you're doing your intestinal inspections.

The First Poop. Before your baby can come home, the docs will make sure that she meets certain requirements, such as not losing weight too fast. But one of the tests you may not know about is this: A baby must poop in the hospital. That signals that there's a clear path from mouth to anus. If the baby doesn't, it could mean there's some kind of obstruction or underlying problem.★

★ In Hirschsprung's disease, kids are missing some nerve endings in their bowel wall that get the colon to work in a coordinated fashion. These infants may not pass stool on their own for weeks. Other problems can also keep a baby from passing stool, like bowel obstruction or the hereditary digestive disease cystic fibrosis. A bowel obstruction hurts—the baby will be bringing her knees up to her abdomen—while cystic fibrosis makes those first poops especially sticky. The latter disorder is characterized by a deficiency of vital digestive enzymes produced by the pancreas.

RASH DECISIONS

If there's a whole lot of poopin' going on, or if it's summertime and your child likes to sit in the sandbox and sweat, there's a good chance that your baby's tush is going to end up redder than a steamed lobster. You have lots of options for taking the hurt away. You can try A+D ointment, Pinxav (pronounced "pink salve"), Desitin, Balmex, and many other brands of creams that act like a slippery or gluey barrier to keep acid in stool and urine from breaking down the skin and stinging like an angry ray. (See more on treatment for diaper rash on page 225.)

At the same time, you should also be on the lookout for a yeast infection. Yeast lives in our intestines, so it's not unusual for a diaper rash to be yeast related. This is marked by angry-looking little red bumps. If it is yeast, you'll need a special prescription antifungal cream (like nystatin) applied four times a day, to go along with the other gluelike ointments. If you find that your child always has diaper rash, she might be allergic to some chemical in that brand of diaper or wipe you're using, so it's worth trying others to see if they cause less of a reaction. You can't go wrong wiping with plain water and a soft paper towel. Or she may have a food 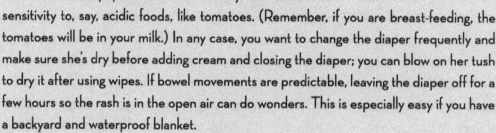 sensitivity to, say, acidic foods, like tomatoes. (Remember, if you are breast-feeding, the tomatoes will be in your milk.) In any case, you want to change the diaper frequently and make sure she's dry before adding cream and closing the diaper; you can blow on her tush to dry it after using wipes. If bowel movements are predictable, leaving the diaper off for a few hours so the rash is in the open air can do wonders. This is especially easy if you have a backyard and waterproof blanket.

Now, once that first poop comes, it will probably be unlike any poop you have ever seen. Called meconium, it's sticky, greenish black, and thick like tar. Meconium comes from the baby swallowing blood along with amniotic fluid during the last phase of pregnancy; the blood comes from placental capillaries that break before and during labor. The good news is that it passes in a few days as the baby transitions to newborn nutrition—and newborn digestion and newborn poop.

The Newborn Poop. Changing a baby's diaper can be like opening a present: You often have a pretty good idea what's going to be inside, but every once in a while, something's going to surprise you. The truth is that babies have at least as many different poop patterns as adults do, but there are some general rules that they follow.

Breast-fed babies tend to make more poops than formula-fed ones: two to five a day, maybe even after every feeding, compared to one or two a day for formula-fed infants. Why? Breast milk contains immunoglobulins, substances produced by the body's immune system, which also work as natural laxatives. This is especially helpful for clearing meconium, while also contributing to frequent pooping and a lack of constipation in nursing babies. These poops tend to be less smelly than poops from kids drinking formula; nature's way of saying thank you, perhaps, for using breast milk. But breast-fed babies may vary their patterns; what you eat and drink gets passed along in the milk, and that may or may not agree with your child.

Newborn stools are also nature's way of clearing out the baby's bilirubin, the yellowish pigment that, in excess amounts, causes jaundice (a condition signaled by yellowing of the skin; see page 235 for more). That's another reason we want to make sure a baby's pooping like a champ before sending him home. If the bilirubin won't

HE WHO MAKES THE MESS DOESN'T HAVE TO CLEAN IT

In a few years, your child will be responsible for cleaning up the toys and wiping up the spills. But for now, those dirty jobs are all yours. You have lots of options: Baby wipes can work well for spit-up or poop stains, as do such products as Shout, OxiClean, Totally Toddler, and Mother's Little Miracle. You can also try products that clean pet accidents, such as Nature's Miracle. For getting poop or vomit smell out of the carpet, use a combination of white vinegar and water with a little mild dishwashing liquid. Don't rub, just let it soak in, then blot with a clean rag and rinse, blot, rinse, blot with water.

clear from his bloodstream, he'll be placed under special lights or a "biliblanket," which help breakdown the pigment.

Some additional things to watch for in this early period:

Color: Stools should be brown or a seedy yellow-green; formula-fed babies will have brown stools faster, and the poop will stink. If the stools are black after the first four days, there may be blood in there from a location upstream, and it's worth a call to your pediatrician to check it out.

Frequency: It's not uncommon for babies to go long periods without pooping. That doesn't necessarily mean they're constipated (more on that in a moment). But if your baby goes more than ten days without a poop, your doc may recommend an over-the-counter glycerin suppository. Slide it in, and it helps poop slide out.

Weight (of baby, not diaper): If you feel like your baby is pooping more than your coffee-drinking and bean-eating uncle, it's not necessarily a bad thing. As long as she is growing normally and gaining weight, it's okay; it just means that her GI system is running efficiently. If you are particularly concerned about your baby's weight gain, you can buy a home baby scale.

The Toddler/Preschooler Poop. By this time, you're probably most concerned about trying to get the poop into the city sewer system rather than in the pants. (See our toilet training tips in chapter 3.) But just because you're focused on *where* doesn't mean that you can ignore the *when* or the *what*. Toddlers' poop patterns vary in frequency; it's not uncommon for a child to go twice a day, or once every two or three days, or even just once or twice a week. It may still be mushy, or it may begin to appear more formed. What's important is that poop should come out smoothly, without excessive pain or strain (see constipation, below).

The biggest thing that will likely scare you is color: Kids are what they eat at this age, and Technicolor poops are usually more a sign that they just ate some funky-colored yogurt or cereal than anything else. Blueberries can be quite dramatic; beets will dye both poop and pee red. Streaks of red may simply be a sign of small anal fissures, or breaks in the tissue, rather than anything serious (see below). But the biggest thing you typically need to worry about at this age is keeping track of any foreign objects or toys your child may have swallowed, so that you can dig through his poop later to make sure the Lego came out the other end.

Strains, Pains, and Stains: Problems of the GI System

Now that we've spent a few pages dissecting the ins and outs of a child's GI tract, it's time to look a little more closely at the most common intestinal issues for children.

Constipation. You've just learned a bit about bowel frequency, so now you understand that docs don't get too wrapped up in specific numbers—as in, how many days since her last poop? While ten days of unsoiled diapers signal classic constipation in a toddler (not so much so in an infant), docs are more concerned with quality than quantity.

Constipation happens when the muscles at the end of the large intestine tighten, preventing the stool from passing (see Figure 5.2). That slower passage allows more water to be drawn off from the stool through the bowel wall into the bloodstream, making the stool harder and more compact (and thus more painful). Relatively rare

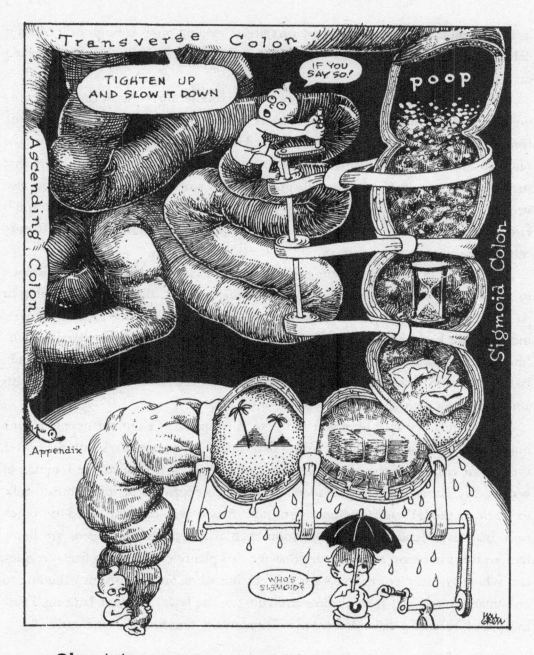

Figure 5.2 **Slow Motion** The colon is responsible for squeezing fluid out of poop so it can pass through the digestive system. To treat constipation, you can speed things along with Karo corn syrup.

in newborns, it can occur if the baby isn't breast-feeding often enough or if Mom is dehydrated. Stool that looks like rabbit pellets tells you that too much water is being drawn off.

The pain of constipation can lead the average toddler not to want that stuff coming out at all and not to want to eat, either. Clinically, we call that withholding stool. (Freud calls it being anal retentive.) As he holds in the stool, more water gets drawn out, and more poop keeps filling the space, stretching out his rectum. In turn, that stretching sends pain fibers firing. To make matters worse, passing the big mass also stretches the anus, occasionally causing microscopic tears called anal fissures. You'll know your kid has one if you see streaks of blood around the stools. An anal fissure warrants a call to the pediatrician.

All of this can be very upsetting for a child and can become a major roadblock to toilet training. So the goal here is to get things moving, allowing the big plug to pass. Sometimes some liquidy stuff will also form around it. Natural food "looseners" include fruits such as prunes, apricots, plums, raisins, cherries, and blueberries; high-fiber veggies, including peas, beans, and broccoli; and whole-grain cereals and breads. Extra water also helps for toddlers on up. However, too much water for newborns and infants can get their electrolytes out of whack.

For a baby, a doc may have you add ¼ to ½ teaspoon of Karo corn syrup to one bottle of formula or stored breast milk a day, which draws water back into the bowel. Or if your child is four months old, the doc may ask you to give her 1 ounce of water a day, either separately or added to a bottle of formula or stored breast milk, to lubricate the GI tract. One important note: A two-year-old who is fed too much milk may experience some constipation even if her nutritional needs are being met, so it is important to make sure that she eats plenty of fiber-rich fruits, veggies, and whole grains. (See chapter 4 for our nutritional recommendations.) Tending to constipation early can avert chronic stretching of the lower intestine later on. That's important, because a distended colon will eventually function less efficiently.

Spit-Up/Throw-Up. The most common spit-up problem in babyhood is gastroesophageal reflux. This happens when the junction between the stomach and the esophagus isn't as constricted or angled as it should be, and some of the stom-

HOW TO HANDLE COLIC

Colic, a condition in which an otherwise healthy infant is crying, fussy, and irritated for more than three hours a day and more than three days in any given week, usually goes away within a few months. But it can be upsetting, frustrating, and hard to handle. Some of the crying may be GI related, but that's not always the case. Here are some strategies for dealing with it. Unfortunately, sometimes you just have to wait the crying and screaming out.

- *Stay cool.* Babies pick up on cues from their parents. If you're temperamental because he's temperamental, he's only going to get more temperamental.

- *Stretch him.* Flex your baby at the knees and hips to see if you can relieve some trapped gas.

- *Move it.* Many babies with colic are soothed simply by getting up and going. Put him in a stroller or baby carrier and take a walk, go for a drive, or strap him into one of those vibrating seats for a fifteen-minute break. However, we don't want the kid *living* in the vibrating seat.

- *Change your diet.* You can try to relieve some discomfort by eliminating dairy, onions, garlic, spicy food, chocolate, caffeine, cauliflower, and even all wheat from your diet if you're breast-feeding. Play detective: Try eliminating one food at a time every four days to see which one is the offender. Or eliminate them all, then add one food back every four days to see if it's a keeper rather than a culprit.

- *Get some support.* Whatever you do, do *not* shake your baby to get him to stop crying; his delicate brain can be permanently damaged. If you feel yourself reaching your limit of frustration and exhaustion dealing with a colicky baby, enlist a support person—partner, friend, neighbor, relative, sitter—to give you a break.

ach's contents wash back up into the esophagus. While most babies spit up a little when they burp after a feeding, in babies with reflux, the quantity and frequency can be significantly greater. Now, you can usually get some signs from your child that there's a problem, depending on the age. Babies may arch their backs, trying to "get away" from the acid. They may also wheeze, cough, or have a hoarse cry, as acid is irritating to the throat and the voice box.

Toddlers, of course, can communicate more directly; they may complain of pain in their upper stomach, experience heartburn, or burp more frequently than a beer-guzzling frat boy. If behavior and lifestyle modifications don't work (see our YOU Tips), docs may try medicines like antacids, histamine-receptor blockers, and proton pump inhibitors. H2 blockers and PPIs both work by reducing the production of gastric acid, albeit through different mechanisms.

Thankfully, kids usually outgrow reflux by the time they're eight or nine months old, when they are spending more time upright and the esophageal sphincter tightens up. In babies, there's no cause for concern or treatment unless she is in distress or not gaining weight. A lot of times, a baby's spit-up may look like the whole meal of milk he just ate, but it's really only a fraction.

Projectile Vomiting. Any parent who's seen her child shoot vomit across the room onto a wall or relative's blouse knows full well the power of the *Exorcist* hurl. It can be darn scary, because it is hard to believe that a tiny baby could have that much strength. Projectile vomiting may be confused with reflux spit-ups; the difference lies in how far the stuff flies. Projectile vomit projects; spit-up merely bubbles up like lava from a volcano.

In infants, projectile vomiting happens when a baby has a condition called pyloric stenosis: an overdeveloped pylorus muscle at the bottom of the stomach. When the muscle tightens, it causes the entire contents of the stomach to empty, going "up and out," which can lead to dehydration. It usually happens in firstborn males, at around four to six weeks of age and tends to run in families. To a doctor conducting a physical exam of the abdomen, an overgrown pylorus will feel like an olive, and he can see it using ultrasonography. Pyloric stenosis can be fixed surgically.

Diarrhea/Vomiting.

As an adult, you know all too well what it feels like when you've got a bug. You spend half the night sitting on the toilet, half the night kneeling in front of it, and the time in between vowing to never again eat a fourteen-day-old mayo-based sandwich. So when your child is going all geyser on you, you can certainly feel her pain. It's not uncommon for infants to have loose stools regularly, but as they get older, we become concerned when loose turns to leaky—that is, when some kind of bacteria or virus is wreaking intestinal havoc. Here are some of the most common causes:

Rotavirus. This ugly virus is very foul, very green, and very contagious. An oral vaccine given at two, four, and six months is effective. It's also safer than the previous injectable vaccine, which was associated with intestinal lymph nodes leading to something called intussusception; more about this on page 159. Taking a probiotic—an oral supplement or other preparation containing beneficial healthy bacteria to replenish the gut—seems to help reduce diarrhea associated with the rotavirus in older children and adults. To treat infants, breast-feeding moms should take the probiotic, too, as children populate their guts with bacteria found around and in their mothers' breast milk. As that bacteria becomes popular in and on the mom, that decreases intestinal infections in your baby.

Norwalk virus. This virus causes the same symptoms as rotavirus: nausea, diarrhea, and the like. Because of its incubation period (ten to fifty-one hours) and because it can survive the heat, it's a hearty bug that can hide out in foods, meaning that it can find its way onto, say, cruise ships, then decimate the ship's passengers after the carrier is long gone from port. While it usually resolves itself in a day or two, this virus is one of the reasons why we preach wash hands, wash hands, wash hands.

Salmonella. Oooh, the ol' food-poisoning bug that makes news every time there's a significant outbreak. It also has a long incubation period (six to seventy-two hours) and can hide out in pets such as iguanas and turtles, as well as in the more traditional places like livestock and poultry. The treatment is usually supportive: lovin' and liquids. Skip the antibiotic (it prolongs the time that the bacterium is carried), but follow with a probiotic. Carefully washing foods is essential to help prevent outbreaks. Also, cook meat thoroughly, avoid consuming raw animal products like eggs (no licking the beaters when you're making cookies), and wash your child's hands after she feeds the pot-bellied pigs at the zoo.

Irritable Bowel Syndrome. Whoever decides to name medical diseases has two choices: Use medicalese (see pyloric stenosis) or call it as you see it. Irritable bowel syndrome is exactly what you'd think it would be: It's classified by a crampy pain that occurs at least once a week for two months combined with a bothersome and frequent stool pattern. Kids will often experience constipation, diarrhea, or the all-frustrating combo of both. If that's not enough to make one irritable, we're not sure what is.

Irritable bowel syndrome happens when the bowels are literally irritable, or trying to move things through faster than is comfortable. Actually passing the stool makes some people feel better and can relieve the cramping. The downside is that stools in IBS come more often than usual and are usually harder or softer than normal. You should also note that irritable bowel syndrome is different from a class of diseases called inflammatory bowel disease, which is marked by—you guessed it—inflammation of the bowels. Crohn's disease and ulcerative colitis fall into this category.

To treat IBS, docs will help you identify triggers that irritate your child's bowels. The symptoms of IBS are one way your child may manifest stress, anxiety, and behavior issues; it occurs more frequently in school-age kids who have more homework and other stresses than younger ones. A high-fiber diet can help, and some families swear by peppermint oil: Just drops a day can soothe the savage bowels. Other treatments include antidiarrheal meds and drugs called anticholinergics (to slow things down) to let your child's gut feel the benefit of his own homemade serotonin before his body takes it up and breaks it down.

WHAT'S A HERNIA?

Kids on the playground like to use the words *innie* and *outie* to describe their belly buttons, but if an outie is a "way outie," that's called an umbilical hernia (pictured here). It happens when the abdominal muscle doesn't completely fuse around the umbilicus at the time of delivery. Though umbilical hernias can extend up to 5 centimeters in diameter (about 2 inches), docs usually won't perform surgery on them because as Baby grows, the hole does not—meaning that the intestines are less likely to sneak out of the hole. (The intestines—not all, just some—are actually what are in an extreme outie belly button.) If a child still has this by age five, then docs may stitch the bowel tissue in place, using general anesthesia.

An inguinal hernia is a similar defect in which part of the small intestine bulges through a weak spot in the inguinal ring, located in the groin. These tend to need surgery to keep the bowel in place. They can come in two forms:

- ⊃ In boys, an indirect inguinal hernia slips through the inguinal ring and into the scrotum, making the testicle on that side look, shall we say, generous. The condition is rare in girls, but when it does occur, tissue from the small bowel or the female organs slides through a vulnerable area of the abdominal wall and into the groin.

- ⊃ A direct hernia, exclusive to boys, will look like a little bulge in the crease of the groin, right at the lower end of the abdomen.

Gluten Sensitivity. Gluten, the gluey substance found in wheat, rye, and barley, gets a lot of play in the press these days, and rightly so. Gluten intolerance (affecting 1 in 8 kids), allergies (1 in 30 kids), and celiac disease (1 in 250 kids) are associated with the body's inability to digest gluten. For kids, the problem with these conditions is not only the raft of symptoms that comes with them (including gas and abdominal pain) but also the fact that, in the case of gluten allergy or celiac disease, the inflammation they cause in the intestinal lining can make it difficult to absorb important vitamins and nutrients.* While you need a doc to give you a definitive answer on whether a child has a gluten sensitivity and, if so, which kind, you can certainly sense and see whether your child acts differently after eating certain foods. That's usually the first sign that something is up. There's a whole host of foods that are gluten free, and if your child develops an allergy or intolerance, you quickly learn which foods will give your child optimum nutrition and make him feel well. See our list of tips at the end of this chapter.

Bowel Emergencies. At the time, it may seem that vomit on the Tibetan rug is an emergency, but for us docs, there are two major GI emergencies that require immediate attention. They are:

Appendicitis. When the appendix† gets inflamed, it can burst, potentially poisoning the abdomen and bloodstream, which is life threatening. So it's important to know the difference between appendicitis and suffering from an overdose of birthday cake. With appendicitis, which is rare in youngsters under two, your child may feel pain around the belly button. Over a few hours, it will move to the lower right part of the belly. He won't want to move at all, because any kind of movement will hurt. Ask him to jump up and down (or help him if he's younger); if he absolutely

---

* The difference between an allergy and an intolerance is that an allergy can cause an inflammatory reaction in the skin, mouth, and lungs, while an intolerance does not involve the immune system and produces symptoms such as gas, diarrhea, and abdominal pain. Celiac disease is a permanent intolerance to the chemicals associated with gluten or wheat protein.

† The appendix used to be thought of as a useless organ appended to the large intestine, but now it is believed to store good bacteria that can repopulate the gut following a nasty infection.

can't, it's likely an inflamed appendix, and you need to get to the hospital. Surgery is typically done laparoscopically (with a small incision) and calls for a one- to two-day hospital stay.

Intussusception. Intussusception isn't what happens when a cornerback picks off a quarterback's pass; it's when the bowel acts like a telescope, folding in on itself. Frankly, this hurts like the dickens, and your child will be drawing her legs up to her abdomen. It happens most commonly in kids from three months to six years, and the condition also comes with a side order of fever, vomiting, and the passing of currant-colored, jellylike stool.

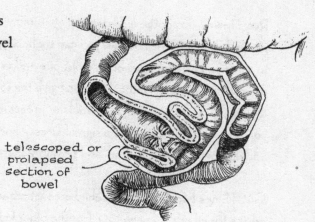

telescoped or prolapsed section of bowel

To treat it, a doc will push an enema (either air- or barium-based) into the anus and up the bowel, to help untelescope that part of the colon and relieve the pain. If the enema doesn't work, surgery may be necessary.

• • •

While one of our aims in this chapter is to help you minimize the mess of all of these issues, we also have loftier goals in mind. By paying attention to a child's digestive patterns and irregularities, you'll gain valuable insight into her overall health. As is the case with adults, happy bowels equal happy person. So use these strategies to keep things running smoothly.

YOU TIPS

Rub Down. To soothe a garden-variety tummy ache, you can try rubbing in circles out from the belly button. With babies, you can try flexing them at the hips and also bicycling their legs to see if you can get a gas bubble out one end or the other. For older toddlers and children, peppermint tea can soothe. But don't give tea to a baby under age one; you may be giving him too much water in relation to formula or breast milk. Stomachaches, headaches, and other body complaints can definitely be a sign of stress—and also of sexual abuse. When the story does not add up, visit your pediatrician and privately share your concerns.

Get Things Moving. If your child is constipated, you can help move things along. See our advice for infants on page 150. For the older kids, try these tactics:

- ⊃ Loosening foods: prunes and/or prune juice, bran (with plenty of accompanying liquid, be it water or milk), at least five servings of fruits and vegetables a day.

- ⊃ Make sure kids aren't eating binding foods, like oatmeal, bananas, and rice.

- ⊃ Perfect time for the playground: Exercise speeds the digestion process, whereas lying in bed when you do not feel well can induce constipation.

- ⊃ Just add water. Have them drink an extra cup or two a day.

- ⊃ Try prune juice in a bottle or boiled with water later on.

Consider Reinforcements. As babies learn to push out a bowel movement, they can grunt and strain with the force of an Olympic power lifter. (They may even draw their legs up; the baby, not the power lifter, that is.) A well-timed glycerin suppository, available over the counter, can help ease the passage. Insert a rocket-shaped suppository into your baby's rectum just enough so it's not visible and hold the buttocks together for a minute to dissolve the glycerin.

After you insert, wiggle it a bit to relax the muscles in the area. In no time, you'll be singing "Slip Slidin' Away." If this strategy doesn't work, it means the poop is not down far enough in the rectum or the anus to slide on out. Try repeating in four to six hours and see if things are closer to the end, so to speak.

Rehydrate as Needed. If your child has been suffering from a bug or virus, you should be concerned about dehydration.

With all that pooping and vomiting going on, there's a good chance that she's lost a lot of water. Nursing babies can be rehydrated with breast milk, but formula-fed ones and older children should drink Pedialyte or a similar rehydration liquid to prevent them from having to go to the hospital for intravenous fluids. Clear juices—apple, white peach, and white grape—can also help get some much needed calories and liquid back into the system. You can freeze these juices or Pedialyte and serve as Popsicles for the older kids. If you prefer to prepare your own electrolyte solution, try this commonly used formula for what's called oral rehydration therapy: 1 level teaspoon of salt, 8 level teaspoons of sugar, 1 quart of boiled water (cooled). Stir until the sugar and salt dissolve.

Be careful when rehydrating with liquid: No big gulps, or they'll just recycle it again. Aim for small amounts, about 1 ounce every fifteen minutes. You can get a good sense of whether hydration is an issue by keeping track of how much fluid seems to be getting in, whether the child is urinating, and seeing if his tongue is dry. Tinkling even twice a day means something is successfully getting in; fewer times than that warrants a call to the doc.

Minimize the Acid. Some docs will prescribe meds for children suffering from reflux, but you should also try some at-home tactics to help minimize the discomfort. In infants, be sure to burp your baby frequently during feedings (every 1 to 2 ounces or every five minutes when breast-feeding if he or she is a spitty baby) and prop up your baby after meals to allow gravity to work;

backwash can happen more easily when an infant is lying down flat. If you're breast-feeding, you can also help by minimizing your own consumption of gassy foods such as onions, cruciferous vegetables (for instance, cabbage and cauliflower), and dairy. With toddlers and preschoolers, try adjusting their diet to see if certain foods trigger acid.

Other strategies:

⊃ Have your child eat smaller meals more frequently.

⊃ Don't let her eat two to three hours before bed.

⊃ Raise the head of your child's bed by placing blocks under the mattress to help gravity do its work.

⊃ Not that your child is consuming carbonated drinks, chocolate, caffeine, and high-fat foods, but these can trigger acid reflux. Avoid tomatoes and citrusy foods with a lot of acid.

Go Pro. If your child is having a lot of GI issues, it might be worth exploring the use of probiotics—that is, organisms that live in fermented foods that help colonize the gut with good bacteria. While it's not clear how probiotics work (they may calm the immune system or help the immune response in other ways), it is clear that they do help relieve irritable bowels. Get them in the spore form. That's because acid in the stomach can kill the live form of bacteria, and we need to recolonize those.

Go G-Free. If your child has gluten allergies or intolerance, you'll have to watch what you feed her (see below). But for those times when you won't be there to monitor her every bite, it's also important to teach your child and those interacting with her about how to manage her condition.

Our suggestions:

⊃ Cook and bake together to help your child learn to take ownership of her diet.

⊃ Take your child grocery shopping and teach her which foods are okay for her body and which are not. Older children can be taught to recognize the words *gluten free* on food labels.

➲ Talk, talk, talk. Teach your child what gluten sensitivity is, what foods she can eat, and why it's important. The more she knows, the more she'll be able to advocate for herself.

➲ Be sure that your child's grandparents and other caretakers understand the serious-ness of her condition—there's often a generation/cultural gap in understanding about these issues, and indulgent grandparents sometimes find it hard to believe that "one little cookie" will hurt.

➲ Talk to teachers and ask if you can give a presentation to parents, so they understand your child's dietary limitations. While you're at it, you can lobby to change cafeteria standards to include more G-free foods.

➲ Get involved with other parents who are dealing with the same things. Besides there being power in numbers, there's also great value in having a strong support system.

➲ If the whole family isn't going to go gluten free, come up with gluten-free alternatives to whatever you eat, especially for snacks and dessert, so your child doesn't feel deprived.

➲ Use this sample shopping list. Here are some examples of healthful G-free foods that you can introduce into your child's diet:

Fresh fruits	Corn	Eggs
Unflavored milk (no chocolate)	Brown rice	Popcorn
Dried beans, lentils, peas	Fresh pork	100 percent fruit juice
Most yogurts	Fresh poultry	Plain nuts, seeds
Fresh vegetables	Fresh fish or seafood	Cocoa
Tofu	Canned salmon or tuna	Jell-O
White or sweet potato	Natural, organic peanut butter	Spices and herbs
		Pudding
		Canola and olive oil

THE GI CHEAT SHEETS

Use these quick-reference guides to help diagnose your child's digestive discomfort.

DIARRHEA	
SYMPTOMS	CAUSE
Green and foul smelling	Rotavirus, salmonella
Yellow-brown, watery	Irritable bowel syndrome
Cramping	Irritable bowel syndrome
Post-antibiotics	Normal, no worries
Chronic	Infection, disease, too much sugar or fruit juice

PAINFUL STOOLS	
SYMPTOMS	CAUSE
With bloody streaks	Anal fissure: small tear around anus
No blood	Constipation

VOMITING	
SYMPTOMS	CAUSE
With fever	Infection or inflammation (see doc)
Bloody	Small tear in stomach lining or rupture in GI tract (see doc); blood may also be from cracked nipples of breast-feeding mom
Yellow, bilelike, profuse	Blockage or obstruction; call doc and go to ER

VOMITING (cont.)	
Belly distended, severe pain	Obstruction; call doc and go to ER
Longer than twenty-four hours	Risk of dehydration; go to doc or ER
Projectile	Pyloric stenosis (see doc)
Nonprojectile	Reflux
	After head injury (call doc)
	Extra fluid in brain; go to ER or doc

ABDOMINAL PAIN	
SYMPTOMS	CAUSE
If child can jump up and down	Not an emergency; try BRAT diet and call doc. If constipated, do the CRAP diet (page 161)
If child can't jump up and down	Appendicitis (go to ER)
Bringing knees to abdomen	Intussusception (see doc)

6

Bug Out

Get the Lowdown on Infection Detection

In this lifelong journey of raising a child, parents assume a heck of a lot of different roles. Sometimes we're life coaches, sometimes we're boo-boo fixers, sometimes we're short-order cooks, and sometimes we're rule enforcement officers. It's just the nature of parenting: We wear many hats (often at the same time) with the ultimate goal of raising a happy, healthy, and well-adjusted child.

One of our most challenging jobs is that of Secret Service agent. Our mission: Protect our VIC★ at all costs. We arm ourselves with equipment (car seats, sunblock, words of wisdom) to help our kids avoid any threatening mishaps. Unfortunately, every enemy we face isn't as obvious as an unprotected electrical socket. Enemies come in the form of microscopic buggers that think it's funny to watch a kid test the absorption capacity of Pampers. Every child, no matter what steps a parent takes,

★ Very Important Child

will come face to face with invaders that make her sick, miserable, and cause her to shriek like a novice roller-coaster rider.

Fortunately, you can minimize the damage, and you don't even need a fancy earpiece, dark sunglasses, and shoe phone to do so.

Our bodies are equipped to handle all kinds of invaders. Because our skin, mouth, and nose interact with the outside world, those are the areas that tend to show symptoms. They're also where most of our defense mechanisms are located. While there may be some collateral damage sustained along the way (fevers, runny noses), even young children's developing immune systems can handle many biological threats.

In this chapter, you'll get your first glimpse into how the immune system works and how it defends the body against all kinds of foreign invaders. Once you understand the immune response, you'll realize how important it is for you to take the steps that will amp up your child's immune cells and help him stay healthy.

War and Peace:
How Immune Battles Are Fought

Maybe it's because we're anatomy and biology freaks, but we're constantly amazed at all the cool stuff bodies do. Brains think, hearts pump, skin serves double duty as body armor and bearer of goose bumps. Truly amazing stuff. In the pecking order of miraculous processes, immunity has to rank right up there. Here's the primer:

A newborn baby isn't a perfectly packaged toy ready to go right out of the box. During his time in utero, he developed a bit of his own immune system, but he also relied on Mom's immunity to help protect him from toxins. Both those immune cells and antibodies, or protective proteins, were passed to him through an equally miraculous process involving the placenta. By six months after birth, a child's immune system is mostly all his.

The immune cells come in a few different forms and perform a few different functions (see Figure 6.1). While they're all part of the same foreigner-fighting army, they certainly can't all do the same jobs. After all, no military operation would be successful if everyone were a Navy SEAL, or if everyone were a commander, or if everyone specialized in tank repairs. You need specialized people and parts, as well as a complete team, to work well.

In your body, the first soldier on the ground you need to know is a type of white blood cell called the macrophage. When your body spots some type of intruder such as a bacterium or virus, the macrophage moves in, finds the offender, engulfs, and digests it—sort of the way a soldier would take a prisoner of war hostage. But the macrophage isn't equipped with all the tools necessary to finish the job, so it radios for backup; that's when other helper cells arrive to assist in the operation.

While the macrophage waits for the other immune cells to speed their way through the bloodstream, it takes notes about the intruder, or antigen: who it is, what it is, and any identifying characteristics. That's important, right? Your body needs to be able to recognize this bad boy the next time he invades your territory, so it can respond quickly and flush it out of your system.

Now, back to the action. Thankfully, reinforcements arrive in the form of other white blood cells known as T cells and B cells. Both play a role in actually killing the invader. The T cells, which in infants mature in an organ called the thymus*, directly attack the invader (think hand-to-hand combat). The B cells create chemicals called immunoglobulin antibodies that act like bullets against the foreign substance. *Die, antigen!* After a successful battle, the foreign cells do, in fact, die. But the interesting part here is that the T and B cells die as well, in a cellular process that's called apoptosis, or programmed cell death. The reason? If they didn't die, the T and B cells could attack

* The thymus is much bigger in children than in adults because their immune systems haven't been exposed to much, so they need a larger defense system to handle so many unknown invaders.

healthy cells after they've finished their primary job—sort of like soldiers suffering from post-traumatic stress disorder who may confuse wartime with peacetime.

This process typically works just fine, especially in the case of very simple and

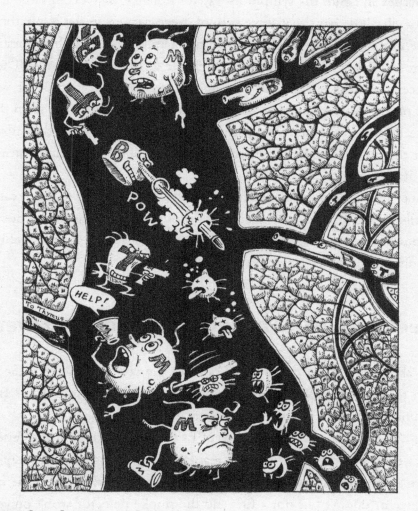

Figure 6.1 **Fight the Good Fight** When a child gets sick, immune cells take action. First responders are the macrophages (m), who call in the SWAT team—specifically B and T cells, who come to the rescue to fight off invaders, whether they come in the form of bacteria or viruses. Symptoms from colds, flu, and other immune-related conditions are caused not only by the germs themselves but also as collateral damage from the battle between immune cells and foreign ones.

straightforward bacterial and viral infections, which we'll discuss in more detail in a few pages. When the immune system tackles an invading agent such as a virus, the invader triggers body reactions that cause symptoms, then the immune system fights off the invader and ends the symptoms. Say, for instance, that a cold virus attaches to respiratory cilia: little hairs that serve as mini street cleaners in the respiratory system. When the immune cells are alerted to the problem, they start an inflammatory process that forces the nose faucets to turn on in the form of a runny nose. Then, as the immune cells do their job and kill the offender and then kill themselves, we see the remnants of the battle: more snot. So we experience reactions both from the body's attempt to defend against the foreign invader, as well as from its battle with the antigen. After the battle is won, the symptoms begin to subside, the faucet turns off, and the child starts feeling better.

As you can imagine from the intricacies of this microscopic process, it can't always work perfectly. We'll be discussing some of those malfunctions in the next chapter on allergies and asthma, but for now, let's take a closer look at how a child's body handles some common contagious conditions.

Feel the Heat: The Biological Role of Fevers

Look up above you. What do you see? No, not the cobwebs. No, not the silverfish scurrying to the corner. We're talking about the smoke detector. Why? Because it helps us understand how to interpret a fever: as a warning sign.

When our children get fevers, many of us focus on "bringing the fever down." And that's okay. But the fever isn't the real problem. The fever is the *beep-beep-beep* of the fire alarm alerting you that there might be a fire elsewhere in the body. The smoke detector doesn't put out a fire, and the smoke detector won't prevent a fire; what the smoke detector does is alert you that something needs your attention. The alarm may be sounding for a minor reason such as a drained battery, or it may be wailing to alert you to something potentially catastrophic, such as roaring flames in the next room. The alarm detects and alerts. And that's exactly what a fever does; it acts as a first-line detection system. Once you understand that big principle, it will help you take a more holistic view of what happens when your child gets sick.

It probably won't surprise you that fevers are one of the most common reasons that kids visit the doctor. That's because most parents are pretty darn good at hearing the alarm go off and then deciding to investigate the cause of the fire. Here's how it happens biologically:

When a child's body encounters a virus or bacterium (we'll explain the difference between the two in a moment), that rendezvous kick-starts the immune response. The body raises its internal temperature, which acts as a sort of call to arms for the immune cells.

Now, there are lots of reasons why our body digs the heat during the immune process, and here's where a fever outperforms a smoke alarm. For one, heat actually breaks down the bacteria, weakening them. Two, heat stimulates our body's immune cells to release special chemicals called cytokines, which put a biological bull's-eye on foreign invaders. This improves the accuracy of our immune response and minimizes collateral damage to other cells.* Finally, heat works by activating chemicals that

> **FACTOID:** The reason why moms kiss their babies is to show affection, as well as to get a surge of the feel-good, we-are-the-world hormone called oxytocin. (Mom doesn't pick up oxytocin from her baby; the act of kissing her baby stimulates her own production of oxytocin.) But you can also pass along this little tidbit at your next cocktail party: Subconsciously, when a mom kisses her baby, she's sampling pathogens that are on the baby's face and in danger of being ingested. Mom unconsciously scoops up these pathogens, and her immune cells produce antibodies, which then get passed along to her baby through her milk. Wow! More evidence that the body knows best. On the downside, kissing a child on or around the mouth can transmit your oral bacteria to your child, which can lead to cavities for her down the road (see page 100), not to mention the type 1 herpesvirus, or cold sore.

---

* Further evidence that heat is a necessary part of the immune response: Lizards climb on rocks to sun themselves and absorb heat. If you introduce infection to lizards and prevent them from getting on top of the rocks, the infection is more severe, even life threatening.

protect some of our body's important proteins. So in some ways, fever is both smoke detector and sprinkler rolled into one.

Fever is an adaptive response that decreases microbial reproduction and increases the inflammatory response. Inflammation and heat go together like peanut butter and jelly. With a cut, for example, you'll see redness and swelling to go along with inflammation and heat in the area of the cut. But when there's inflammation of internal organs—via a virus or bacterium—that inflammation is internal and systemic and the heat can come in the form of a fever. In a child without other inflammatory problems (such as chronic diseases like juvenile rheumatoid arthritis), fever alerts you to the fact that you're most likely facing an infection and need to find out what kind of infection it is, how sick the child is, and what your plan of action is.

That's all well and good, you might be saying, but what you really want to know is what exactly you're supposed to do when your child starts burning up like a black-leather seat in a Florida-registered convertible. Excellent question. First off, it's important to know that for children, there's no set "normal" temperature. A child's temperature can vary depending on the time of day (it's nearly 2 degrees lower in the early morning than in the late afternoon or early evening), how much food she has eaten, how much sleep she's gotten, or whether she has a fast or slow metabolism. The range of typical temps for a kid is between 96 and 100.2 degrees Fahrenheit (or 36 to 38 degrees centigrade), but that also depends on how the temp was taken:

○ Temp taken in the tush: Accurate.

○ Temp taken in the mouth: Add ½ degree.

○ Temp taken under the arm: Add 1 degree.

○ Temp taken in the ear: Accurate, theoretically (depends on the thermometer used).

So if your child has a low-grade fever of 100, you might not need to do a thing—except make sure that he's had enough sleep, fluid, and his daily multivitamin. It likely isn't anything that warrants the pediatrician's attention. However, once the fever exceeds 100.2, it indicates that something else is going on. Use the chart below to help you navigate your next steps:

DO NOT PUT TOO MUCH ANGST INTO BABY'S FEVER IF . . .

She is over three months old and she's smiling, playing, and doing a good job of eating, pooping, and tinkling, unless the fever rises above 105.

She's under three months and the fever is under 100.2.

CALL YOUR PEDIATRICIAN IF . . .

She's under three months with a temp of 100.2 or higher.

She's eating poorly or not pooping and has a temp over 100.2.

She looks a little listless or acts especially fussy.

She's had a febrile seizure in the past and her temp is on the rise.

She had a fever and doesn't seem the same afterward.

CALL YOUR DOC *AT ONCE* AND GO TO THE ER IF . . .

She's unresponsive, listless, and hasn't produced tears or urine in eight hours.

She has difficulty breathing.

She has a fever of 105 or higher.

While it might be your immediate impulse to try to bring down the fever, the truth is that you don't need to rush to the medicine cabinet if (1) the fever is not bothering the child; (2) she has no history of febrile seizures, mitochondrial disorder*, or other chronic metabolic disease; and (3) she shows no other symptoms.

* Mitochondrial disorder limits or inhibits the ability of the mitochondrial cells to convert oxygen and the substances you eat into energy for essential cell functions.

THE GERMIEST PLACES AT HOME

Well, that would be your kitchen and bathroom: the former for all those food remnants that can be left on the counter; the latter because of the toilet. We're not talking about what goes *in* the toilet, but rather what comes *out* when you flush. Toilet spray can travel a long way, with the bacteria in the bowl landing squarely on soap, towels, your child's toothbrush. Teach your kids to shut the lid before they flush. It also makes sense to thoroughly clean pillows, towels, binkies, teddy bears, and sheets after someone has been sick. And toss out Typhoid Mary's toothbrushes, too. Other things to disinfect: toys, remote controls, computer mouse, telephones, doorknobs, light switches, toilet flush handles.

Fever has protective benefits, as we mentioned, so sometimes no action can be the best action. But if she is showing discomfort, by all means talk to your doc and take the following steps to bring down the fever and improve the way she feels. Note: A child should stay home from school or day care until she's been fever free without meds for twenty-four hours.

Start with the recommended doses of acetaminophen (Tylenol) or the nonsteroidal anti-inflammatory drug ibuprofen (Motrin, Advil) every four hours or alternating the two every two hours if your child experiences febrile seizures or has mitochondrial disorder or another condition where fever can pose a problem. Be sure to read the label carefully. (See p. 274 for advice on giving over-the-counter medication to your child.) The doc will want you to wait a day or two to see if other symptoms develop or if the fever has come down. The point here: Look at your child, not just the thermometer, when deciding how to treat. Some kids can be playing like a sea lion puppy with a temperature of 104, while others will feel miserable at 102. So you need to use your instincts, common sense, and sleuthing skills to determine your best course of action, along with talking to your doctor.

Because their immune systems aren't mature, infants are more prone to serious infections, especially during the first three months, which is why it's important to see your doc if your newborn has a fever. But please don't assume that a baby has to have a fever for something serious to be going on; sometimes their smoke alarms have been unplugged. If your child doesn't look right or you just have a feeling something is up, it's never—repeat, *never*—wrong to call your doc. We welcome those kinds of false alarms. Mothers' instincts have saved many young lives.

FACTOID: Scary thought of the day: A science experiment showed that ice found in fast-food restaurants was actually dirtier than toilet bowl water 70 percent of the time. Now, if that's not a reason to stay away from these places, we don't know what is! Oh yes, we do: the food!

Most Unwanted:
The Scoop on Bacterial and Viral Infections

If we think about germs in everyday terms, we tend to think of the places we find them: the toilet, the kitchen sponge, the sixteen-day-old kung pao chicken that hubby buried in the back of the fridge. But the reality is that it's very hard for us to truly visualize what a germ is and what it does.

In this section, we'll be discussing the specific contagious conditions that most often affect kids. And it should be noted that we rarely see the most dangerous contagious diseases anymore thanks to vaccinations. (See our section on them starting on page 392.) Before we get to the specifics, let's take a step back to make sure you're clear on the two main categories of contagious enemies:

Bacteria: Bacteria are one-celled organisms that feed on substances in the body, and when they do, they sometimes release toxins that trigger the outward symptoms of illness. Now, there are plenty of good bacteria that live in our bodies (we actually couldn't live without them), and you can cultivate more of them by taking probiotics (see page 162). Bad bacteria can be fought with antibiotics. Most antibiotics just injure the bacteria; you need your army of white cells to finish off the bad guys.

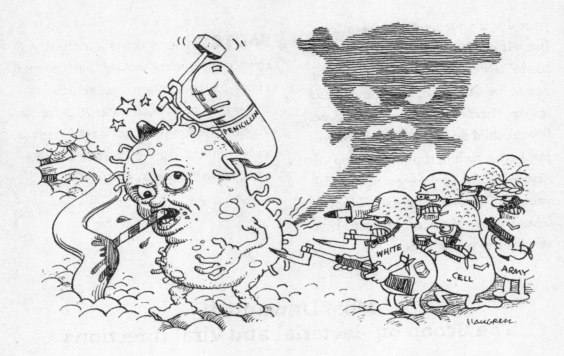

Viruses: Much smaller than bacteria, viruses are not independent organisms; they need one of your body's cells, or host cell, to reproduce, unlike bacteria, which can reproduce on their own. A virus invades a host cell, switches out the host's genetic code with its own, then uses the cell's equipment and resources to pump out lots and lots of new viruses, which go off and invade other host cells. The distinction between the two: Antibiotics are typically ineffective at killing viruses, but antiviral medications help fight some viruses by inhibiting them from either entering or exiting the host cell.

Now, let's take a spin through some of the more common infections your child might encounter. (Infections of the digestive system are discussed in chapter 5.)

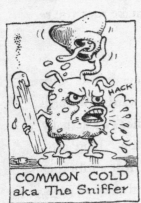

COMMON COLD
aka The Sniffer

Perp: Common Cold

AKA: The Sniffer

Weapons: Runny nose, sore throat, cough

Not surprisingly, the common cold—caused by a viral infection of the upper respiratory tract—is the most common contagious condition in the United States. Most kids get an average of three to six colds a year; double if they're in day care. Children catch colds when the cold virus (called the rhinovirus, of which there are more than one hundred different types) penetrates the lining of the nose and throat. At that point, the immune reaction kicks in, triggering all of the annoying symptoms, including a runny nose. The invaders, which prefer a moist environment, attempt to stay as long as they can in those conditions, whereas your body treats mucus like an ejection capsule to rid itself of the buggers.

Since over 90 percent of respiratory infections are viruses, using antibiotics doesn't help. While you can't cure a cold, you can help relieve some of the symptoms by making sure that your child drinks plenty of fluids to replace some of the fluids lost during the immune response. You can also make him more comfortable by giving him the recommended dose of ibuprofen or acetaminophen for pain and fever reduction. But stay away from any over-the-counter decongestant drugs or cough medicines for children under two, or combination acetaminophen-decongestant or ibuprofen-decongestant medicines for children of any age. That's for a couple of reasons: One, because there are more episodes of overdosing by well-intentioned parents than we care to count, and sometimes with serious consequences. Two, because they can induce side effects, including respiratory symptoms that may make it harder for asthmatic babies and children to breathe. Try chicken soup if Junior can tolerate it: The ingredients seem to help activate fighter cells in the immune system to make secretions less tenacious, plus soup helps with hydration.

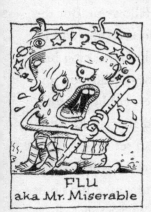

FLU
aka Mr. Miserable

Perp: Flu

AKA: Mr. Miserable

Weapons: Fever, chills, muscle aches, dizziness, sore throat, cough

If the common cold is a criminal who commits misdemeanors, then the flu is the one who commits felonies. The symptoms may be similar to that of the common cold, but they are much more severe. Caused by any number of strains of virus, the flu can make a child feel bad for up to two weeks until the virus clears the system. Again, since it's caused by a viral infection, you can't cure the flu per se, but you can make your youngster feel better by making sure that she drinks lots of fluids, rests, and takes pain relievers to reduce fever and aches. It's always worth calling the doc to talk about your child's symptoms, and call immediately or seek medical attention if the fever is running above 100.2 in children under three months or 105 degrees if older than three months.

If your child is six months or older, we recommend that she have an annual flu shot or—for kids over two who do not have asthma and are not immunocompromised due to, say, cancer chemotherapy or the HIV infection—the flu nasal mist vaccine. The flu vaccine will not only help protect her but also those around her, especially if she comes into contact with anyone in a high-risk group, such as infants, grandparents, or young asthma sufferers. Unlike other vaccines, the flu vaccine has to be repeated annually because each year brings a different strain of the virus. More on our vaccine recommendations on page 392.

In kids with asthma or kids with an impaired immune system, influenza can be life threatening, leading to bacterial pneumonia. In fact, half of all childhood deaths from influenza occur in otherwise normal, previously healthy children. The antiviral medication oseltamivir (Tamiflu), given in the first twenty-four to thirty-six hours after symptoms develop, can be a useful treatment if your child has asthma or other cause for concern. Your pediatrician can perform a twenty-four-hour test for influenza and start the medicine if your child tests positive. Now, Tamiflu has side effects, and overusing it can breed resistance to the med when your youngster really needs it, so we don't recommend that it be handed out like candy at Halloween. But the moral of the story is this: If it's flu season and your kid hasn't had the shot, and he looks like he's coming down with a cold, don't wait a few days before taking him to the doctor. In that first day, influenza testing will likely be positive already, and by thirty-six hours, you can be starting Tamiflu if necessary. When cold symptoms and fever resolve only to return, that is also a time to see the pediatrician ASAP, as that is the exact setting in which a dangerous bacterial invader can set up camp on the heels of a viral infection. If you delay, you and your asthmatic child will be stuck toughing it out with asthma meds and supportive care only. You are your child's best advocate. Don't be afraid to call the pediatrician early and often. That's what she is there for.

WHAT IS MENINGITIS?

THE CONDITION: Inflammation of the three-ply membrane around the brain and spinal cord (called the meninges).

THE KINDS: The bacterial form, which is most serious and life threatening, is rare and is caused by a number of different bacteria, while the viral form looks a lot like the flu symptomwise and is more common.

THE SYMPTOMS: They can be the same as a cold or the flu (runny nose, vomiting, fever, headache, feeling and looking sick). But a child can also experience a stiff neck, sensitivity to light, seizures, and skin rashes. In infants, it's a little harder to tell, with the main symptoms being hard-core irritability, jaundice, fever or low temperature, or a bulging fontanel (the soft spot in the skull).

THE SELF-TEST: Lay your child flat on a bed or couch or on the floor, and lift her knees up. If her head pops up too, she is instinctively trying to relieve the pressure off her meninges by curling her spine. The same thing happens if you lift her head up: Her knees will pop up, so her spine stays curled rather than extended. (The child automatically moves to relieve the pain.) This is a useful sign, but if it's not there, your child still could have meningitis. Use your parental instinct here. If the kid just does not look right, call your doc.

THE TREATMENT: Viral meningitis resolves itself within a week or ten days with no treatment or complications, but bacterial meningitis needs immediate attention. A doc who suspects meningitis will order blood tests and a spinal tap to collect spinal fluid; that will determine whether a virus or bacteria is the root cause. If it's bacterial meningitis, the doc will start IV antibiotics right away to help prevent any of the serious complications associated with the disease, such as brain damage or hearing loss.

THE PREVENTION: All forms of meningitis are contagious, so it's crucial to follow our infection-prevention steps throughout the chapter, and please see our vaccine recommendations on page 392.

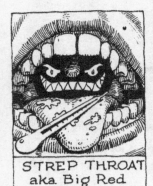

STREP THROAT
aka Big Red

Perp: Strep Throat

AKA: Big Red

Weapons: Blazing red throat (perhaps with pus and white patches), headache, fever, general discomfort

Even if you're not a doc, you can get an inkling of the difference between strep throat and a sore throat just by taking a quick peek into your child's mouth. Strep throat—a bacterial infection caused by the streptococcus bacterium—is typically diagnosed by a red throat with or without pus. Moms and docs also tend to note a distinctive odor—"strep breath"—that smells different (and worse) than when Junior has a cold. If the sore throat is present without nasal dripping, then it's most likely strep and not a cold or other infection. Your child may feel a little more lethargic, have a fever, and even stomach pain, or none of the above.

If you suspect strep, you'll want to have your child's throat swabbed and the cells cultured to ID whether the bacteria are present. This laboratory test, the gold standard, takes twenty-four hours to confirm the presence of the virus, but many docs do a preliminary rapid antibody test (or rapid test) that recognizes strep, and takes only five minutes. If the rapid test is positive, your doc will prescribe antibiotics to fight the infection. If it's negative, she will still order a throat culture or a DNA probe (a more specific test) to definitively rule out strep throat. The results usually come back the next day.

If either test is positive and you have, say, a major family event coming up, you may ask the doc for a shot of antibiotics, rather than the usual ten-day oral course.* The injectable penicillin can help your child feel relief within as little as twelve hours. Many of us remember the days when, if you had strep, down came the pants, in went the shot, and you were back to school in two days feeling *much* better. While less cost effective and more tear producing than antibiotics, it is still always an option in your pediatrician's office—with the added benefit of reducing the risk of

---

* Azithromycin (Zithromax) is a three-day or five-day course, but it's not recommended for strep unless the child is allergic to everything else.

WHAT'S THE DIFFERENCE BETWEEN . . .

Strep and a cold?	Strep is more likely if a child has a raw throat and difficulty swallowing minus the drippiness. A cold causes a drippy nose and throat. Also, strep rarely hits a child under one year old, while a baby can get a cold or flu in the first few months of life.
Strep and mono?	Strep and mono (infectious mononucleosis) can go together, but the mono test will not turn positive until a week after symptoms begin. So if she has a raw, red throat, get the throat culture. A raw, red throat with golf-ball size tonsils, tiredness, and it's not going away after a week? Check for mono.

contagion in the household. If you choose the oral option instead, you need to ensure that your child takes all ten days of the medicine to clear the infection—even if she feels like a million bucks after three days. Failing to do so will make the bacteria "smarter" and harder to eliminate or encourage the development of rheumatic fever (see below). If you don't think you'll be able to get your child to take the full course, opt for the shot.

If your kid is getting more than five or six strep infections a year, it's worth a visit to the ear, nose, and throat doc, or pediatric otolaryngologist, to see if she needs to have her tonsils taken out, as they may be hiding grounds for the little strep buggers. Evidence suggests that removing the tonsils doesn't always fix the problem unless there is a pocket of pus, or abscess, chronically living there, but this is a good reason to talk further with your pediatrician about options. Although untreated strep is highly transmissible, once your child has been on antibiotics for twenty-four hours, she's no longer contagious and can return to school or day care.

Now, if you simply can't get your child to the doctor, and five or more days go by, he will likely clear the offending agent on his own. But in the process of getting rid of that strep, your child's immune system can empower a permanent defense battalion known as antistreptolysin antibodies, or ASOs, that can then attack other parts of his body. These antibodies can cause rheumatic fever, which can permanently damage heart valves and requires monthly shots of penicillin to control. So, when in doubt, get the strep test within the first three days, so as to avoid activating the whole squad and setting up the permanent perimeter guard.

Scarlet fever just means strep with a rash. Scarlet fever used to be associated with more drama—and more childhood deaths—in the days before penicillin. Now it is an easily treatable problem, like any strep, and simply requires a penicillin shot or the ten-day course of oral antibiotics (remember, no missed doses, please!). More on scarlet fever on page 230.

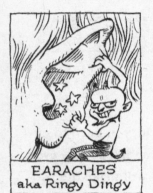

EARACHES
aka Ringy Dingy

Perp: Earaches
AKA: Ringy Dingy
Weapons: Painful ears (look for ear tugging), fever

The reason why kids tend to get a lot of earaches has nothing to do with how loudly they're watching those goofy Wiggles, but with their aural anatomy. In the first year of life, a child's ear canal (the tubes that connect the nasal passages to the middle ear) are narrow and almost horizontal, without much of a downward slope. So? Well, that means that fluid behind the eardrum has less of a chance of having gravity drain it out. Add that to the fact that babies tend to spend

IS IT SWIMMER'S EAR OR AN EAR INFECTION?

If your child's ear hurts, tug on the earlobe on the painful side. If a gentle tug elicits an "ouch," it is likely swimmer's ear (called otitis externa), and it's worth seeing the doctor for antibiotic eardrops. Your child should stay out of the water for the next five days. Inner ear infections hurt more on the inside; he'll likely have a fever and feel lousy. See your doc.

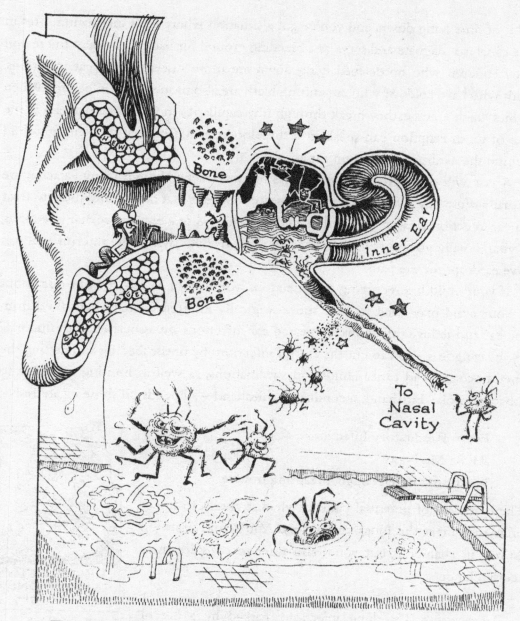

Figure 6.2 **Ear Ye** When docs look into your child's ear, they can look at the thin membrane between the bones and wax in the inner ear. In children, the thin and flexible eustachian tube between the inner ear and nasal cavity often collapses and fails to drain an infected ear. This is also why kids have more trouble in airplanes.

a lot of time lying down, and you've got a situation where fluid that accumulates in the canal can stagnate and serve as a breeding ground for bacteria. It's also the reason why children who bottle-feed lying down are more susceptible to ear infections. Kids who have colds or who are cutting teeth are also prone to ear infections. When babies' teeth emerge, they break through tiny capillaries in the gums. Bacteria at the site of tooth eruption can sneak into the bloodstream, find that nice yummy fluid behind the eardrum, and set up camp.

A doc will often prescribe antibiotics for an earache, though many earaches are actually caused by a virus. And recent research suggests that taking antibiotics to treat an ear infection is associated with a higher likelihood of a recurrence. Ear infections, if viral, usually go away by themselves in three to five days. In the interim, you can give eardrops for the pain.

If your child has recurring ear infections, you'll want to talk to your doc about it. Your child may need to have tubes surgically inserted to help drain fluid from the ear and reduce infections. Repeated ear infections are associated with fluctuating hearing loss. You can cut the risk of infections by breast feeding and getting the pneumococcal and other childhood vaccinations, as well as limiting exposure to tobacco smoke. Firsthand, secondhand, thirdhand—all hands off those cigarettes!

Perp: Respiratory Infections
AKA: Mr. Nasty
Weapons: Fever, cough, breathing trouble

There are lots of potential culprits when it comes to infections that affect the lungs and airways. You'll find more on asthma in chapter 7, but you'll also want to consider these acute offenders:

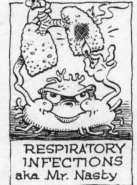

RESPIRATORY
INFECTIONS
aka Mr. Nasty

◌ *Pneumonia.* This lung infection, marked by a big ol' cough and fever, can be viral or bacterial, and it makes kids feel like they've been walloped by a ten-pound boxing glove over and over and over. Bacterial pneumonias typically cause children to get sick suddenly (and they usually follow a bout of strep), whereas kids who get viral pneumonia tend to slide into it more gradually. And here's one symptom you may not recognize: Abdominal pain or neck pain can be a sign of pneumonia because of referred pain from above the diaphragm toward the bottom or top of the lungs. Most cases of viral pneumonia resolve themselves within two weeks, but oral antibiotics should be prescribed when a bacterial one is suspected. To help relieve chest pain, a warm pad on the area of discomfort may help. A regular vaccination schedule can help prevent some cases. (More on vaccines on page 392.)

⊃ *Croup.* This is a viral infection that narrows the airways (into the shape of a church steeple) and comes with a cough that sounds scarier than it actually is. At about the time that inflammation of the airways occurs, your child will develop a seal-like, barky cough. A runny nose may be the first sign, and the cough usually sounds worse at night. When you hear this, put him in the bathroom, turn the shower on steamy, and let him breathe in the steam. (Neither of you has to be in the shower.) After twenty minutes or so, take him out back for a minute or two; the cold air hitting his lubricated lungs will further decrease inflammation. Next, back into the shower steam for twenty minutes, then back outside, back and forth, until he can breathe again without coughing so hard that he throws up. Yes, that happens, but it's not dangerous as long as he's upright.

⊃ *Epiglottitis.* This whopping bacterial infection comes out firing all guns. You'll have a very sick-looking kid with a high fever sitting forward in what we call tripod position—leaning forward with his body, both hands leaning on a table or bed in front of him—looking anxious because somehow, intuitively, he knows his airway might close at any second. This happens when the epiglottis, the part of the throat that closes when you swallow so food doesn't get into your lungs, becomes infected. If he looks like this, get him to a pediatric emergency room immediately. Epiglottitis is life threatening, which is why we strongly recommend the Hib (*Haemophilus influenzae* type b) vaccine, which protects against its most severe varieties.

Besides these common infections, there are many other intruders that can make your child sick. The fact of the matter is that unless you want to hole your child up in

THE HARM IN HOSPITALS

Though we don't wish it on anyone, chances are that every parent will while away at least some time in an ER. Doesn't matter if you're there to check out a fever or a suspected broken bone, the hospital can be one of the worst places for getting an infection. (Hospital-acquired infections are called nosocomial infections.) While you may not be able to prevent all of them, you can still take precautions by carrying hand sanitizer and keeping a stash of toys and books in your car for your kids. It's also imperative that you be vigilant in making sure that hospital staff wash their hands before seeing your child—even if they're wearing gloves. The fact is that latex gloves can harbor even more germs than bare hands; also, rings on fingers can harbor extra bacteria, as the germs get trapped between the jewelry and the skin. So a fresh wash is a must for anyone checking out your child.

solitary confinement forever, he's going to get sick every once in a while. Your goal, besides helping soothe him and doing what you can to speed his recovery, is to help prevent as many illnesses as you can. Our tips below can act as your defense plan.

YOU TIPS

Get Her in the Habit. We recently spent a whole chapter talking about instilling healthy habits in your kids. There's one we'd like to repeat here: Wash hands, wash hands, wash hands (with baby wipes or Purell if there's no sink in sight). Coming in from outside, after riding a bus, before dinner, after the bathroom, after playdates, and anytime that your kid will have a lot of interaction with others. We don't want you to become a germaphobe, because there is some value to building up immunity by being exposed to the outside environment. But the easiest way for unwanted germs to pass from one person to another is through touch: Germ lands on your kid's hand (via high-five, sneeze, and so on), she then uses it to rub her eyes, feel her mouth, or (gasp!!) pick her nose. Voila!* Instant transmission. But if you can get her in the habit of killing those germs with soap and water or antibacterial gel, you'll minimize the chance that she'll catch something nobody wants her to catch.

Use the Sleeve. Bet you didn't know that the contents of a sneeze travel at roughly ninety-five miles per hour.† That's what we call high-speed snot. While most people use their hands to cover the contents, that doesn't help a whole lot in decreasing germ transmission if said sneezer goes on to touch Bubby's chubby cheeks a few minutes later. Please, for all of our sakes, teach your child to use the crook of his elbow to cover his nose and mouth when he coughs or sneezes. Instruct him to throw out tissues—and immediately wash his hands!—rather than stuffing them in a pocket to be reused later, because germs will stay on tissues for two to six hours. In this case, we'd prefer that your youngster not save a tree in order to stop germs from spreading.

Go Ahead and Treat. While a fever itself isn't necessarily dangerous, treating it is worthwhile if it helps your child feel better. First check our guidelines for when to call the doc (page 173)

---

* That'll be the last time we use two interjections that close together. Promise.

† And if you did know that, then may we recommend that you find a hobby, because you're spending entirely too much time on Wikipedia.

FACTOID: There's some preliminary evidence that probiotics—good bacteria that coat the GI tract—are not only beneficial for children's digestive systems but can also reduce the incidence of cold and flu symptoms by more than 65 percent. Get them in the spore form, which come in pills that you can mix with formula or baby food, rather than in live culture. The live culture (yogurt-based ones, generally) does not survive the acid in the stomach very well. Also, the protein in yogurt is not well handled by the intestines of children under one; it can punch holes in the intestines if given in more than a few spoonfuls.

and if it's okay, then go ahead and try to bring the fever down with acetaminophen or ibuprofen (use the dosing on the boxes, according to weight—see page 272). One caution: Do not overdo it in the hope of speeding up the process or because you want to see a dramatic change fast. At high doses, both types of fever reducers/pain relievers can accumulate in the blood and cause liver damage. Do not give aspirin to children unless instructed by your doc, for it has been linked to a rare but fatal disease of the liver and brain called Reye syndrome.

Bring Your Own Toys. To the doc's office. To the airport. To any place where a lot of germs may be passed from one kid to another via plastic object. If you're in a place where you have to wait a long time, you should expect that your kid won't be able to do the same. If you bring your own stuff, then you reduce the chances that he'll pick up germs brought there from other children. And ask your child—just this once—*not* to share his toys. You can also wait outside the doctor's office and have the receptionist call you when they are ready to bring your child into a room. Most of the other children at the doctor's office are sick. If your child is also sick, he's more susceptible to pick up pinkeye from the other kid he's playing with in the waiting room.

Use the Rule of Two. We have pediatrician colleagues who like to use this rule to determine whether or not they would call a doc for their own children's sickness. If a child has one symptom, it may be something you can wait out. But if there are two or more things going on, it's usually worth a call. So if a child throws up just once but is acting normally otherwise, you might wait to see how she does. Or if a child has a fever with no other symptoms, you can try acetaminophen or ibuprofen. But if a child has a fever and belly pain, or has a fever and a headache, or throws up and feels lethargic, then it's a good idea to call the doc. Of course, please know that we're not discouraging you from calling your doc. Anytime you feel like you need to, make the call. Another good idea is that if your doctor's office is closed on Saturday and it is Friday afternoon at four o'clock and you're unsure if your child is "sick enough" to call the doctor, err on the side of overcautious and make the call. Sitting in the urgent care clinic on Saturday morning with the other sickies is never a fun way to spend the weekend.

Use the DIY Model. For years, many people have used do-it-yourself remedies to help lower fevers and improve immune defense systems. Here are a few that certainly won't hurt your child and might (repeat, *might*) just help:

- The Wet Socks Treatment. The theory behind this is that if you put wet socks on kids with fevers, their bodies will work to raise their internal heat to warm their feet and thus allow their immune system to kick in. You can also put a cool, wet towel on large surface areas of the body, like the belly. But do not do supercold temps: That causes the baby to shiver and raise the temperature more than is helpful to fight infection, as shivering generates unneeded heat.

- Fluids. Drinking lots of cool fluids can lower body temp and help replace any fluid lost during an illness.

- A lukewarm bath.

- Apple cider vinegar. Apply the vinegar mixed with water to the baby's feet. It seems to help reduce fever because the acid helps draw heat out of the skin. Why on the feet? Because our feet contain a higher concentration of sweat glands than the rest of our bodies, aiding in the release of heat.

Get a D. In a few years, you won't like it too much if your child brings home a D, but now is a good time to be thinking about D in the vitamin form. Vitamin D_3 protects against infections, and it seems to be one of the nutrients lacking in breast milk. You can make sure that your baby gets adequate amounts by giving her 1 milligram daily of a liquid baby multivitamin like Poly-Vi-Sol up to age two, and then change to a chewable multivitamin after that. Always take the proper amount listed. Just because a little is good doesn't mean that a lot is better; for instance, fat-soluble vitamins A and E are dangerous in high doses.

Be on the Lookout. When you're traveling, you can take precautions to help protect your babe against easy-to-transmit germs found in confined spaces. For instance, if you're flying, drape a loose blanket over your baby's mouth and nose, so that spew from a selfish sneezer doesn't wind up on her face. And turn off the air nozzle above her head, so that everyone else's breath doesn't get blown back onto her. Also, it's not a bad idea to carry a travel-sized container of disinfectant or baby wipes that you can use to wipe down remote controls and other things that your child may play with in hotel rooms.

Finish the Job. If your doc prescribes your child antibiotics or other infection-fighting meds, it's imperative that you finish the dose and not stop early—even if symptoms subside. Stopping early or taking the wrong amount can help the little buggers develop resistance and avoid treatment next time.

YOU TOOL

TAKE A TEMPERATURE

If this is your first child, the last temperature you have taken is probably that of the turkey on Thanksgiving. While the principle is the same (stick it in and read the number), the process is a little more delicate than the flesh puncturing that goes on with the ol' Butterball. Here's how:

Rectal Temps: Use the thermometer with the short, round bulb, which has less of a chance of breaking than the oral thermometer with the long, skinny bulb. Carefully, shake it and make sure that it reads under 96 degrees Fahrenheit or 35 degrees centigrade. (No need to shake a digital thermometer.) Put a little Vaseline or K-Y jelly on the bulb end, put Junior belly down on a firm surface, and hold him down so he can't crawl away. Insert the bulb about a half inch to an inch into his rectum, leaving it in for a full two minutes. *Very accurate.*

Aural (Ear) Temps: Angle the thermometer toward the eardrum, which lies at the end of the external ear canal. Gently tug on the ear to open it up. Press down and get a reading in seconds. *Fairly accurate.*

Oral Temps: We don't recommend that oral temperatures be taken until a child is six years old, when there's less of a chance that he'll bite down on the thermometer and break it. Temperatures taken under the armpit (axillary temp) or along the surface of the forehead (arterial temp) are generally not considered as accurate as other methods.

7

Reaction Time

How the Immune System Falters When It Comes to Allergies and Asthma

et a group of parents together, and chances are that they'll have different opinions on everything from stroller styles to diaper brands. But if there's one thing that all parents agree on,* it's this: We can't stand seeing our kids sick. The upside, if there is one, about many infections is that your kid's immune system (with a little help from modern medicine, in some cases) can fight them off and get Junior back to tossing balls and playing peekaboo in no time at all.

In many kids, the immune system doesn't quite perform the way it's supposed to—leading to chronic immune-related conditions, including asthma and allergies. In fact, about 30 percent of infants are affected by allergies or asthma; that's a heck of a lot of kids.

* Besides the genius of Dr. Seuss

In most cases, children can mount pretty impressive and effective military operations when it comes to handling outside invaders, as you saw in the previous chapters. Their bodies sense the invasion and respond to it, and they stop puking mashed yams relatively soon after the conflict begins. But sometimes there's going to be friendly fire, where the defense system has trouble differentiating between what is foreign and what is friendly, and attacks itself.

FACTOID: Eating local honey—the unpasteurized kind—may help decrease the symptoms of seasonal allergies related to local plants. Like allergy shots, this low-level exposure to local allergens can stimulate the immune system to produce antibodies. Note: Never feed a child under one year of age honey because it may contain botulism spores, which produce toxins that cause a potentially lethal reaction.

A child's immune system is a delicate one, especially as it transitions from including Mom's immune cells left over from the time in utero to being populated solely by its own cells. As you can imagine, it is susceptible to malfunctions that can throw off the entire system. While allergies and asthma can be big problems in and of themselves, the deeper issue—and danger—with any immune errors is this: If your immune system is busy battling things that aren't real threats, like Fluffy's fur, it won't be prepared to attack things that might turn out to be real threats. In this chapter, you'll learn how and why these aberrant immune reactions occur, and how to manage the situation if they do.

Why Ask Why?
The Evolution of Allergies

Talk to anyone who's been around for a few generations about allergies and asthma, and there's a good chance that she'll have a similar observation to the rest of us. "I don't remember this many children having allergy problems back when I was a kid. We played in the dirt, we bathed in pollen, we pet the neighbor's dog, and never sneezed a bit." In fact, there is quite a scientific debate about why we're seeing so many allergies these days and how we developed them in the first place.

One prevailing theory about allergy development stems from a biochemical reaction that occurs when our antibodies react to invaders. Remember the troops called B cells, which shoot at invaders? The bullets they use are called immunoglobulins, or antibodies, and they're specifically designed to target particular threats. In addition to shooting antibodies, B cells also wear them on their surface. The surface antibodies associated with allergies (called IgE antibodies) stick to B cells like green on peas, supercharging them to fight invaders that may not be particularly dangerous. Like Fluffy. How did we end up with this overzealous class of antibodies? Some immunologists believe that way back in the day, a high-octane disease or infection appeared, and those of our ancestors who had IgE were able to survive it because of their powerful immune response. Those IgE antibodies have been with us ever since. The downside is that they can now react strongly to nonlethal stimuli, and that's what causes an allergic reaction.

Other common explanations for the rise in allergies include the "clean" and "dirty" hypotheses. The clean theory says this: We're so hyperfocused on staying germ free that we fail to build up a tolerance to harmless exposures. We clean, we wash, we no longer subscribe to the five-second rule. Without any significant germs to attack, our germ fighters end up overreacting when they're exposed to anything foreign, even if it's perfectly innocuous. Pollen? Dog hair? Mold? Sneeze! Cough!

Ugh! There's even some research to suggest that firstborn children have higher rates of allergies and asthma than younger kids. That seems to support the too-clean idea, if you assume that most parents are hypervigilant about cleanliness with first children and relax their standards a bit with subsequent children. (Or they just don't have the time or energy anymore to fight with their child when he wants to eat a pretzel off the ground.*)

The too-dirty premise, as you might imagine, is quite the opposite, though it has nothing to do with whether you ate a chip that fell on the floor. This theory says that our environment is contaminated with all kinds of pernicious toxins: chemicals, cigarette smoke, all the noxious gunk that's the offshoot of an industrialized society. Essentially, our world has evolved faster than our bodies can keep up with it. The result: The toxins can't be fought off effectively, and we get allergic reactions.

Interestingly, the most common allergies are not to these toxins themselves; rather, the toxins act as chemical adjuvants that stimulate the immune response when you're exposed to an allergen. The two biggest criminals: cigarette smoke and car fuel. In genetically predisposed children, exposure to an allergen (cat dander), particularly in the presence of an adjuvant (secondhand smoke), establishes an allergic sensitivity. Once sensitized, they are at risk for asthma, yet the asthma trigger (say, dust mites) may be completely different from the initial allergen to which they were exposed.

As fascinating as these theories may be (try one out the next time you're stuck in an elevator), what we're most concerned with is the scientific *process*. And that's what we're going to explore next, by walking you step by step through the allergic response so you can figure out how best to prevent and treat allergies in your child.

---

* Here's another too-clean theory about why we've seen an increase in asthma: In the 1930s, the rate of infection with *Helicobacter pylori* (the bacteria that cause stomach cancer and peptic ulcers) started declining with the introduction of antibiotics. Today fewer than 10 percent of children in industrialized countries carry *H. pylori*, as opposed to 90 percent in developing countries. *H. pylori* protects against pollen and mold allergies and reduces the incidence of asthma. Some research has shown a strong connection between antibiotic treatment of children and later development of asthma and allergies.

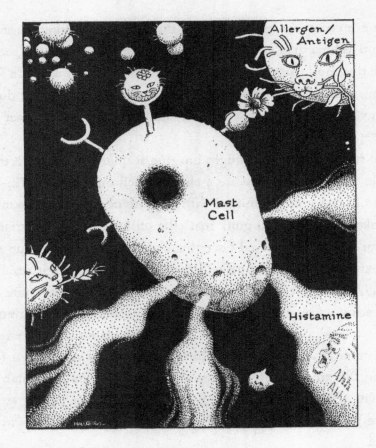

Figure 7.1 **The Act of React** Allergic symptoms—sneezing, coughing, runny eyes, or even more severe reactions—are caused when an allergen such as dust or pollen enters the body via the nose or the lungs. When that allergen interacts with mast cells, the cells release histamine, which causes the symptoms. That's why a child's nose can run faster than Usain Bolt in the 100-meter dash.

The Rebel Reaction: All About Allergies

We all have people in our lives who are prone to overreacting: bosses, spouses, impatient drivers intent on sending vertical finger messages through the air. They're the kind of people who get all hot and bothered over something that the rest of the world would simply shrug their shoulders at. Essentially, that's exactly what an allergy is: an overreaction by the immune system to some type of allergen that the body is exposed to (see Figure 7.1).

When that invader enters the body, often through the nose, the body tries to protect itself by producing those antibodies called immunoglobulin E (IgE). That sets off a chain reaction in which IgE sends a signal to allergy cells (mast cells) to release chemicals that fight the allergen. When those chemicals (some are called histamines; others belong to the cytokine system) are released into the bloodstream, they produce inflammatory reactions throughout the body, not just at the site of invasion. It's those reactions that trigger the itchy eyes, the runny nose, the hives, etc.

In cases of food allergies, a rowdy GI tract attempts to purge the body of the allergen. As you learned just a few pages ago, the immune system takes note of these invaders, and whenever it encounters them again, it defends itself the same way. Sometimes reactions become more and more severe with each exposure; in other cases, reactions diminish, and a child can "outgrow" an allergy as his immune system matures.

A hypervigilant allergic system moves from code green to code red as soon as it's exposed to certain (often innocuous) foreign substances such as dust or pollen. The immune process kicks in, the cells start attacking, and your child starts feeling the symptoms. When your child's body attacks a foreign invader, his immune cells move in to get rid of it. In the case of allergies, the cells pull out Uzis rather than BB guns to fight a minor pest. This kind of overreaction can cause a lot of damage to your child's body.

The range of allergic symptoms is wider than the Amazon River: Some people simply are annoyed by occasional sniffling, while others are at risk of developing a life-threatening reaction called anaphylaxis (see below). The degree of reaction really depends on which systems are activated in the body. Here we'll outline some of the most common allergies in children and what you can do to treat them.

Airborne Allergies. You don't have to be a linguistics scholar to figure out this category: They're allergens that are carried through the air, and they're most strongly associated with the classic allergy symptoms of watery eyes, runny nose, and throat coated with phlegm. Some of the most common:

THE SUSPECT	THE RAP SHEET	THE WHEREABOUTS
Dust mites	Microscopic insects that make up house dust and live in pillows and mattresses, where they feed on dead skin; their feces are what activates the emergency response.	Live year-round in bedding, carpets, fabric, stuffed animals.
Pollen	Gets into the air when trees, flowers, weeds, and grasses release it to fertilize other plants.	Seasonal; depends on pollination times in your geographic area.
Mold	Fungi that live in warm, moist, dark environments.	Can be year-round and found in musty places like damp basements and piles of rotting leaves.
Dander	When a pet licks itself and the saliva dries, protein particles called dander become airborne.	Anywhere that warm-blooded animals or household pets live.

Food Allergies. With as much attention as food allergies are getting these days, it shouldn't be a surprise that nearly 10 percent of all kids are affected by them. The eight most common foods that cause allergic reactions in kids are: eggs, fish, milk, peanuts, shellfish, soy, tree nuts, and wheat.

While it may seem easier to handle food allergies than, say, airborne allergies that are out of your control (just avoid the food, right?), the issue is a bit more complicated than that. Eggs, milk, wheat, and soy are on the ingredient lists of so many foods. What's more, many allergens come hidden in prepared foods, making them much more difficult to monitor. While manufacturers have gotten much better about identifying potential allergens and letting consumers know when food may have been exposed to an allergen in the factory, restaurants are a different story. Accidental contamination can occur if the food your child is allergic to was cooked in the same pan or flipped by the same spatula used to prepare your child's food.

While food allergies can cause a range of allergic reactions (skin rashes are a frequent symptom—see chapter 8), we're most concerned with anaphylaxis. (See details on page 202.) Peanuts can cause one of the most severe reactions. (Please see our sidebar about the increase of peanut allergies on page 203.) In some cases, children outgrow food allergies; for example, most outgrow egg allergies by age two. If you suspect that your child has outgrown a food allergy, reintroduce the food incrementally under the supervision of a pediatric allergist.

Other Common Allergies. You now understand enough about the immune system to know that virtually anything foreign that comes in contact with your child's body can be an allergen. That includes things like insect stings (the allergy is to the venom, not the actual stinger); poison oak, ivy, and sumac; medicine; latex; and various chemicals, such as ones commonly found in popular laundry detergents.

Catching the Suspect:
Allergy Diagnosis and Treatment

In kids, it can be especially tough to catch the allergy perp. First, young ones can't always explain what's bothering them. Second, many of the symptoms mimic cold symptoms. Third, it's often hard for parents to make the connection between a possible trigger (like a food) and a reaction that may not come immediately afterward or may be in a remote location (like diaper rash). So the key for parents who suspect an allergy is to find patterns linking exposure to symptoms. There's no cure for allergies, but a doc can help you pinpoint triggers and suggest solutions to relieve the severity of symptoms.

To help you navigate this often tricky world, here's a cheat sheet for diagnosing and treating many types of allergies in kids. (We'll detail contact allergies in the next chapter, where we talk about skin.)

Symptoms. For airborne allergies, symptoms include sneezing, itchy nose/throat, nasal congestion, coughing, and watery, red eyes. For food allergies, symptoms depend on several factors, including how much the child ate or was exposed to, as well as her sensitivity to the food. Symptoms include hives (raised, red, itchy bumps on the skin), itchy mouth and throat when the food is swallowed, rash, runny/itchy nose, weight gain from swelling in the bowel, abdominal cramps with nausea/diarrhea, and the life-threatening ones—difficulty breathing, and shock.

Diagnosis. If you suspect that your child has allergies, contact your doc, who may refer you to a pediatric allergist to ID them and select the best course of treatment. Two of the ways that docs will try to determine if your child has allergies:

> **Skin Test:** These tests can be performed in infants, but the results are typically more reliable in kids over two. There are two techniques: One, a drop of a liquid containing the suspected allergen is dropped onto the skin. The doc then pricks the area. If the skin turns red and blotchy, that indicates the possible

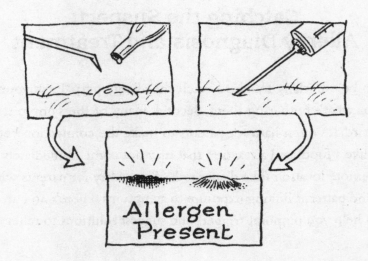

Allergen Present

presence of an allergy. (Note the word possible. Many skin tests yield false positives.) Two, a small amount of the allergen is injected under the skin (comes with a small sting). If a lump appears at the site of the injection, the child is judged to have tested positive for the allergen, and the bigger the lump, the stronger the liability.

RAST Test:* This blood test can detect allergies by testing for markers of eosinophils, a type of white blood cell. An increase in eosinophils indicates an allergic reaction. While this blood test is an accurate gauge of the presence of allergies, a skin test is commonly used in children over two because it's less expensive for surveying a range of potential allergens than performing a blood test for each one.

Treatment. We wish there were treatments that would magically cure all allergies, but as you know now, the immune system is complex and nuanced, meaning that there's no simple solution to erasing allergies. The best line of treatment is preventing exposure to allergens; you'll find preventive guidelines in our YOU Tips. It's also important to recognize signs early on because quick treatment can improve the condition. Elimination is a reasonable course of action for, say, food allergies, but it's hard to avoid airborne allergies unless you live in a plastic bubble. So the next best strategy is to relieve symptoms to help make your child more comfortable when she is exposed. Some options:

Medications. Depending on a number of factors, you have several choices, including:

⊃ Diphenhydramine (Benadryl), an antihistamine, which reduces itching, swelling, and hives. It is a first-line treatment in acute allergic reactions (anaphylaxis). Dose according to the box or your doc's instructions.

⊃ Other antihistamines (Claritin, Allegra, Zyrtec) for chronic seasonal allergies.

* RAST stands for radioallergosorbent test, in case you're curious.

⊃ Nasal steroids, which help stabilize the body's allergy cells (mast cells, the ones that release histamine) to decrease symptoms associated with allergic reactions.

⊃ Topical antihistamines such as hydrocortisone cream to decrease itching and swelling. We suggest avoiding topical creams such as Caladryl or Benadryl gel, as the Benadryl component in each can easily get overdosed if you apply them too generously to the skin. It is safer to use Calamine lotion, oatmeal baths, and hydrocortisone cream.

Allergy Shots. In some cases, a doc may recommend that your child get allergy shots. These are usually given if she is just miserable with allergic symptoms and the doc needs to find some way to improve the quality of her day-to-day life. The way it works is that your child will be given a very small amount of the allergen over a period of time, to help her body learn to tolerate the exposure. Allergy shots are not typically given to kids under five. They can be a positive life changer for a subset of kids.

Anaphylaxis. Children with severe allergies can develop a sudden, life-threatening reaction to an allergen called anaphylaxis. The most common triggers are peanuts and bee stings. Anaphylaxis involves many different systems of the body, but, most severely, it causes airways to close and fluid to leak out of the bloodstream into the tissues of the body (it's like drowning). Those suffering this type of reaction need immediate medical attention in the form of a shot of epinephrine (adrenaline) to help open the airways and stop the leakage of fluid. While some reactions happen immediately, anaphylaxis can also occur up to two hours after being exposed to an allergen.

HOLD THE NUTS

More and more, we're hearing about kids who have severe allergies to peanuts. They don't even have to eat them to have a severe, anaphylactic reaction. They can be in the same room with them or they can touch someone who's had them. Research shows that the number of kids with peanut allergies has doubled over the last few years. It's not exactly clear why, but these are some theories:

- ⊃ Peanuts contain proteins not found in other foods, and they're proteins that trigger very strong reactions from the immune system.

- ⊃ Roasting nuts changes the protein, intensifying the reaction. (Peanut allergy rates are much lower in China, where they tend to boil nuts rather than roast them.)

- ⊃ Processed or genetically modified foods are irritating the delicate lining of infants' GI systems, making them more susceptible to allergies.

- ⊃ We're exposing babies to peanut products hidden in nonfood items such as skin creams and lotions.

It's important to note that anaphylaxis doesn't typically happen in children under age one, although it can, and severe reactions in those under one usually manifest in the form of red rashes. The reason: Young children's immune systems aren't fully developed, so they can't muster the heavy artillery needed to cause such severe inflammation.

Symptoms: Difficulty breathing (ragged, raspy, gaspy breaths), air hunger (low oxygen due to fluid in the lungs); fast heart rate; swelling of the face, throat, and lips; dizziness, light-headedness; hives, often in a ring around the neck; tightness of throat; sudden drop in blood pressure.

⊃ Emulsifiers and other ingredients added to peanuts to make common forms of peanut butter increase the potential for allergic reactions. Kids who grow up in countries where peanuts are boiled and pure peanut butter—made from just peanuts—is used, develop much fewer allergies at a much lower rate.

If your child does have peanut allergies, you already know to follow our advice about vigilance on page 209. But if you are looking to help prevent future children from developing severe peanut allergies, you may be wondering whether avoiding peanuts during pregnancy can help. If you have a strong family history of food allergies, you might consider it; otherwise, eating peanuts during pregnancy doesn't seem to have any effect on children's nut allergies. Once Baby is born, we recommend that you avoid eating foods that she is more likely to be allergic to based on family history and that you do not introduce solid foods until the baby is four months old, as there is some evidence to suggest an increased risk of allergies for kids who eat solid foods in the first four months. And if you have a strong family history of any kind of allergy, we recommend that you avoid giving your child peanut butter and peanut products until after the age of two. That includes avoiding peanuts until after your baby has finished breast feeding; weak but consistent evidence relates moms who eat peanuts and breast-feed to peanut allergies in their children.

Treatment: If your child experiences an anaphylactic reaction, your doc will prescribe injectable epinephrine, which comes in an EpiPen spring-loaded syringe. Upon the onset of a severe reaction, a parent or caregiver injects epi into the child's thigh, and the surge of adrenaline helps ease the allergic reaction by opening arteries and airways and stopping leakage of fluid out of blood vessels in response to the swelling that the inflammation has caused. It's important that parents, teachers, and caregivers of children with severe allergies be trained to give these shots, and that parents make sure that EpiPens are readily accessible at school, day care, in the car, at Grandma's house, in Mom's purse, and everywhere the child is. If it's the first time, before you have EpiPen on hand, call 911 and get to the ER.

Deep Breaths:
The Biology of Asthma

You might think that the only reason that we put asthma in the allergy chapter is because of their first-letter similarity. But if that were the case, you'd also be reading about such kid topics as appendicitis, ADD, and aversion to vegetables. The real reason, of course, is that they share biological similarities: Asthma is a form of an allergic reaction, one that's characterized by breathing difficulties. Now, that doesn't mean that all kids with allergies have asthma or that all kids with asthma have allergies, but there is some overlap.

Recently, we've seen quite an increase in asthma among kids. It's very common in inner cities, where people are exposed to pollution and cockroaches, but much lower in kids raised on farms (possibly because of a protective effect from being exposed to various toxins from animals). Considering that up to 15 percent of kids develop asthma at some point in their childhoods, it's important to learn about the condition, which means a crash course in the structure and function of the lungs.

To start, picture your respiratory system as an upside-down tree (see Figure 7.2). When you breathe in, air goes down the trachea (windpipe): the trunk of the tree that funnels the air into your lungs. Quickly, the trachea divides into two main pathways—the bronchi—which go to your right and left lungs, respectively. These in turn branch out into thousands of tiny tubes called bronchioles.

At the end of each bronchiole are tiny sacs called alveoli, each one of them lined with a thin layer of fluid that keeps each alveolus open. Alveoli, the primary gas-exchange units of the lungs, are surrounded by networks of tiny capillaries. Oxygen from fresh air diffuses through the thin walls of the alveoli into the bloodstream, while carbon dioxide diffuses out of the capillaries into the alveoli for expulsion from the body. The lungs and surrounding structures have several mechanisms to help you breathe clearly and easily. For one, the trachea is lined with millions of tiny hairs called cilia that trap any gunk you might have breathed in. You need such filters. After all, the lungs are one of the few places in your body that interact directly with the outside world—and are directly exposed to toxins from the environment.

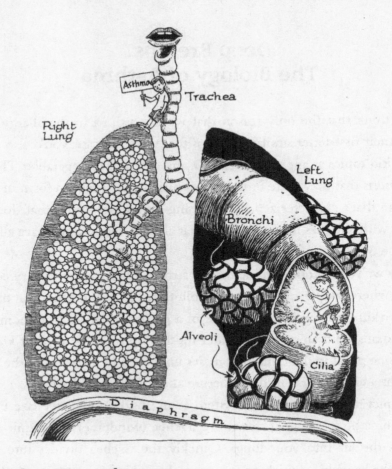

Figure 7.2 **Baby's Breath** The lungs are shaped like upside-down trees with one big trunk breaking off into many branches. Contraction of the diaphragm at the bottom of the lungs helps the breathing motions, and the cilia are tiny hairs that help clean out unwanted particles. Asthmatic reactions—the closing of airways—happen because of a process that's similar to an allergic response.

For another, the diaphragm, a large, dome-shaped muscle at the bottom of the chest cavity, helps you draw air in by pulling down on your lungs and opening up the pathways, and helps you exhale by pushing up on your lungs and squeezing air out through your nose and mouth.

In a perfect world, that system works beautifully. The diaphragm contracts, the lungs open up, we breathe in; the diaphragm relaxes, the lungs compress, we breathe out—all without a second thought. But for kids with asthma, that natural response is far from guaranteed. Here's what happens:

When exposed to some kind of trigger (like smoke, pets, even cold air or exercise), an immune response causes the membranes that line the small airways in the child's lungs to become inflamed and swollen. This narrowing of the airways makes it difficult to breathe. To make matters worse, a child who can't breathe begins to panic, and that releases stress hormones, exacerbating the problem.

The next thing you know, the child is coughing his head off. (Wheezing is more of a sign of asthma in adults; kids with asthma tend to cough.) To treat pediatric asthma, docs may prescribe various medications, including inhaled steroids to open up the airways. These are safe and do not interfere with growth. A physician may also prescribe anti-inflammatory meds to help control inflammation. Short-term bronchodilators to open the airways can give quick relief, but if your child needs to use these three or more times a week, it's a good bet that she needs to be prescribed preventive medicine. In addition to the acute risks of asthma attacks, the disease is also associated with many health risks later in life, such as obesity, high blood pressure, high blood sugar, and heart disease. Hence, the need to get it under control now. Use the following guidelines to help you ID it in your child. At first sign, it's smart to keep a diary of symptoms and possible triggers to see if you and your doc can determine patterns.

In the case of either asthma or allergies, the key is to be on the lookout for behaviors and symptoms that give you clues as to whether your child might be experiencing some kind of inappropriate immune reactions. Below you'll find some preventive tips, as well as ideas that will help a child with allergies or asthma best manage his or her life.

ASTHMA

RISKS	SYMPTOMS	TRIGGERS
• Family history of asthma and allergy	• High-pitched cough and wheezing	• Sinusitis
• Early viral respiratory infection in baby	• Chest wall sucks in with each breath (called retractions)	• Exercise
• Mom smokes (including during pregnancy), or other people in the house smoke	• Grunting at end of each inhalation (this is the body's way of keeping air in the smallest airways so they don't collapse)	• Dust
• Premature delivery		• Smoke
• Mom under twenty at the time of delivery	• Nasal flaring	• Change in weather
• Obesity	• Chest pain and/or tightness	• Viral infection
• Acetaminophen use either by mom during pregnancy or by child under the age of 1	• Fast breathing	• Pets
		• Cockroaches
		• Mice

YOU TIPS

Let Them Eat Dirt. No, not as a meal and not by the bucket load. The point here is that it's better for your children to get messy, get dirty, and come in contact with the natural world than it is for them to grow up in an ultrasterile environment where you scrub every surface with disinfectant. The reason: You need to allow their immune armies to get their basic training. If they don't have an opportunity to practice fighting, then they'll be trigger happy when they encounter a minor intruder. So while we certainly recommend that you be vigilant when it comes to hand washing to protect against those viruses and bacteria that can get passed from kid to kid and from hand to mouth, remember that there's an absolute biological advantage to exposing your kid to all kinds of things in the natural world, including dirt. Note the difference between dirt (organic, such as what's found on a farm) and filth (city grime).

Reduce Exposure. As we said, you can't cure allergies or asthma, but you can minimize the damage by trying to reduce your child's exposure to triggers. Some tactics you can take:

- ⊃ Keep the floor in your child's room uncarpeted, because bare floors don't trap allergens as much as rugs and carpets. Even better, do the same for the whole house.

- ⊃ Use light drapes that you can wash regularly instead of heavy ones, which can trap dust. Even better, install blinds and wipe them down frequently.

- ⊃ Use special 1 micron or latex covers for all pillows and mattresses to keep dust mites from sneaking onto your child. Commonly sold as "hypoallergenic dust mite protectors," they should zip closed, not just wrap or stretch around like a fitted sheet.

- ⊃ After your child plays outside, change her clothes, because they may have picked up pollen. And have her take a shower or bath at the end of a good day of play outside, to minimize exposure to poison ivy and other contact allergens (not to mention ticks: see chapter 8).

➲ If your child is waking up with allergic symptoms, it could be the stuff inside his pillow, either the feathers or the mite poop. Switch from feather to foam and seal with a one micron pillowcase to see if his symptoms improve.

Be Assertive. If your child has a severe peanut allergy or other serious allergy, you will have to be his strongest advocate everywhere he goes—clearly communicating *in writing* the seriousness of the allergy and how to handle it, including prevention, an action plan in case of exposure, and emergency numbers. Many other parents will try to help, some will be aloof, and some will underestimate the severity of the problem, so make no assumptions about what other people know and don't know about allergies. Be clear about the risks and about the parameters: for example, that your child will get reactions even if the peanuts are anywhere in the room. As your child gets older, she'll learn what she can and can't have, but at this stage it takes hypervigilance on your part to educate everyone else around her. Clear up some of the most common rookie mistakes that adults make: like making a sandwich with the same knife that was used to spread peanut butter, or sharing foods that don't overtly contain any peanuts but may have been made with peanut oil. We recommend that you check with the manufacturer of all foods your child eats to make sure that their production lines are nut free. Interesting note: A lot of locally made products are manufactured at small facilities where different food companies rent time, so you don't know whether another food company may have contaminated the equipment. Often, the large national brands are the most reliable.

Get Your Pets First. In an ideal world, you'll want to have the pets before the kids. Why? That way, your newborn will be exposed to the animal's allergens from the get-go, so his immune system will learn how to handle them and thus reduce risk of allergy. If you have a family history of pet allergies, you may have to choose not to have any furry pets at all (fish are nice . . .), or do some research on dogs to find some of the less allergenic breeds, such as poodles and Labradoodles.

Watch the Eggs. We recommend that you avoid giving egg whites to children until they're at least one year old, because exposure to the whites may induce an allergy. A hard-boiled egg yolk is okay after six months of age. By the way, kids typically outgrow egg allergies by age two.

Change Up When Necessary. Since many kids are allergic to the protein in cow's milk, you need to watch out for symptoms that may indicate such an allergy in babies. The symptoms may include bloody or mucousy stools, irritability, and the baby drawing her knees up to her abdomen from cramping. If that's the case, and you are feeding with formula, you can switch to a nonallergenic brand, and the symptoms will usually resolve within a few days. And if you're breast-feeding, you may need to experiment with your own diet. Eliminating milk protein from *your* diet often will do the trick. Children often outgrow milk allergies by age two, so ask your doctor about reintroducing milk in small amounts periodically to see if your child can tolerate it down the line.

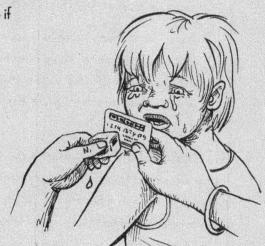

Soothe a Sting. If you ever see a child have a run-in with a bee, a wasp, or a pile of fire ants, you know his reaction: He's hightailing it out of there (and high-screaming it while he's at it). If he does get stung, bitten, or swarmed by an angry insect, then you need to be prepared to run triage when he comes running. Stay calm to help him calm down, and follow these steps:

- ⊃ Brush any remaining insects off him.

- ⊃ Scrape away any remaining stingers, using a credit card or a fingernail. Don't pinch the stinger, because that may force more venom into the skin.

- ⊃ Put ice on the site of the sting and elevate the part of the body that was stung. You can also try applying a penny, which will oxidize (turning a cool green) as it draws some of the ouch out of the sting.

- ⊃ Give your child an oral antihistamine such as Benadryl to control the swelling, relieve any itching, and slow down the allergic reaction. Ibuprofen or acetaminophen can be used alternatively to relieve any pain.

⊃ And, of course, call 911 if your child has any difficulty breathing or experiences severe reactions like those described on page 202.

Help Junior Breathe Free. If your child suffers from asthma, prevention is half the battle. Some actions you should take:

⊃ No smoking, and get rid of all allergy triggers that we discussed earlier on page 208.

⊃ Keep pets out of your child's bedroom—or even better, out of the house.

⊃ Stay calm. When your child is having trouble during an asthma attack, it's easy to panic. But your losing control only exacerbates your child's stress response, further constricting his airways. Having a clear plan for how to respond will help ease some of your anxiety. (See treatment guidelines on page 204.)

See the Animals. If you live near a zoo, take your child there before she turns six months old. While she won't remember the poop-playing monkeys or the sleep-all-day lions, her immune system will. The zoo is filled with a particular type of antigen called endotoxin, which will actually help your child build up her immunity army. Similarly, if you can visit a working farm before your child is six months, you'll reap the same benefits.

Get Up and Go. Children who hang out in front of the TV for two hours a day seem to double their risk of developing asthma. The theory is that TV watching takes the place of physical activity. While the relationships between the behaviors and asthma aren't fully known, researchers believe there's a link between lack of physical activity and a change in the structure and function of the lungs.

And go swimming: Seems like swimming does an excellent job of lessening asthma symptoms in children, although some kids do have reactions to the chlorine.

8

Let's Flesh Things Out

Keep Your Child's Skin Beautiful on the Outside— To Keep Her Healthy on the Inside

There are lots of things we like to describe as being as smooth as a baby's bottom: the marble countertop or the pretty little silk thing you haven't worn since before you had kids, perhaps. There's good reason why the tiny-tush image has become the punctuation point in this popular cliché. Sure, it has a little to do with alliteration,★ but more important, it has to do with the fact that a newborn's skin is just about one of the most magical and magnetizing things a parent can touch. With one brush, pat, stroke, or tickle, parents are awash in baby love.

From a purely health perspective, though, a child's skin is about more than just transmitting love and affection. It's an early warning system for parents; it's there to

★ "Smooth as a baby's armpit" doesn't have the same ring to it.

tell you what's happening on both the outside and the inside of your child. Simply, skin can be a proxy for overall health.

So your precious kid suddenly has red bumps on her face; or thick, greasy scales clumped throughout her hair; or a few spots that look like Grandpa's skin, too. That's the signal that something's going on, and not just on the surface. Behind those symptoms could be an infection, an allergy, or any number of other causes. Those early sleepless nights are difficult enough without wondering why she has more pimples than her teenage cousin. This chapter provides an up-close look at what can go wrong with your child's skin, what it means, and what you can do about it.

The Biology of Skin

Skin is the body's largest organ. At the very basic level, it not only serves as a neat wrapper that keeps our innards in one place but also is our body armor, protecting our organs from all kinds of threats, from UV rays to animal teeth. But skin can be much more than that (including the ultimate artistic canvas). One of the goals of this chapter is to help you think about skin on many different levels—to really understand how skin works and what purposes it serves us as humans. To start, let's take a quick look at the structure of skin, which has several components (see Figure 8.1).

Epidermis. Less than a millimeter thick, the epidermis serves as your body's protective coat, keeping potential toxins out. It's where some molecules are created (like vitamin D₃, from the sun) and others are destroyed (like folic acid, from the same sun). This layer of skin is continually renewing itself; beginning at birth, old skin cells die off and are replaced by new ones.

Dermis. The thickest layer of skin, the dermis is made up of cells that produce two proteins, collagen and elastin, that give your skin both strength and flexibility. The dermis also contains such important skin features as hair follicles, sweat glands,

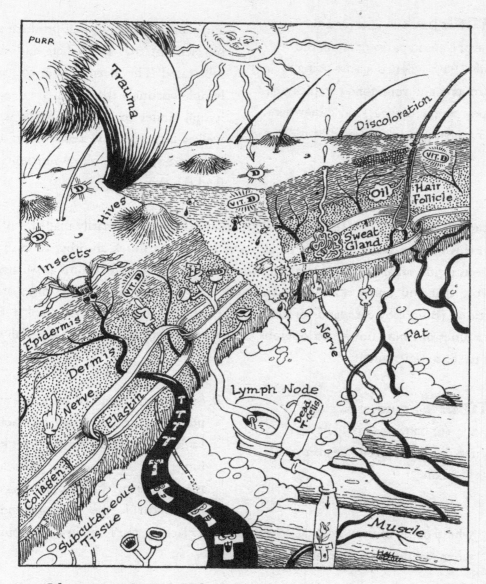

Figure 8.1 **Showing Some Skin** Skin has three levels: the epidermis, dermis, and subcutaneous tissues. They all serve different purposes, everything from providing a barrier to the sun to helping produce sweat to cool us. Capillaries carry blood and lymph carry immune cells. Both cart off waste material to be cleaned. Elastin fibers have not been sun damaged (yet) so the skin is extra bouncy, but a baby's soft skin is especially sensitive and prone to getting rashes, especially as moisture builds up and rubs between body and diaper.

and sebaceous glands that produce the oil (sebum) that keeps hair and skin lubricated. The dermis also contains lymph channels that drain to deeper lymph nodes to help clear toxins, as well as little blood vessels that act as a transport system to allow nutrients to feed the skin.

Subcutaneous Tissue. This innermost layer of skin is primarily made up of fat that helps insulate your body. The fat also acts a bit like a shock absorber to cushion precious inside organs from the outside world. This is the layer that thins as we age.

Now that you know skin's basic structure, you can probably guess some of its functions. (Bingo! Sweat glands produce sweat, which keeps your body cool.)★ But other functions may not be so obvious. Some of the important ones, especially as they relate to your infant:

⊃ Since skin is one of only a few places in the body that interact with the outside world (think lungs and GI tract), it plays a major role in the immune system. Skin is the battleground where many immunological skirmishes take place, as you'll see in a moment when we describe specific conditions.

⊃ Skin communicates with your child's brain when it comes to pain. The classic example is the hot stove: Finger touches stove, nerve fibers in skin

---

★ Babies often sweat a lot from their heads, especially when they're sleeping. Excessive sweating should be checked out; it could be a sign of a heart defect, metabolic disorder, or infection, or nothing.

THE SKIN RULES: THE SIMPLE VERSION

⊃ If it's wet, dry it.

⊃ If it's dry, wet it.

⊃ If it's black and dead looking, cut it off (not you, a professional).

send a message to the spinal cord and brain: "Get your cute little hands off the stove unless you want them fried up like a tater!" If those pain fibers in your skin were dead or didn't exist, your brain wouldn't get the message that there was a problem, and you wouldn't be able to heal properly (assuming that at some point you did, in fact, remove your finger from the stove). It's one of the ways that kids learn. Remember the learning landscape from chapter 1? We process information gathered by all our senses from the world around us to make decisions about what to expect—and what to do next based on those expectations.

⊃ Skin builds bonds. While touch is important for any loving relationship, it's really important when it comes to parenting. Touching in a loving way reduces levels of the stress hormone cortisol and increases levels of the feel-good hormone oxytocin, which is also the molecule that makes us feel bonded to other people. Remember, kids are constantly exposed to stress—maybe not the kind of stress we know, but stress that comes with the uncertainty that all kids experience (such as the stress of Mom leaving the room, the stress from not being able to cover his face from the sun, or the stress of not knowing if someone will ever change his stinking diaper). That's why we recommend infant massage, holding your baby against your skin while feeding, even if you're not breast-feeding, and snuggling up for a good story.

Those are big jobs the skin does, for sure. As smooth as it is, a child's skin is working hard all the time to protect her. Now, let's a look at some of the signs you may spot along the way.

Rash Decisions:
The Skinny on What Can Go Wrong

From time to time, things are going to pop up on your child's skin. Some may scare you. Some may concern you. Some may even amuse you: How did chocolate end up *there*? Our overriding message is that you should regularly inspect your child's skin with the scrutiny of an airport security guard. Check it thoroughly and pay special attention to anything that changes or looks suspicious. While there are many variations of skin problems, we like to think of them in five big categories:

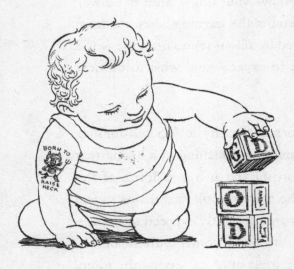

1. Immune function fallout

2. Mechanical problems (part of the structure isn't working properly)

3. Infectious issues

4. Hazards of the great outdoors

5. Congenital issues (spots and stripes that your child was born with)

For an overview of the dermatological things that can go awry in children, see the cross section of skin shown on page 215. For specifics, check out our Most Wanted list of skin suspects on page 230.

IT'S IN THE SHOES

Contact dermatitis, a common skin rash in kids, often gets mistaken for athlete's foot. It starts over the top part of the big toe or on other toes or the back of the feet, becoming red, thick, and possibly even oozing or crusting. Caused by an allergy to all sorts of materials used to make shoes (cements, rubbers, dye), contact dermatitis can be treated by simply giving the kid's foot some air. Let her go barefoot or wear flip-flops or open-toed sandals.

Immune Issues

If you read chapter 7's discussion about the immune system, you'll remember that as invaders infiltrate the body, the immune system sends out warriors to defend your child's turf. That battle often takes the form of sneezes and sniffles, but it's also very common for immune battles to be played out via the skin. Some common immune-related skin issues:

Eczema

The Basics. Eczema, which affects 10 percent to 20 percent of all infants, is an allergic reaction of the skin that shows up in babies as dry, scaly, red patches—first on the face, then on the elbows or knees. It's often found in those beautiful creases where milk and sweat can hide. In toddlers, the itchy rash moves to the crook of the elbow, the back of the knee, the face, and the neck. In babies, eczema may lead to fussiness or irritability (wouldn't *you* be upset if you couldn't scratch the itch?). The symptoms are made worse by certain foods, bacterial infections, reduced humidity, excessive sweating, and irritants such as wool, soaps, and detergent. Eczema is most common in babies two to four months old and children over four years old, and can be triggered by allergic reactions to any number of things. Sometimes it takes a little sleuthing to figure out what may be the cause. (Regarding laundry detergent: Check the label carefully, as the formula may change even if the name on the box stays the same.)

Now, the term *eczema* usually refers to atopic eczema, or atopic dermatitis (*atopic* means "allergic"), which is a complex genetic disorder that results in defective skin barriers, reduced innate skin immune responses, and exaggerated immune (T cell) responses to environmental allergens that lead to chronic skin inflammation. Atopic dermatitis can be the first step in an "allergic march," as infants who develop atopic dermatitis are more likely to go on to develop allergic rhinitis (hay fever) and asthma. Eczema is also used to describe nonallergic skin disorders that are characterized by oozing, scaling, and itchiness, which we call *contact* dermatitis. This often comes from a known irritant, such as a particular brand of diaper wipes, pacifier sucking, or detergents.

The Diagnosis. Think of eczema as an itch that rashes. Children with eczema usually start out with dry skin, which gets worse in the winter, when the air is dry, or if they take frequent baths. That dry skin itches, then turns red and irritated looking. When the area is repeatedly scratched, it will thicken like lizard skin. (Experts call this lichenification.) Continued itching just makes it worse. Those red patches will get blistery, ooze, and crust over.

Here's a trick you can use to diagnose eczema: "Draw" on your child's arm with a fingernail. After about ten seconds, the red line will turn white. Really allergic kids will get a "wheal and flare" response, where it goes white first, then gets red and puffy like a linear hive along the line of the scratch.

The Treatment/Prevention. Use this checklist to help minimize and prevent flare-ups:

⊃ Laundry detergents can cause eczema. We recommend Dreft and other hypoallergenic brands for clothes washing in the first year, especially if your family is prone to eczema. You don't have to wash baby's clothes separately; the whole family can use hypoallergenic products.

⊃ Don't dress your child in wool or rough clothes, which can irritate itchy areas. Choose soft or cotton clothing.

⊃ Wash your child with a mild moisturizing soap (like Dove or Neutrogena) and *lightly* pat her dry before slathering on a water-based lotion (like Aquaphor) or non-water-based (like Eucerin or Moisturel; good ol' Johnson & Johnson's baby lotion also works if you prefer that smell). Do it within three minutes. You can also give your child oatmeal baths, which can soothe itching. Don't bathe your child every day—every two to three days is plenty—and spot clean the diaper area. Also make sure you get in those creases between the legs, under the chin and behind the foreskin of your son's penis where *schmutz* can hide and bacteria can grow.

⊃ For medications, you can use steroid creams to relieve the itch (apply after bath, prior to moisturizer) or antihistamines to quell the allergic reaction (prescription ones can be nonsedating). Try to avoid using steroid creams on the face or diaper area; they can thin out sensitive skin there. If treating the symptoms isn't helping, you may want to talk with your doc about other medications that interrupt the inflammatory process.

⊃ Relieve some of the pain of raw rashes by using wet compresses soaked in a soothing solution of aluminum acetate. Most drugstores carry Domeboro astringent solution or Burow's solution, which are available as tablets or powder packets that get mixed with water. A wet handkerchief works better than gauze, since gauze can stick and irritate a spot further. Washcloths and towels may be too heavy, preventing the moisture from evaporating.

⊃ No bubble baths! And keep bathwater warm, not hot, because hot water stimulates blood vessel dilation, which makes itching worse.

⊃ Make sure to wash off chlorine immediately after swimming in a pool or hot tub; it's very drying.

⊃ Manage asthmatic conditions, since kids with asthma are more prone to developing eczema. Smoking makes asthma symptoms flare, as can pets, stuffed animals, and feather pillows (see page 208).

⊃ Foods can cause allergic reactions in the form of eczema. We recommend introducing a new food or not serving an existing food four days in a row, so you can better ascertain whether that food may be responsible for the reaction. Some of the foods that tend to trigger rashes: citrus fruits, tomatoes, wheat products, fish, and nuts.

⊃ If your infant is at high risk for eczema because of a family history and your bottle feeding, consider switching from a cows-milk-based formula to a partially hydrolyzed whey formula. It can reduce the incidence of eczema by 45 percent.

Cradle Cap

The Basics. Cradle cap, the most common newborn rash, is technically called seborrheic dermatitis. It tends to start between weeks three and four and clears by eight to twelve months, though it may resurface at puberty in some kids. Some docs say it's related to an overgrowth of an otherwise innocuous skin bacteria.

The Diagnosis. Cradle cap is a greasy yellow or salmon-colored scaly eruption. Unlike eczema, it doesn't itch. In addition to the scalp, it often appears in the folds of the neck and behind the ears, and can extend to areas where your baby has lots of sebaceous glands, such as the forehead, eyebrows, sides of the nose, middle of the chest, belly button, armpits, and diaper area.

The Treatment/Prevention. A baby shampoo and a mild 1 percent hydro-cortisone cream can help, but use it sparingly. Or try putting warm baby oil or mineral oil on the area to loosen the thick, sticky scales. Leave on for twelve hours, then use a fingernail or brush to remove the scales. To prevent cradle cap, keep your baby clean and dry, especially in the folds of his chubby neck, arms, and legs. Also, try raking your baby's head with a plastic comb two or three times a day for the first couple of weeks after birth to stimulate his sebaceous glands.

Psoriasis

The Basics. Contrary to popular belief, psoriasis is an autoimmune reaction, not an allergy, that brings about inflammation and excess skin cells. When new skin cells are produced during an immune battle, the old ones die and slough off, leading to the scales and patches. It's most likely to be found on the elbows and knees, and usually on the outside of the joint—unlike eczema, which is often on the soft inside skin.

The Diagnosis. Here you'll see well-defined red lesions with a silvery bit of scale on top. It tends to crop up on elbows, knees, scalp, and private parts, and can also spread to the fingernails and toenails, causing small pits in the nail.

The Treatment/Prevention. Treating psoriasis is hit or miss, so docs typically try a number of approaches to see what works. Some common treatments include using moisturizers, mineral oil, or petroleum jelly to help reduce the dryness that comes with the buildup of skin cells. Docs may also use medicated topical agents to help not only minimize the appearance but also quell the immune reaction, reduce the inflammation, and stop the overproduction of skin cells.

GOT THE LOOK

Skin decisions that may have health considerations

Ear piercing	We don't recommend doing this. Kids can tug on the earring and cause a nasty split in the lobe.
Fingernails	You may want to polish them for fun, and that's okay as long as it's in a well-ventilated area. Avoid products with toluene, which is the most toxic chemical found in nail polish. For basic nail care, trim the nails straight across to avoid ingrown nails, and do it right after a bath when nails are softest. (You can also do it when children are asleep, to avoid the fear and discomfort.) Do not bite your child's nails, as you have less control and may peel off too much, which can cause an infection.
Lips	Use Chapstick, Blistex, Carmex (menthol, camphor, phenol, lanolin, and cocoa butter), or Vaseline in cold weather to avoid chapped, cracked lips.
Play tattoos or face paint	Generally fine, but a small number of kids may have allergic reactions to them. Best to try them first on the inside of the arm before tattooing or painting the face.

Mechanical Issues

When you think of mechanical issues, you may think of a car, washing machine, or refrigerator breaking down. Something is wrong with the equipment. The same is true for the body: Mechanical issues occur when certain pieces of hardware don't quite work right—as opposed to chemical or cellular reactions. In the case of skin, this can happen in several ways:

Milia. These skin growths come in the form of tiny pearly white or yellow cysts, usually thousands of them. Milia can affect up to half of all newborns (and usually right at picture time). They commonly appear on the cheek, nose, chin, and forehead but can also pop up on the upper trunk, limbs, and other areas. Milia usually exfoliate spontaneously in one to four months. Washing with baby soap and water may quicken the process. For the face, try using just a wet washcloth. As much as you may want to, resist popping or squeezing the milia.

Milaria (aka Prickly Heat or Sweat Rash). This rash, which looks like a series of blister packs akin to what you might see with chicken pox, forms when immature sweat glands become obstructed. To treat it, avoid sweaty, humid environments, and have your child wear lightweight clothing, take cool baths, and get plenty of air-conditioning.

Infant Acne. It's unclear whether infant acne is related to hormones, but kids with lots of leftover placental estrogen appear to get acne. We know this because they also have breast buds, which go away by four months. Another cause is blocked hair follicles from overgrowing skin. To treat: Wash with baby soap and water, or try Aquaphor topically. A water-based lotion, it doesn't block the pores and exacerbate the process.

Diaper Rash. A form of contact dermatitis, diaper rash typically comes from the friction that's generated between diaper and skin. It can also be caused by sensitive baby skin reacting to the acidity of urine or something she ate that came out the other end, such as tomatoes. Diaper rash is often confused with yeast infection. The latter is marked by angry red bumps in the creases of Baby's tush and legs, with satellite red bumps away from the main red area. Yeast should be treated with a topical antifungal medicine such as nystatin four times a day. There are combination antifungal-steroid creams available, but the risk is that overusing steroid cream on sensitive private parts or the face can lead to a thinning out of the skin permanently, with what are called "atrophic changes."

It's worth avoiding, and if you can get away with no steroid but just antifungal medicines for yeast infections, that is safer for Junior's bottom.

Better than treatment: prevention! The best way to treat and prevent diaper rash is to create a barrier between skin and the offending poop and pee: Petroleum jelly/zinc oxide, Desitin, Balmex, Pinxav, and Boudreaux's Butt Paste will all do the trick. Just be sure to dry the area completely first. You can use a hair dryer (on low heat), too. Let your child run around without diapers and, if he doesn't poop at night, let him sleep without diapers. (Just make certain that you have a plastic cover for the crib mattress.) Things we don't recommend include baby wipes (they're wet and if used too much, they can make rash worse); corn starch (can keep skin dry, but talcum powder is harmful if inhaled); baking soda (also keeps area dry, but can feed a yeast infection and be harmful if absorbed by skin).

Infectious Issues

Infections comes in three forms: fungal, bacterial, and viral. Each has a distinctive look. You can figure out which is which using the hints below:

Ringworm (Fungal). It's also called tinea corporis when on the body, tinea capitis when on the head, tinea pedis when on the feet, and tinea cruris when on the groin. Forget all the Latin words unless you want to impress the other parents; what you need to remember is that ringworm is caused by a common skin fungus and can be identified by a raised red area with defined edges. It's easily treatable with a topical antifungal medication like clotrimazole (Lotrimin) four times a day, or once a day with expensive prescription-strength oxiconazole (Oxistat) cream. If the ringworm is on the scalp, then it requires an oral antifungal medication called griseofulvin to make it go away. If your child needs griseo, you can tell him he gets to eat ice cream, fish oil, avocadoes, or DHA pills (it's better digested with fat) for at least a month. (Then make sure to read chapter 4.) Griseo has its own risks; it can wreak havoc on the liver, so if your child needs to be on it for four to six weeks, and he starts turning yellow (meaning jaundiced), call your pediatrician ASAP.

Impetigo (Bacterial). This is a contagious skin infection that's caused by strep or staph bacteria, or both. It appears as honey-colored crusty lesions and can be treated with topical antibiotics like Bactroban (mupirocin—prescription-strength bacitracin) four times a day or oral antibiotics like amoxicillin-clavulanate (Augmentin) or erythromycin. Gently wash the lesions to remove the crusts and drain the pustules; warm baths can loosen them up. Impetigo is often found around insect bites, as scratching abrades the skin and allows bacteria to enter. Scratching at bites spreads the infection all over the body.

Strep (Bacterial). We most often associate strep with the throat, but an angry red area around the anus that itches and feels tender can be what's called a perianal strep infection. It can often make it difficult for the child to poop, or cause little fissures that can crack and lead to blood in the stool. Oral antibiotics will treat it, as will Bactroban (but not bacitracin; you need the prescription strength) four times a day topically. And if it's not perianal strep, think about pinworms (see below).

Chicken Pox/Varicella (Viral). The classic diagnosis is made when you see three types of lesions at once: red bumps, blisters, and scabs, all coming out in crops. Chicken pox is contagious until all of these lesions are crusted over, which is usually within a week in kids who have had the vaccination but still get it (which happens about 10 percent of the time), and ten to twenty-one days for those who didn't get the vaccine. Chicken pox is highly contagious, so your child will have to be quarantined until she is fully scabbed over. It is especially dangerous for infants, fetuses, seniors, and immune-compromised individuals to risk exposure.

Coxsackievirus (aka Hand, Foot, and Mouth Disease) (Viral).

This virus causes ulcers and blisters in the mouth, on the hands, feet, trunk, and everywhere else. And it usually comes with an unpleasant side order of high fever and general achiness. Unfortunately, HFMD is contagious until it's gone. Pregnant moms should stay away from this one, especially in the first and third trimesters. (If you are pregnant and have a child with hand, foot, and mouth disease, you can be the Masked Mommy and wear a surgical mask when within three feet of your child.)

To treat mouth ulcers and to make for less painful swallowing, have the child swish and swallow a cocktail containing 1 milliliter each of Mylanta, Maalox, and Benadryl, every four to six hours. The two liquid antacids coat the painful blisters in the mouth, and the Benadryl numbs the area. (See chapter 6 for ways to treat other symptoms, like fever and pain.) Be sure to keep fluids coming in to avoid dehydration, so make sure you have a chaser of your child's favorite beverage. For blisters elsewhere, it's best to leave them be; topical lotions don't help, though a soak in an oatmeal bath may provide some relief.

Warts (Viral).

Though they're more common in the older-kid set (and on fictional witches), small kids can also get warts, which are caused by the human papillomavirus. They commonly settle in on the fingers,

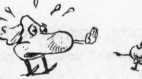

hands, elbows, and bottom of the feet. If a child has them on the soles of his feet, avoid letting him walk around barefooted, or the whole family may become infected, as they're very contagious. About a quarter of the warts will fade on their own within six months, and half within two years. But if they persist, or if you don't want to wait that long, you should seek treatment.

To kill the wart, you have to kill off the cells that have the wart virus in their DNA. Here's how: Soak the affected area, file down the dead skin, then apply wart medicine. Most over-the-counter preparations, such as Compound W, contain 17 percent to 18 percent salicylic acid. Then cover the wart with a bandage. Do this nightly for several weeks. If the wart persists, you can go to the doc for a stronger concentration of salicylic acid or to have it frozen off or burned off with laser therapy. (Both of those options do hurt a bit.) Or you can try the old-fashioned way: Cover the wart completely with duct tape and leave it on for a week. Some swear that the tape will suffocate the wart, and it will come off when you remove the tape. Others also recommend using topical vitamin A, and some anecdotal evidence shows that alcohol sanitizers can do the trick too.

Molluscum Contagiosum (Viral). Kids can break out with just a couple or many hundreds of these flesh-colored or pinkish bumps with a central pearl. The virus lives within the pearl, so you have to get rid of the pearl to get rid of the virus. Docs can remove them by numbing the skin, then "de-pearling" them, or dissecting out the pearl with a straight-edge razor. If your child has lots of bumps or if they're on the face, a doc may use a 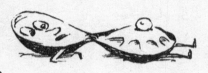 prescription-strength acne medicine called azelaic acid to reduce the risk of scarring. As the name suggests, molluscum contagiosum are extremely contagious and can be spread when children share clothes, towels, or even bathe together.

THE QUICK-REFERENCE GUIDE
TO SKIN SPOTS

CONDITION	WHAT YOU'LL SEE
Eczema, infant	Rash on face first
Eczema, toddler	Rash first appears on inside of elbows, backs of knees, neck, behind ears
Psoriasis	Rash first appears on trunk
Contact dermatitis	Rash where sensitive skin hits offending material
Cradle cap	Scaly skin on head and back of neck
Poison ivy	A line on an extremity with little blisters and bumps
Chicken pox	Bumps, blisters, and scabs—everywhere (even on eyeballs or privates!)
Hand, foot, and mouth disease	Sores in these places, as well as all over body; other than syphilis, it's the only rash that shows up on palms and soles
Measles	Fine red bumps that form red blotches or patches, starting on the face and moving to the body (for more info, see our section on vaccines, starting on page 392)
Scarlet fever	Sandpaper red rash that starts on trunk; caused by the same bacterial species responsible for strep throat (scarlet fever means strep with a rash)

Bugs and Other Hazards of the Great Outdoors

At one level, everything we talk about in this chapter has to deal with attackers, be they allergens or viruses. But in this category of skin issues, we'll look at the attackers that are a little bit more tangible than the microscopic ones we've referred to earlier. (Note that we'll handle more serious forms of trauma like burns and bruises in our next chapter.)

Bug Bites. Doesn't matter whether they're from bed bugs, flies, spiders, sand fleas, or mosquitoes, the bottom line is that these little bites itch. You can try to relieve the pain with cool compresses, antihistamines, hydrocortisone cream, or Calamine (or similar) anti-itch lotion. (Of course, it's a different story if your child has an allergic reaction; see page 204 for how to treat an anaphylactic reaction.) Skip the topical antihistamines such as Caladryl, Benadryl gel, or other skin-soother-plus-antihistamine combinations, as you can easily overdose your child, especially if you're also giving him an oral antihistamine. And take preventive measures like avoiding infested areas (Oscar the Grouch from *Sesame Street* is the only one who belongs near the garbage), keeping kids inside at dusk, eliminating standing water around the house (or where your kids play), and making sure that windows have screens. Feel free to use insect repellant with DEET (it's enormously effective); just be sure to apply it outdoors if you're using a spray and wash your child's skin thoroughly with soap and water at the end of the day.

Ticks. If you live in an area known for ticks, it's smart to check your kids every night. Baths are an especially good way to find ticks, as they are easier to feel on a youngster's body when she's in the water. Key spots to check: inside elbows, inside knees, under arms, between toes, crotch, neck, behind ears, head.

A deer tick (the ones responsible for Lyme disease) is the size of a pinhead, while dog ticks are about the size of a pinkie nail. Don't try to scrape the tick off, because you'll only get part

4 mm — Deer Tick

4 mm

4 mm — Dog Tick

of it. Instead use flat-edged tweezers and try to get the whole little blood-sucking bugger off your child in one pull. If you're worried about Lyme disease, you can take the tick to your doc to have it analyzed. The deer tick needs to be attached to the skin for at least twenty-four hours to transmit the virus, which is why you should religiously check your child once a day. Take him to the pediatrician for a blood test if (1) he has coldlike symptoms after an extended tick bite, (2) there is a red ring around the bite, (3) your child complains of exhaustion or achy joints, and (4) you live in a deer-tick-infested area.

Lice. These tiny insects live on humans and feed on blood, infesting up to ten million schoolchildren a year. Head lice are usually found in hair or on the back of the neck or behind the ears. They spread from one person to another through direct contact or via shared clothing on which lice have laid eggs. To treat lice, use a medicated cream rinse containing permethrin on the hair for ten minutes and then rinse off (do not use if your child has allergies to ragweed). It will leave a residue—that's the point. Repeat in two weeks. A new oral one-dose, anti-lice medication looks promising; ask your pediatrician. Benzyl alcohol lotion is also effective in treating lice, although some of our team still prefer the tried-and-true shampoo method. In addition to treating the hair, you will want to comb out the dead nits and eggs. (If lice are on the eyelashes, put Vaseline jelly on the eyelashes twice a day for eight days, then remove the bugs.) Olive oil smothers lice and prevents nits from sticking to the hair shaft. Your kid's head will smell like salad, but it does the trick for getting out those eggs, often better than shampoo. Contrary to popular belief, dead nits are not contagious, and once treated, your child can be in school, at play, and not avoided like the plague. But be warned that some schools do have a no-nit policy.

Make sure to wash all of your child's sheets, clothes, and stuffed animals in hot water and detergent after treatment. For any items you can't wash, like baseball caps or some stuffed animals, put them in a sealed bag for seventy-two hours or throw them out. And vacuum all the floors, furniture, and bedding. In little kids, transmission is commonly through shared hair ties, headbands, and dress-up clothes, so make sure that you wash/seal/throw out those too. In general, don't let your child share hats or helmets with other children.

Scabies. Look for lines from the little buggers' burrows in between fingers and toes and in the armpits and creases of the groin. The infected area will itch, itch, itch. A lot, lot, lot. Just like lice, scabies is treatable with a topical medicated cream called permethrin. An older version of this medicine, lindane, has more toxicity, so stick to permethrin.

Pinworms. Just when you thought it was safe to go to bed, your child tells you that his tushy itches, and he's scratching his behind more than a ballistic baboon. Your flashlight reveals the intruders: pin-sized, white, stringy things peeping out at you from around the anus. Pinworms come from spores that are in dirt and the environment (think: sandbox) and that find their way from a kid's hand to his mouth. Treatment is easy: A single dose of a prescription med called mebendazole will kill the little guys quietly. Make sure to wash all bedclothes, pajamas, and underwear in hot water with detergent after treatment. A good idea is to change your child's diaper and/or clothes after coming in from the sand or dirt. "Everybody gets naked in the laundry room" is a good rule for getting rid of a lot of pests and keeping a sandbox's worth of sand out of your living room.

Poison Oak/Ivy/Sumac.* All of these leafy plants contain an oil called urushiol that is irritating to 50 percent to 75 percent of us. When kids who are sensitive to urushiol come in contact with it, they break out within eight hours. The rash causes itching, redness, blisters, and eventually scabbing, often in

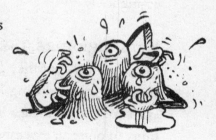

* Poison ivy has three leaves and a red stem, and the leaves turn red in the fall. It grows as a shrub or vine. Poison sumac grows as a shrub or a tree (never a vine) and has seven to thirteen leaves arranged in pairs along a central stem, with a single leaf at the end. It grows in woody and swampy areas east of the Mississippi River. Poison oak grows in an upright shrub and is found on the West Coast.

a line where the skin has been scratched. It usually resolves within three weeks. The best prevention method, besides avoidance, is to have your child wear long sleeves and pants if he's hiking, playing, or exploring an area that you think may be infested with the stuff. Also, make sure to hose off any pets who may be running through infested areas, so they don't carry it back to the family. If your child does have skin-to-plant contact, wash the affected area with soap and water as quickly as you can—within ten minutes, if possible. You may also want to try dishwashing liquid, which removes the oil. Wash his clothes, too. You can use an anti-itch lotion such as Calamine or oatmeal baths to soothe the itch. Oral antihistamines like Benadryl can also quell the reaction. Steroid creams can help, and in extreme cases, your kid's doc can prescribe oral steroids in a tapering-dose pattern. After the initial exposure, a child who is allergic will develop a *systemic* reaction, and the rash will pop up in places that did not necessarily touch the plant, especially the abdomen or face. The lesions are not contagious to others.

Congenital Issues

As you can guess, these skin conditions are ones with which your child may be born. They can arise for any number of reasons, and many of them are harmless medically, but you may need to make decisions about whether to do something about them cosmetically.

Hemangiomas. These benign growths on the surface of the skin may not be apparent at birth, but they grow pretty quickly during infancy. The good news? Hemangiomas stop growing by about a year or so and then start diminishing at about age two. They can vary in the way they look, from a tiny raised red fleshy-looking thing to quite an extensive bump that seems to extend above and beyond the surface of the skin. Strawberry hemangiomas (they look like strawberries) are made up of capillary cells; about 12 percent of kids have them by the time they're one. They usually develop a few weeks after birth on the head, neck, or trunk. Hemangiomas are harmless unless they are too near the eyeball, impairing the child's vision so that her

THE JUICE ON JAUNDICE

WHAT IT IS: Yellowing of skin and eyes in newborns, usually within the first five days. May be associated with breast feeding. (In older children, jaundice is quite rare and may be a sign of liver disease or a medicine toxicity.) Untreated jaundice can lead to nerve damage.

THE CAUSE: When the baby's body tries to break down and get rid of old red blood cells (from, say, a little bruise on the head or from swallowing blood in utero), the breakdown product of those red cells is bilirubin, which causes the skin to turn yellow.

CAUSE FOR CONCERN: If it happens within the first twenty-four to forty-eight hours or after ten days, call your pediatrician. If your baby is yellow from the head to the chest, that's a milder bilirubin level, but you need to let your doc know if the yellowing affects a larger area of the body—say, from head to belly button or the entire body. A small sample of your child's blood can be tested for bilirubin levels to help gauge seriousness, which depends on a number of factors, including your child's age and if there are other, preexisting conditions.

TREATMENT: Phototherapy—putting the child under special blue fluorescent "bili lamps" (with the eyes covered for protection) helps break down bilirubin. More frequent feedings also can help infants pass excess bilirubin through stools. Some jaundice can be caused by breast-feeding, so you may be asked to stop for a bit; you can still pump, though, so you keep producing milk and can then nurse once the jaundice has cleared.

brain stops using the eye. They can be treated by laser, which is a smart option if the marks are on the face and you want to avoid cosmetic issues for the child. They're also easier to treat when you start early and they're smaller; otherwise, delay treatment, since they often shrink substantially by age two.

Port-Wine Stains. Usually present at birth, these deep red skin stains are made of dilated capillarylike vessels. If they are present around the eye, they may be part of Sturge-Weber syndrome, which is associated with glaucoma. Laser treatments can help remove the stain with minimal scarring and pain. If you choose not to have them removed, as your child gets older, you may have to deal with esteem issues. Many families choose to use education as a first-line defense—talking to teachers and parents of classmates to explain why their child may look different. Other parents and older children may decide that medical makeup, which hides the stains, is a preferred route.

Congenital Nevi. A subset of moles, these dark-brown spots are typically not a problem unless they're greater than 1.5 centimeters in diameter (what's known as giant congenital nevi). They can be present at birth or develop after. If the nevus is someplace where it would be easy to remove or if it's in a cosmetically sensitive spot, a doc may recommend removal, especially since there's a risk of it developing into malignant melanoma later in life.

Salmon Patches. Salmon patches are benign, small, pink, ill-defined dilatations of blood vessels found in 30 percent to 40 percent of newborns. They're affectionately referred to as "angel kisses" when on noses or eyelids or "stork bites" when on the back of the neck. Those on the face usually disappear between twelve and twenty-four months, while those on the neck or back of the head may persist longer, although some still fade. The ones around the eyes often result from the pressure of the baby resting his face on Mom's pelvic bones in utero.

Mongolian Spots. These are blue or slate gray spots found on the back of the trunk, legs, or arms. About 80 percent of black, Asian, and East Indian infants have them, and fewer than 10 percent of white infants. They usually fade in the first two years.

Café au Lait Spots. These spots are actually hyperpigmented lesions that come in various coffee colors, from light brown to dark brown (hence the name, "coffee with milk"). They're caused by an increase in melanin, the natural substance that's responsible for the darker colors of our skin, hair, and eyes. There's generally no need to worry about these spots, which are very common. However, if your child has more than five of them larger than 5 millimeters, or about half the size of your thumbnail, she might be at risk of developing neurofibromatosis, a condition in which nerve tissue grows tumors.

YOU TIPS

Lotion Up, Part 1. To keep your baby's skin soft, beautiful, and as smooth as it's supposed to be, use water-based moisturizing lotions rather than ones that are lipid-based. That way, the lotion won't block your baby's pores and won't dry out her skin, which is one of the risks of using a non-water-based lotion. Try Aquaphor for the face, and use Eucerin or Johnson's baby lotion for the body.

Lotion Up, Part 2. The next thing you can do to preserve your child's beautiful skin is to protect it from the sun. The best line of defense is to stay in the shade. But if you are going to be in the sun, then make sure to put a tightly woven wide-brimmed hat and sunglasses on your child and to use SPF 30 nonparticle zinc-oxide-based sunscreen. You may have to try out a number of different hats to find one your child will tolerate. If he's really good at getting the hats off, try one with a foolproof strap for under the chin and try to distract the baby until he forgets it's on. In the first six months, use a sunblock with titanium dioxide, which acts as a barrier; other blocks may get absorbed through the skin.

After that, you can continue with the zinc oxide—our preference, because it has the least potential for long-term toxicity—or use your favorite sunscreen, making sure to apply it thickly and to wash it all off with soap and water at the end of the day. Sunscreen should protect against both UVA and UVB rays and have a minimum SPF (sun protection factor) of 15, but we recommend SPF 30 to provide the greatest protection. When getting ready to go out in the sun, don't forget to hit easy-to-miss spots, such as the ears and along the line of the part in the hair. Reapply frequently, especially after swimming. It's not a bad idea—in fact, it's quite a good idea—to get your child a tightly woven long-sleeve water shirt that has SPF protection. The kids think they're cool, and you have less lotion (and less sun exposure) to worry about. Also check out sunshade options for your stroller. The fewer auxiliary chemical products you need to deal with and your baby needs to tolerate, the better. And avoid the sun between 10 and 2, when it's most likely to cause burns.

Give Good Hair Care. Children's hair doesn't get greasy like adults' hair does, because their sebaceous glands do not produce significant amounts of oil until puberty. So you only need to wash it every few days. We recommend a gentle, tear-free shampoo. If your child has long hair, conditioner or spray-on detangler can help you avoid knots. Use a soft brush for fine hair. African American babies definitely don't need a hair wash more than once a week, since their skin and scalp are quite dry, and washing it can make it even drier.

Make Rash Decisions. Besides following the guidelines above for treating rashes, there are a number of home remedies that may be worth a try. A compress soaked in milk and water (half and half) can help reduce inflammation. Some also recommend soaking in a bath that includes a half cup of baking soda. Supplements and medications that show antirash promise include witch hazel to cool and soothe skin, or meds (lotions and creams) containing coal tar to relieve itching.

Add Salt. For kids with lots of skin infections, you can add two teaspoons of household bleach to a large bath (no more than that!), along with a cup of table salt. This has been shown to help reduce the incidence of skin infections. Be sure to swish the bleach around in the water before your child gets in the tub.

9

Crash Course

Minimize the Risks Associated with Common Childhood Accidents

As a parent, you'll be many things to your child. You'll be teacher, hero, playmate, body washer, chef, coach, milk cleaner-upper, banker, chauffeur, and on and on and on. Heck, parents have more hats than a Kentucky Derby grandstand. But starting from the moment you knew you were having a baby, one job has trumped all: protector.

Parents are protectors.

When your babe was in utero, Mom's body served as the biological Secret Service, protecting her against all threats from the outside world. And then after she was born, the job expanded and became much more complex. Your urge—really, your instinct—is to do anything you can to protect your little one from harm, whether that threat comes in the form of a slippery staircase or a bully's nasty words.

Keeping a child safe can be one of the most delicate balancing acts a parent has to perform. On the one hand, your responsibility is to provide a safety net, but on the other hand, you know logically that you can't bubble wrap your kid for life (as funny a Halloween costume as that might be). As we said in our early chapters, you have to let them explore the world—discovering, creating, taking risks—because that's how they're going to learn and grow. But this is hard to do. At some point, they're guaranteed to get hurt, even if it's only a scrape or a bruise.

Children are prone to accidents because of a subconscious seesawing within them. They usually underestimate the risk level of a situation, often because they haven't experienced it yet. Makes sense, right? Why else would they try to climb a slippery piece of playground equipment? Kids are hardwired at an early age to act, not to think, reason, or calculate. That's a good thing, most times. Otherwise, they'd never explore or learn, and they'd be content spending their whole lives sitting and not doing.★ And there's even an evolutionary reason for it: Risk-taking behavior can lead to innovations that improve the chance of survival. Essentially, we're wired to make mistakes and learn from them.

So where does that leave you? With some frightening moments, for sure. While you know that kids are at risk of severe injury from accidents, the number one cause of death and hospitalizations among kids, you also know deep down that you're putting them at even greater risk down the line if you don't allow them to take risks and understand what consequences may mean. The key is to expose your child to developmentally appropriate risks and provide sufficient support until he masters skills. Think of providing safety as giving your child training wheels for life: You let him ride all kinds of metaphorical bikes but provide training wheels until he learns how to ride on his own. For instance, when he first explores stairs, you follow behind

★ It's interesting to note gender differences here, as boys are often more likely to be the danger-seeking ones. While toddler girls tend to be content observing the universe at this age, boys are often trying to change it. There seems to be some science to the stereotype. Besides being endowed with more testosterone, the male sex hormone, boys are later in responding to verbal cues than girls are, so the warnings that parents send boys may not register as quickly as they do with girls. Evolutionarily, they're more of the risk takers, because many of them weren't expected to make it to reproductive age, as they had to take risks (angry beasts needed to be caught and killed) to provide for the tribe.

him; when she first jumps off the edge of a pool, you catch her. It's better to teach your child to climb the stairs with you as a safety net, so that if you are looking the other way and he sneaks over there, he's better prepared.

Another approach to safety is to always keep your child within reach, not by the apron strings, but by a visual leash. That means you're always keeping an eye on your child, even when you're encouraging exploration and some reasonable amount of risk taking. You're there when she needs you and can monitor situations so that they don't become too risky; at the same time, you're also giving her room to breathe and to develop a sense of independence and self-reliance. If you hover over her every move and don't let her try new things, she'll never attain the sense of mastery that is the basis for healthy self-esteem.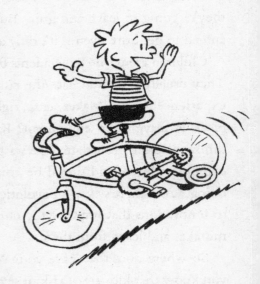

In this chapter, we're going to take you through some of the major threats to a child's safety and give you some basic tips about how you can create a safe environment at home. But the reality is that your home is only one environment in which your child will live. He'll live on the playground, at friends' houses, in the supermarket aisles, at day care, in a garden, around pets, and many other places. And despite your best efforts, you're never going to be able to cover the world in baby bumpers and pillows. So your most important job early on is this: Teach your child to understand your warning signals.

From an early age, your child should be able to read your tone of voice and understand that there's a huge difference between a "You're my sweetie" tone and a "Danger! Danger!" tone, even if she has no idea what the actual words mean. Of course, you can overuse your DefCon 5 tone of voice, so save it for true red-button emergency situations, so that your child knows you mean "Stop immediately!" Oh, she'll test your limits, especially as she gets older (see chapter 3), but one of the keys to success and safety is establishing your signals early.

THE FAMILY PLAN

⊃ In addition to a visual leash, having a family whistle or call that your child recognizes is a good idea. It's the family equivalent of the ol' "Olly, Olly, In Come Free!" We don't suggest using that particular one, as your child may deliberately pretend not to know you . . .

⊃ Have a fire escape plan and rehearse it with your kid; teach him "Stop, drop, cover your face, and roll." Make it a game at first.

⊃ Be vigilant not just in your own home but in any home where your child is likely to play or spend time. If necessary, quiz parents about their safety standards in a nonjudgmental way.* Also, ask whether they have guns and, if so, how they store them.

* For example, you can say, "I never even thought of having Bob screw the TV into the wall so it doesn't tip over." A friend's reaction may give you a clue about how they approach childproofing a house, which will give you a clue about how much time your child will spend at that home.

The Ouch House: Childhood Injuries

Kids are like car doors: Inevitably, they're going to get dinged, nicked, dented, and scratched. As a parent, your hope (and plan) is to prevent as much damage as possible, especially serious damage.

The biggest help you can give your youngster when she gets hurt is to stay calm; children feed on our emotions. (Remember those mirror neurons?) So if you're panicked, she will be too. When talking to your child, try to remain calm and use a soothing tone of voice. The emotional anesthesia you provide complements the medical kind. The best way to control your own stress is to be prepared.

Here are brief descriptions of the most common childhood injuries and accidents, so that you can take steps to prevent them from happening and deal with them if they should occur:

Broken Bones. Broken bones typically aren't a frequent problem at early ages; that's because very small children don't fall with enough force or have enough body weight to really break a bone. And bones are tough; they can take a fair amount of bending before they actually break. But as children enter the playground age, their risk increases. One way you can tell if there's a break at the point of an injury is if your child can pinpoint one exact spot where there's much more tenderness than other spots around the area. He may also complain of nausea, though not always. Sometimes a child with a broken bone can continue to play, and you may not realize it's an issue until a few days later. One hint is if the child avoids using that limb.

Common broken bones include: collarbones and wrists, from falls and bracing for falls; fingers, from being slammed in doors; and toes. The most common orthopedic injury in kids under two is called nursemaid's elbow, in which the elbow gets tugged out of its socket by a caregiver holding a child's hand and yanking the elbow. ("Hurry across the street, dear.") This injury is not a fracture, but it sure can mimic one in the way that the child holds her arm—as if it's in a sling—and won't use it.

You can treat nursemaid's elbow yourself by holding her elbow in one hand and then rotating the arm in the proper direction. If you're not comfortable in the role of amateur orthopedist, take her to the doctor for a three-minute visit: one minute for telling what happened, one minute or less to pop the elbow back in, and another minute to get a sticker for being so brave!

If you suspect a broken bone, you'll need an X-ray to confirm it, of course. On your way to having it checked out, apply ice to help ease your child's pain and reduce the swelling. Depending on the location of the break, that part of the body will be immobilized, giving the bone time to knit itself back together. For most typical childhood breaks, bones will heal within three to six weeks, and you need to follow your doc's directions on activities that your child can and can't participate in not only when he's in the cast but also when he comes out.

The best ways to increase your child's bone strength are making sure he gets enough calcium and encouraging weight-bearing exercises—that is, moves like running uphill and jumping, which stimulate bone growth. (You can see some of our suggestions for games and activities on page 376.)

Head Injuries. Chances are, your child is going to spend some time (other than Halloween) looking like a unicorn—with a prominent bump on his head. Many times, that's okay; the goose-egg swelling is a sign of normal blood clotting beneath the skin at the site of the injury. Nevertheless, you'll need to keep a close eye on your child during the forty-eight hours after a head injury because it can take that much time for damaged veins to leak and cause swelling in the brain. You may also want to see a doc to rule out a skull fracture, because a fracture can tear underlying blood vessels and place a lot of pressure on the brain. Because the skull-encased brain has nowhere to expand when it gets inflamed, an untreated skull fracture can lead to decreased brain function.

After a head injury, be on the lookout for a whole range of symptoms in your child: prolonged headaches, dizziness, vision disturbances, nausea, impaired balance, ringing in the ears, general confusion, irritability, tiring easily, and a change in eating and sleeping patterns. Of course, making it more difficult is the fact that young children and kids with head injuries can't always communicate those symptoms easily. So it's never wrong to have a head injury checked out. You also want to hear an immediate cry after a head injury (you'll never be so happy to hear your child cry, because at least it means he's conscious), and wake him a couple times during the night after a head injury to check for any unusual symptoms.

Seek medical attention immediately if your child loses consciousness, if he wobbles while walking (more than usual), if his pupils are dilated or of different sizes, if his eyes aren't in sync, if there's blood anywhere in the eye or ear, if the bump was near the temple, or if you feel an uneven part of bone in the lumpy area.

While you're not going to be able to prevent every fall, there are some basic preventive strategies you can take to minimize the chances of serious injury. When your child graduates to a big-kid bed, put rails on the sides so she doesn't roll out; put gates on the stairs as soon as she's mobile; install window guards; and be vigilant about making your child wear a helmet anytime she's biking, blading, scootering, skating, skiing, boarding, etc. If you get her in the habit early, it will become second nature. A helmet can be a fashion statement, so let him pick out his own! And be a model: Wear one yourself; remember, kids follow *your* actions.

Drowning. You cannot be too vigilant around pools, lakes, oceans, and bathtubs. If you have a pool, make sure that it's surrounded by sturdy, unclimbable fencing and that your child cannot release the latch on the gate. (Be on the alert: Other people's pools may not be as securely enclosed.) Never leave a young child in the tub or around any water without adult supervision, and never run to answer the phone while a child is in the tub, not even if a sibling is watching. A child can drown in just two inches of water, so buckets and toilets are also hazards. If you forgot the towel during bath time, it's better to get your child out, get all wet yourself, and hustle to get your child warm. We'd rather your child get a few goose bumps and you have to do an extra load of laundry than the alternative. And always use smart sense around water: that means life vests in boats and never taking your eyes off a child who is swimming, even if he has a floatie or water wings. If you do find a child in water, immediately call 911 and turn him on his side. Vigorously rub or pat his back to help him cough out any water and clear his lungs.

Burns. Any burn that covers more than 2 percent of a child's body (that's about twice the size of his hand) needs medical attention. And if a burn of any size comes from an electrical cord or is in a sensitive area, such as near the eyes or genitals, see a doc. If the burn is small, then run it under cool water for about five minutes. You can use a mild soap to clean the area, but don't use alcohol, because that will hurt. And don't pop any blistered areas, so as not to increase the risk of infection. After you rinse, gently pat the area dry, then cover the burn with a topical antibiotic and a gauze pad. A doc may also give you a topical medicine called Silvadene cream or, even better, pure unadulterated honey such as Medihoney; the antimicrobial power of silver and intrinsic bacteria-killing properties of polyphenols in honey help heal the area. The only downside is that both silver sulfadine and honey are goopy. Silvadene turns yellow, which makes many parents think that there's an infection; we'd go with honey.

HOLIDAY HORRORS

Nothing like the holidays when it comes to joy, laughter, and creating memorable moments for children. Let's just be sure to stay safe out there, okay?

HOLIDAY	RISK
New Year's	Clean up all glasses of leftover alcohol, so your child doesn't come across them the next morning (we guarantee he'll be awake before you) and sneak some sips. Alcohol can be fatal in large quantities, and you may not notice your little one has had too much till it's too late; he'll look like he's sleeping peacefully.
Easter	Lilies are poisonous. Keep them out of reach.
Fourth of July	Fireworks can burn off or blow off fingers; keep out of reach.
Halloween	Whole-head masks should not be used, as they restrict vision and have suffocation risks. If trick-or-treating house to house, accompany your child and have her wear reflective clothing.
Thanksgiving	Hot stoves. Somebody watch the kid while you're watching the bird.
Christmas	Poinsettias = poison. If you must use sharp and breakable tree ornaments, hang them high (and make sure kids can't get hold of or tangled up in strings of lights). No candles in the tree, either. And secure the tree so it doesn't tip over.

STRANGER DANGER

By age five, children should be taught their parents' real names, address, and home and/or cell phone numbers (also how to dial 911). They should also know not to give this info to anyone who isn't a teacher or official (in uniform). If they get separated from you for any reason, they should ask for help from a uniformed official, a shopkeeper, or another parent (with children), not another random adult. They should know never to get into cars or accepts gifts or food from strangers.

The family dog would also prefer honey; either way, keep all mouths off the wound. You can also give your child Benadryl to help minimize any inflammatory reaction.

One note: If a kid's clothes are smoldering from a burn, get him in the shower and rinse him off before removing the clothes. If you remove the clothes while they're smoldering, you risk spreading the burns all over the body.

Of course, as soon as your child is old enough to understand, it's also smart to teach him about general fire safety (no playing with candles!), make sure he knows the fire escape plan for your house, and practice the famed "stop, drop, cover your face, and roll" technique. Burns from hot liquid can be as damaging as from flames. Always test the temperature of bathwater with your own hand before putting your child in the tub. Turn all the handles of your pots and pans toward the wall when you're cooking and do not leave hot drinks where they can be knocked over by rambunctious children—or babies using furniture to cruise around the house. And forget about tablecloths for a few years.

Cuts. If it's a superficial cut, you can just clean it with tepid water or saline and mild soap and cover it with a bandage. Add a topical antibiotic ointment or Medihoney if you like. If you observe jagged edges, like puzzle pieces, or if you can see underneath layers of skin, it's worth having a doc check it out. And do it within six hours, because if you wait, it'll be harder to suture; the rule is, the sooner the better. A doc may use sutures or skin glue to pull the skin together. Skin glue is nice

IF YOUR CHILD SWALLOWS POISON

⮌ Stay calm, act fast.

⮌ Get the item away from the child and have him spit out anything that's left in his mouth. Save the container so the docs know what was swallowed.

⮌ Call 911 if your child is unconscious, not breathing, or convulsing (having seizures).

⮌ If your child does not have these symptoms, call the Poison Control Center at 800-222-1222. If the poison is very dangerous or your child is very young, you may be told to go straight to the nearest hospital. If not, you will be given instructions on what to do. In most cases, you are usually told to head immediately to your doctor's office or the local ER. Ipecac (or syrup of ipecac), which helps you vomit, is no longer recommended for *any* ingestion, because of the risk of throwing up and having vomit go down the wrong passage into the lungs, where it is highly inflammatory. If a toxin gets in the eye, you may be told to flush the eye with water but not to let the child rub it.

because it minimizes scarring, but it's not strong enough to be used on areas where the skin is stretched tight, such as the chin, knees, and elbows. If the cut is on the face, ask whether a plastic surgeon is available to do the suturing to reduce the risk of scarring—though, of course, they're not always available depending on the time of day and location of the hospital.

Bumps, Bruises. You can use the same treatment method you'd use for an adult: the RICE method (rest, ice, compression, and elevation). For icing, you can wrap an ice pack, frozen veggies, a plastic baggy full of ice, or even the cooler from the kid's lunch box with a clean dishcloth or paper towel so the ice doesn't sting so much. (Double-bag frozen items with plastic bags to help prevent accidental leakage.) Compress with an elastic bandage, but not so tight that the area beyond the

ACE turns blue. The RICE method works by reducing the inflammation that occurs after an injury. An OTC anti-inflammatory pain reliever like children's ibuprofen (Motrin) may help too.

Foreign Object in Eye. Try flushing it under water for five minutes. You can use one of the medicine droppers that you have left over from when you had to give Junior antibiotics for his first ear infection (wash first with saline or water). If that doesn't help, see a doc. Eye injuries are nothing to mess around with. Most common eye invaders: chemicals and sand. Not a bad reason to get your child in the habit of wearing shades at the playground and on the beach.

Choking. If your child is choking, take two fingers and sweep through his mouth to see if you can remove the object. If that doesn't work, you can turn a baby upside down and pat her upper back fairly vigorously. Around age two, you can start performing the Heimlich maneuver. If you try to do that when they're too young, you risk cracking their ribs. The most common foods that kids choke on: peanuts and buttered popcorn. We recommend that they don't get a chance to eat them unsupervised until they're five years old. The reason isn't just because of their size and shape but because the fat in them is inflammatory to the lungs if the food should go down the wrong pipe.

Dental Trauma. If your child loses a tooth slamming his mouth on the pavement or by way of any other kind of trauma, throw the tooth in milk and take it and your child to the dentist. Milk will keep the tooth at the correct pH level so that the dentist can put it back in your child's mouth. It's important to try to reimplant even a baby tooth that gets knocked out because losing a tooth early can change the spacing of teeth and affect how adult teeth grow in and are aligned.

The Bathroom

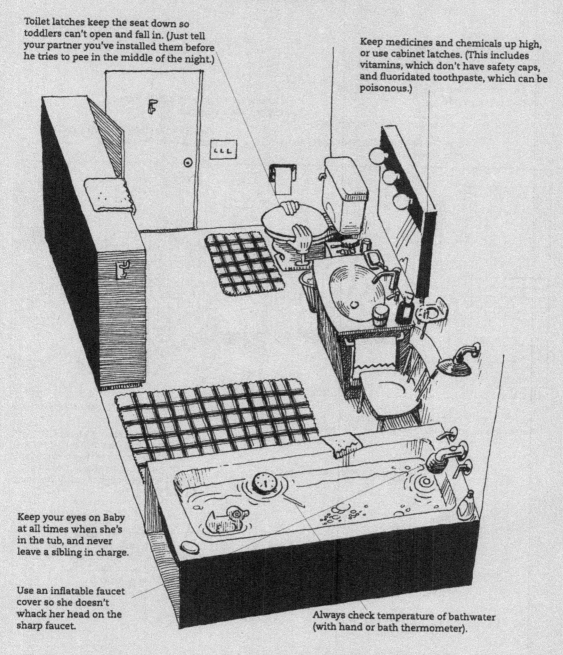

Toilet latches keep the seat down so toddlers can't open and fall in. (Just tell your partner you've installed them before he tries to pee in the middle of the night.)

Keep medicines and chemicals up high, or use cabinet latches. (This includes vitamins, which don't have safety caps, and fluoridated toothpaste, which can be poisonous.)

Keep your eyes on Baby at all times when she's in the tub, and never leave a sibling in charge.

Use an inflatable faucet cover so she doesn't whack her head on the sharp faucet.

Always check temperature of bathwater (with hand or bath thermometer).

Set water heater to 120 degrees F (50 degrees C)

Baby's Bedroom

Window guards on windows. There should be no greater than a five-inch opening in any direction (mandatory in some cities, but advisable even if not).

Window shade and curtain cords kept out of reach.

If you use a humidifier, clean it regularly with bleach.

Door handle covers prevent a child from heading outside on his own

No toys with small parts, like stuffed animals with button eyes.

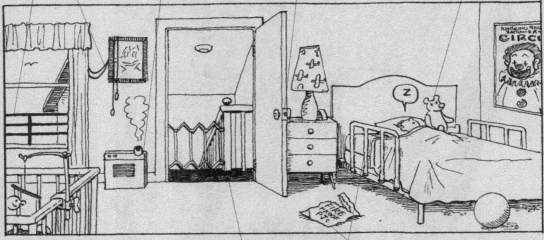

No suffocating items in crib. (See more crib safety tips on page 319.)

Baby sleeps on back.

Outside room, use stair guards or safety gates.

Flame-resistant PJs are a good choice, but they can contain toxins (and some have been recalled because they don't meet the flammability standard). Cotton pj's that fit well and are not overly loose are a good alternative.

Bed rails can keep kids from falling out of big-boy or big-girl beds. (Some parents choose to just use a mattress on the floor.) Crib tents can safeguard a toddler just learning to climb out of his crib.

The Kitchen

Counters are for food, not for little ones to sit on. That includes in a bouncy seat.

If an older child is watching you cook, make sure he's covered up in case oil from the pan spatters.

Put covers on oven dials, even if your toddler thinks she can whip up a grilled cheese herself.

When cooking, point pot and pan handles in, so your toddler can't reach up and grab.

Keep all plastic bags out of reach.

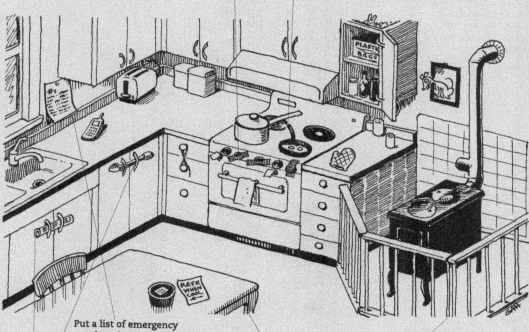

Put a list of emergency numbers in plain sight. Don't forget to include your Poison Control Center, 800-222-1222.

No tablecloths. They can be pulled by kids—and hot drink spilleth.

Don't leave out foods that kids can choke on, especially nuts.

Install gates around fireplaces and woodstoves.

Use latches to lock cabinets containing chemicals, alcohol, and cleaning supplies, as well as drawers with knives, scissors, and matches. Keep all poisonous materials out of reach.

The Living Area

All of your smoke detectors working? Check 'em. Even better, get combo devices that include carbon monoxide detectors.

Outlet covers everywhere!

Use door stoppers to prevent doors from closing completely and pinching a child's fingers. And cover corners of furniture, especially glass tables, so there are fewer sharp edges for Junior to bump into.

Always keep an eye out for choking hazards. If it can fit through a toilet paper roll, it's too small!

Tether standing lamps so they can't be pulled down.

Bookcases should be screwed to the wall, and TVs need to be secured. (Flat-screen models can be especially tippy.)

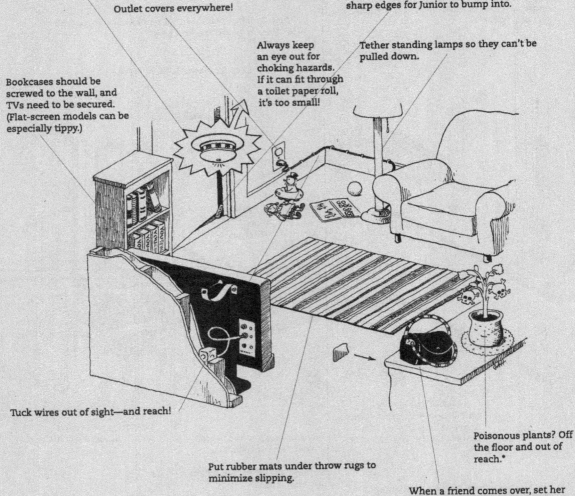

Tuck wires out of sight—and reach!

Poisonous plants? Off the floor and out of reach.*

Put rubber mats under throw rugs to minimize slipping.

When a friend comes over, set her purse out of reach so your kid can't dig around and find meds or choking hazards.

Take wheels off any walkers or get a stationary ExerSaucer instead.

* Remember, just because something is natural doesn't mean it's safe. (Tornadoes and hurricanes are also natural.) Common poisonous plants include buttercup, hyacinth, amaryllis, hydrangea, morning glory, holly, mistletoe, wisteria, lily of the valley, and juniper. For a more complete list, check the following websites from the Oregon Health and Science University (www.ohsu.edu/poison/youAndYourfamily/plantSafety.htm) and the Cornell University Department of Animal Science (www.ansci.cornell.edu/plants).

Yard and Garage

Use soft materials such as sand or wood chips underneath playground equipment.

Do you really need the trampoline? It's a huge source of accidents. The mesh walls are better than nothing but will not prevent all injuries.

Use fencing around the pool 100 percent of the time.

Keep all lawn equipment and chemicals locked up and/or out of reach. The same goes for guns, if you have any: Keep 'em locked up. Also, don't be hesitant to ask playmates' parents if they have any guns and if they're locked up.

Routinely inspect your son or daughter for poison ivy and ticks.

Teach your kids about how to approach animals, even the neighbor's dogs: cautiously, with a closed hand from below (so a dog does not expect to be hit), and never when the dog is eating and only with your supervision.* Make sure they know to ask the dog's mommy or daddy, "Does your dog like kids?" before they start petting.

That barbecue can be hot. Supervise kids while supervising salmon—and for a long time after, since the grill stays hot for quite a while.

If you decide on installing an at-home playground set, make sure to get one with manufacturer instructions that give you the lowdown on safety and installation. Avoid models with pressure-treated wood, to avoid toxins. There's a lot to look out for, with moving parts, screws, and so forth, so make sure that you have all safety checks in place.

---

* On your trip to the petting zoo, teach your kids to feed the goats and horses with a flat hand rather than with their little fingers holding the apple or other food. Animals can mistake a child's tiny fingers for tiny carrots.

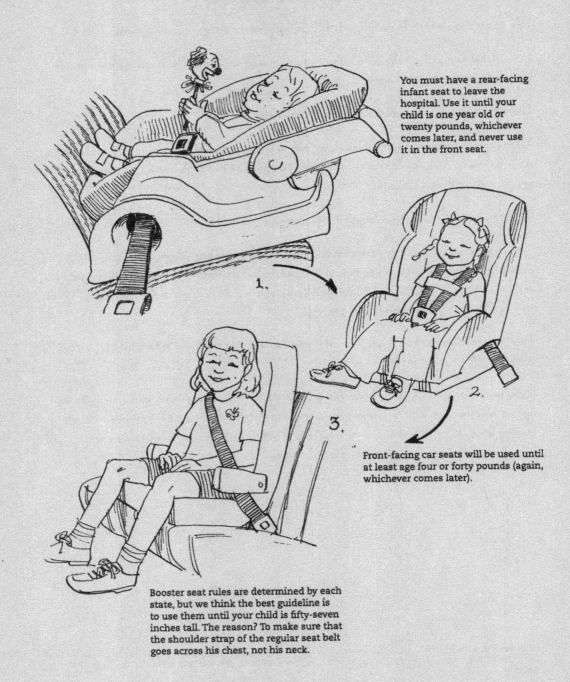

You must have a rear-facing infant seat to leave the hospital. Use it until your child is one year old or twenty pounds, whichever comes later, and never use it in the front seat.

1.

2.

3.

Front-facing car seats will be used until at least age four or forty pounds (again, whichever comes later).

Booster seat rules are determined by each state, but we think the best guideline is to use them until your child is fifty-seven inches tall. The reason? To make sure that the shoulder strap of the regular seat belt goes across his chest, not his neck.

The Car Seat

The biggest mistake made with car seats (besides not using them): Not securing the seat in the vehicle properly, which is the case an estimated 80 percent of the time. It actually can be quite difficult to get a snug fit, so it's worth having yours checked or installed by a pro. Local fire stations will do it. You can also find certified car seat technicians in your area who will install the seat; visit the website of the National Highway Traffic and Safety Administration at www.nhtsa.gov. While you're there, check for any car seat recalls.

Kids under five should never ride in the front seat. Being close to the windshield drastically increases the risk of injury, and the force of deploying airbags can severely injure or even kill a child. Most states don't allow children to ride shotgun until they're thirteen. If you have no choice and have to put a child in the front seat, disable the passenger side air bags or, if you can't, move the seat as far back as it goes to minimize the impact of the air bags should they deploy.

The recommended angle for a rear-facing car seat is tilting back 45 degrees. At 45 degrees, the back of the seat absorbs most of the forces in a crash. If the seat is overreclined, those forces go to the child's shoulders and neck instead of the car seat. Plus, the angle helps keep a newborn's airways open. You can test the angle by making an L with your thumb and index finger, then lining up the seat in between the two. If the seat angle juts out in between those fingers, it's 45 degrees.

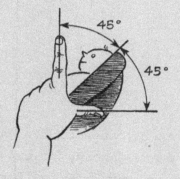

It's best if your car comes equipped with metal anchors that attach directly to the car seat. (All cars manufactured after 2000 are required to have them.) If not, you need to thread the seat belt through the car seat and pull as tight as you can. Then pull tighter. And even tighter. Get a couple of friends and all pull together. The seat must be rock solid to be fully effective.

Never leave your child in the car alone, due to the risk of heatstroke and other accidents.

10

Let's Get Medical

How to Navigate the Often Confusing
(and Sometimes Scary!)
World of Docs, Hospitals, and Emergencies

f you know us at all, then you may think of us as the DIY Docs. Do it yourself. Take responsibility for your own actions and behaviors. Take control over your health and your life. Eat real berries, not Frankenberries. That goes for you as well as for your child. So much of what good health is all about comes down to making good decisions on the front end so you can avoid the treatments and miseries on the back end.

But we'd be DIY Dingbats if we thought that every single health issue could be handled with a few ounces of prevention, a couple words of advice, and three rolls of duct tape.

Your child is going to need docs. Your child is going to need organized medicine. Your child—as much as we hope it's not the case—may need a stitch here, a cast there, and maybe even a medical mystery or two solved by a pro. And that's what this chapter is all about: providing everything you need to know about finding a pediatrician, getting the most out of checkups, and navigating the ER and hospital if it should ever become necessary.*

In this chapter, we offer more nuts and bolts than The Home Depot, and we hope that you will use these insights to help you and your fellow caregivers figure out what works best for your child and your family. No doubt, some of the issues we'll be dealing with in this chapter can be scary: one, because you're concerned about the health of your child; and two, because if you haven't been through it before, there are a lot of unknowns. Besides, we know that if it were a choice, you would rather that you be sick than your baby. So we hope you use this chapter as the ultimate weapon against fear: knowledge. After all, a smart parent is a prepared parent. And a prepared parent can handle medical issues calmly, coolly, and wisely, which is exactly what your child needs from you. Having a calm and confident attitude—rather than being anxious, which your child will pick up on—will go a long way toward helping your child get better.

What's Up, Doc? Finding the Right Pediatrician

We're sure there are millions of ways you *could* find a pediatrician. There's the ol' finger-in-the-phone book trick. Or you could just choose the neighborhood pediatrician's office because it's five minutes away from your home—which can be a great choice *if* that doc and you share the same views on health and wellness. But if the neighborhood doc seems more like Cruella De Vil, not such a good move. Or maybe you just pick the one that Aunt Joanie used two decades ago, hoping that he kept up with his CMEs (continuing medical education, in doc lingo). Sometimes, but not all the time, the easy way to go isn't always the smart way to go.

That's especially true when it comes to identifying a doc for your child. It may

---

* Special thanks to Jennifer Trachtenberg, M.D., and the Joint Commission, for their insights into the subject. Trachtenberg is author of *The Smart Parent's Guide to Getting Your Kids Through Checkups, Illnesses, and Accidents.*

take a little legwork and even some in-person interviewing to find a doctor who matches your approach to parenting and health. But once you ID a doctor that you like, you'll realize that the prep work was well worth it. And besides, sometimes it really is easy, especially if you live in a medically saturated area, or if you already know and trust the judgment of several parents near you.

So whether you live in rural Iowa or midtown Manhattan, how do you begin?

Step 1: Identify which docs are in your insurance company's network. That will automatically narrow the list.

Step 2: Scour your area for recommendations—from families with kids a little older than yours, neighbors, anybody you or your partner works with who has ties to the health care field. Which names keep popping to the tip of people's tongues? And do the folks recommending them share your approach to parenting and health care? Those docs should make your short list. If your situation is special (special needs, multiples, international adoption, and so on), you may want to focus your search on those with specialized expertise if they're available in your community.

Step 3: Take that short list and do a little online investigating. Start with a basic Google search to check out a hospital page or an online bio. You may happen upon affiliations with local organizations or charities, which is a positive sign. Other good sites include:

➲ The American Board of Medical Specialties (www.abms.org), to make sure that the doc is board certified and specializes in the area you want, like pediatrics or family medicine. In some areas, the family practice doc may be the most knowledgeable for the whole family but keep in mind that family practice training only includes three months of training in pediatrics, compared to three full years for the pediatrician.

➲ The Federation of State Medical Boards (www.fmsb.org), to see if the doc has had any serious disciplinary action against him or her. In most states, the information is free and public.

⊃ The Joint Commission (www.jointcommission.org), a private, nonprofit organization that leads the way in patient safety and health care quality. You can check any health care organization that the doctor is affiliated with to see if it gets a Gold Seal of Approval, denoting that it complies with rigorous safety standards.

Step 4: Once you've narrowed the list to the few pediatricians that you like, based on info gathered from the three previous steps, it's time to turn to in-person investigation. Most pediatricians routinely offer consultations—either prenatally or at a later stage in the game—to allow you to see if they are a good fit for you. Meet with your top choices and ask them (and their office staff and colleagues) about their views on breast feeding versus formula, child-rearing principles, and other topics that could be important to you. But also ask about how their offices work. Your goal is to find someone whose principles, temperament, and logistics agree with yours. Often, the doctors whose names keep coming up as the town favorites are no longer taking new patients. You have to decide if you want to try to pull out the connections, beg, or possibly look for someone else in the same practice. Below we're going to suggest some good questions you may ask, but we're not going to give you the answers, because there are often no "right" answers. Ultimately, you have to be the one to determine whether the answers the doc gives you feel right to you, so you can make your own decision.

• • •

Now, the funny thing about pediatricians isn't the fact that they have limitless Elmo bandages, it's the fact that there can be as many differences in docs as there are in musicians. Every doc conducts his or her medical orchestra in his or her own way. You'd think that kid ailments are all pretty standard in how they're treated. But the differences, well, make a difference. You'll find that some pediatricians take an aggressive, high-tech approach, wanting to treat every symptom, while others are more mellow and take a watch-and-wait approach to nonurgent issues. Some will answer email; others will not. Some are open to complementary medicine; others aren't. Some are willing to modify the American Academy of Pediatrics (AAP) vaccination

PAGING DR. JUNIOR

Your kid needs surgery? If you get a chance, ask if the hospital has tours or Child Life programs designed to put your small person at ease. Most children's hospitals have special dolls with IVs that can be put in them (no needles, of course), videos of what to expect, and lots of time for questions and explanations. This little bit of prevention can greatly ease a child's fear of the unknown—not to mention relieve his parents' anxiety.

schedule, while others insist on following it to the letter. (See our take on the hotly debated topic of vaccines on page 392.)

Ultimately, your goal during the doc interview is to feel a connection on a personal level. You're trusting this person to care for your little chickadee, and you want to feel that the doc is warm, smart, and really cares for kids—especially your kid. It may be important to you that she be a leader in the field; then again, brilliant with no bedside manner may not cut it for you. Since it's a doc's job to give advice, many dislike it when you don't take the advice they give. For example, a pediatrician may say, "Absolutely no pacifiers!" If that's something you cannot deal with, move on and find another doc.

In your interview, you can ask the office manager some of the basics; you should save the big-picture questions for the doc. Here are some questions you might consider:

Questions for Yourself

⊃ Is the office convenient? Can you park right up front so you don't have to lug the car seat a half mile? Or are the tolls more than the copay? In the first year, you'll be visiting the pediatrician fairly often; hopefully less so after that.

⊃ Is the office clean, cheerful, and comfortable, and does it have a separate sick-child waiting area? Or does it feel more like a tense courtroom awaiting a capital sentencing? Having a lot of toys is less relevant; we recommend bringing your own (see page 188).

○ Is the staff friendly? Or did you run into more than one Nurse Ratchet?

○ Did the doctor and staff seem concerned, caring, and friendly? Or did you not even get to meet the doctor?

Questions for the Office Manager
(If You Can't Find the Information Online)

○ Is the doc board certified? He should be proud enough to display the certificate.

○ What is the doc's education, training, and experience? How long has he been in practice?

○ What hospital(s) is the doc affiliated with? Is it the best hospital for children in the area?

○ Does the doctor accept your insurance? Does his hospital(s)?

○ Is the doc a solo practitioner? If so, who covers on evenings and weekends or when the doctor is away? How does the physician covering for your doc learn about your child?

○ Is the doctor part of a group? If so, will you visit your doctor exclusively, or will you see whoever is available (including, perhaps, a nurse practitioner)? Make sure to meet the partners or at least check their credentials.

○ Does the doc have early morning, evening, and/or weekend hours to accommodate your schedule?

○ Does the doc encourage email communication? Or maybe she wants u 2 text and is gr8 abt it?

○ How long can you expect to wait for a response when you email or phone with a question? Is it within a day, or would a transatlantic cruise deliver a message faster?

➲ How long is the response time for after-hours questions?

➲ Does the doc use electronic prescriptions? Most will now, as they reduce dosage and drug errors (because the doc's handwriting won't be an issue).

➲ Does the pediatrician's office have electronic medical records so that when Junior graduates from high school, his records are complete?

➲ Is this doc older than Methuselah and likely to retire before your child reaches kindergarten?

➲ Does the doc's journal *Pediatrics* ever get read? By the doc? Or is it used as a coloring book in the waiting room?★

Questions for the Doctor

➲ What is your attitude toward breast feeding versus bottle feeding? Most pediatricians will favor breast feeding, but if you choose to bottle feed, you don't need a heavy dose of doc-laden guilt to add to your own parental worries.

➲ How do you treat ear infections? This is a good litmus test for how interventionist she may be: Some dispense antibiotics liberally, while others encourage you to watch and wait, as most suspected ear infections resolve themselves within three days.

➲ What are your views about various parenting preferences (such as cosleeping and circumcision)?

➲ What are your feelings about complementary medicine? Ask more specifically about herbal remedies. This does not determine whether the doc is good or bad, but rather how open minded she is to modalities that she may be uncomfortable with. You want someone whose sensibilities match yours.

★ "Now, honey, try to color within the lines of this epiglottis diagram."

GETTING A SECOND OPINION

We know that second opinions can be as awkward as ill-timed burps. Patients worry that their doc will think they're questioning her competence. But, really, any good doc welcomes your seeking a second opinion—especially when you're dealing with something serious. Many docs actually like them, because it's one of the ways they learn about new things from other specialists in their field. The truth is that about 10 percent of people get second opinions, and one-third of the time, those second opinions change the diagnosis and/or the treatment. Here's a tactful way to bring up the subject without coming off as accusatory or offensive: "This sounds serious to me. I'd like to get a second opinion. Who would you take your child to?"

And this goes both ways: If you've joined the Anti-Reiki Revolution, then you do not want to pick a pediatrician who supports all things complementary with unquestionable faith. Or maybe there's some middle ground that makes you and your doctor most comfortable.

➲ What is your standard protocol for vaccinations? What are your thoughts on the timing of vaccinations and the administration of optional vaccinations?

The Office: Visiting the Doctor

Some kids never get sick. Some kids seem to spend more time in the doctor's office than they do in their own playrooms. No matter the case, at minimum your child will visit the doctor regularly for "well" checkups several times in the first year, tapering off to an annual physical by age two. That's the time for you and the doc to confab about your child's development, for you to ask about any concerns you have, and for your doc to get baseline measurements and impressions of your child. In this section, we'll outline some of the basics for handling these well visits and also give you some insight into what goes into a checkup, so that you can understand what your doc may be looking for.

To start, let's take a look at the basic checkups your child will have:*

Visit at Two Weeks. Unless there's a feeding problem or jaundice, you won't see the doc until ten to fourteen days. At this first visit, he will make sure that your baby's weight has returned to where it was at birth. Then he will conduct a physical exam that includes measuring head circumference, to make sure your baby's brain is growing; looking to make sure that your baby's eyes can focus on a face; checking your baby's hearing; and making sure that all the organs and systems are present and accounted for—including heart, lungs, nervous system—via a head-to-toe physical. The doc will inspect your baby's private parts to see whether the testicles are in the scrotum or hiding in the canal, or whether there are any labial adhesions. (That's where the lips of the vagina are fused together, a not uncommon condition that's easily treated by applying an estrogen cream.)

Baby's reflexes will also get checked: the Moro (startle) reflex, the grasp, the tonic neck reflex (think swordsman stance), the step reflex ("Look, Ma, I can walk!!). The doc will also be happy to hear about all the sleeping, pooping, and fussing that's been going on (with the baby!).†

Visits at Two, Four, and Six Months. Doc will take measurements (height, weight, head circumference) and tell you how your child fits on the growth chart. She'll ask about how your baby is doing with regard to various developmental milestones. At each visit, the doc will ask about what's going in and what's coming out: how much, how often, breast milk or formula, and how are those poops going?

At two months, the doc will also check for the two soft spots: one on top of

* If you choose the vaccination schedule devised by Dr. Robert W. Sears, you'll be going every month, rather than every two months in the beginning (see pages 408–9).
† Actually, a good doc will also ask about how you're doing—and look for signs of postpartum depression or baby blues.

the head and one midway down the back of the skull. They're called fontanels, and they're the membrane-covered openings at the points where the plates of the skull haven't yet fused together yet. Both should feel soft.

At four months, you get to discuss transitioning to solid (a relative term) food, and by six months, most kids are eating some supplemental food to receive adequate protein. At each visit, the doc will have a thorough once over, feeling the soft spot, checking reflexes, and so on.

At each visit, she'll review safety (like don't leave the baby on the couch or bed; by two months, many can wriggle off the edge, and by three months, some are already rolling. See our tips for baby-proofing your home on pages 251–55). At six months, the doc will discuss your baby's mobility in terms of sitting up and precrawling, as well as any sleeping or teething issues. Each visit comes complete with a head-to-toe physical, three shots and a squirt in the mouth of a fourth vaccine if you subscribe to the standard immunization schedule.

Visit at Nine Months.
This is an easy visit: no shots unless it's flu season! That leaves lots of time to discuss development, safety, stranger anxiety, feeding (wow—we get to start chicken! It's a bit allergenic before then), motor skills such as cruising, climbing, walking, and other fun topics. The pediatrician will check to see if your baby is ready for walking by checking his parachute response: Lift your baby up, then aim him toward the ground; the baby who is getting ready to walk will start to put his arms out to break his fall, whereas the baby who is not ready to walk will still be angling headfirst toward the ground. When he is ready to walk, he will also start standing flat-footed instead of up on his toes. Those are hints the pediatrician uses to tell if walking is imminent. And don't forget that whole head-to-toe physical thing, too, with the height, weight, and head circumference.

Visits at Twelve, Fifteen, and Eighteen Months.
At these visits, the doc will again get vital statistics such height, weight, and head circumference, and she will ask about language development and interactions with others. At twelve months, your baby's weight should be three times his birth weight. The doc will ask about feeding, the transition to whole milk (happens around twelve months), pee-

ing and pooping (always favorite topics), safety and exploration, and developmental milestones. By twelve months, most kids have mastered the fine pincer grasp: the art of picking a small object up between finger and thumb. First steps usually occur at about a year, but anywhere between nine and eighteen months is normal, and the doc will look for that toddler gait: tummy out, butt out, toes often out but occasionally in, and flat feet. (The fatty pad under toddlers' arches subsides by around two years.) With heightened mobility comes greater safety concerns, and the pediatrician will make sure you really have childproofed high and low. Plus, he'll be getting shots (see pages 406–7). And, somewhere between twelve and eighteen months, he'll have a blood test for lead and another for a hemoglobin or hematocrit (measurement for anemia). This is an easy blood draw that may cause you more angst than him; he'll cry for a second, then forget about it. If your baby is African American or of another ethnicity where sickle-cell anemia is a risk, he may need a sickle prep.

Visit at Two Years (and Annually After That). Every year, the doc will do a whole physical exam, although she'll stop measuring head circumference after two years; it will stay at that percentile and follow the growth curve as your child continues to grow. Most head growth occurs in that first year. Every visit will include a check for vision and hearing (done by observation until four to five years, and then using fun equipment in a separate room). In high-risk areas, your child may need an annual "snake bite" or "bubble" TB test (see vaccination schedule) and yearly flu and possibly H1N1 shots, but otherwise the two- and three-year-old visits are free of shots and sticks. The next big round of shots is at four to five years old, as a child prepares for kindergarten. Developmental screening continues at each age (looking for age-appropriate development of motor and language skills), making those milestones important and giving you the chance to have all your questions answered about why the kid next door can do this, but your small one can only do that. Sensory development issues can be big clues into all kinds of development issues. If you have any concerns, bring them up—an ounce of prevention is worth a ton of cure. (See page 46 for more details.)

• • •

While the docs and nurses will be taking the lead at your office visits, that doesn't mean that you should be a passive participant. In fact, the more you're involved, the more you'll get out of the visit. Here are some things you should consider:

Don't Save the Best for Last. It's smart to come to any doctor's visit (your own included) with a list of questions, but don't make the mistake that many parents make, by saving the most important questions for the end of the visit, when the doctor may feel that she has the least amount of time. Instead, open with the big questions (after pleasantries, of course), so that they're at the forefront of the doctor's thoughts when she's examining your child. Take notes, and leave room on your question list for them. (You'd be surprised how few give space on their papers to write down doctor comments!) And repeat the answers back to the doc to make sure you understood them correctly, or ask if you can use an audio recorder to make sure that you capture every word.

Prep Your Child. As your kid gets older, it's normal for him to be a little apprehensive about going to the doctor's office. (Needles ain't so fun, after all.) Tell him the reason why you go: Doctors want to see how children are growing and help healthy kids stay healthy; they also help sick kids feel better. At the same time, it's a good idea to tell your child what he can expect (see our discussions above), explaining that the doc may feel his tummy, tap his knee, and look in his eyes, ears, and mouth, and that you'll be right there every step of the way. You can even practice by playing doctor at home. (By the way, make sure to explain to your child as he gets older that a doc will have to glance at, and sometimes even touch, private parts. Since you've probably told your child that people shouldn't touch his private parts, you'll need to explain that docs are an exception because their job is to keep kids healthy.)

Be Prepared. On sick visits, you'll save the doc and nurses some time if you bring a list of symptoms (including when they started, how long they've lasted), as well as any medications that you may have given your child. Be sure to include over-the-counter drugs, vitamins, herbs, and homeopathic treatments. If you've found something on the internet that seems relevant, it's better to email or fax. It's unrealistic for a doc to be expected to know everything on the web about children's health, but they don't want to be overwhelmed with too much material.

HEADLINE PARENTING

Many parents get excited or inquisitive when they see the latest health news. Some other ways that you can handle headline parenting, after talking it over with your doc: Email the study author directly (most study author email addresses are listed on the front page of the journal abstract). You can also look for a second source to see if any other docs are supporting a new finding or technique, and if something appears in your local paper, it might be worth checking some national papers to see if their health sections are also covering it. By the way, since there's a lot of health information swirling out there, it does make sense to have some go-to sites that you trust. Our faves include the American Academy of Pediatrics (www.aap.org) and the Centers for Disease Control and Prevention (www.cdc.gov).

Bring Your Own Toys. Not only can they comfort a scared child, but they're also a better choice for the waiting room. Better to have your daughter play with her own toys than the ones that may be covered in germs from sick children. You may be waiting a long time too, so make sure you bring snacks and drinks just in case.

Follow Up. If you forgot something that was said at your appointment or didn't quite understand it, it's quite okay to send an email or make a phone call to clarify. It's better to get it right than to take a guess.

Medicine: Myths and Mysteries

Throughout this book, we've recommended various medications for treating specific conditions, but we also believe that it's worth spending a little time talking more generally about giving your child meds. Our overriding principle: In many, many cases, kids don't need medicine to get better; nature will run its course, and your child will soon feel better—and get better—on his own. There are risks associated with both prescription and over-the-counter meds, so don't take medicating your child lightly. Here's where finding a doc whose principles mirror yours is especially important; you'll want to feel comfortable following her lead when it comes to medication recommendations. Below are some of the major things you need to know about doing drugs:

Don't Push for Unnecessary Meds. When your child is coughing, sneezing, and downright miserable, the temptation is there: Just give me something that will help her feel better, Doc. The fact is that 90 percent of colds are from viruses, not bacteria. Antibiotics generally kill bacteria, not viruses, so nine times out of ten, that medicine will do nothing to help kill the offending invader. But that's not the most serious reason why prescribing an antibiotic for a virus is so bad. Unnecessary use of antibiotics increases the chances that bacteria will get used to them and eventually become resistant to the drugs. That increases the odds that super bugs (like MRSA, or methicillin-resistant Staphylococcus aureus) will spread, and these resistant strains can be especially dangerous because they are untreatable by common antibiotics. So here's a case where you need to really follow your doc's lead, and if she says your child has a virus that needs to run its course and can't be treated with antibiotics, then do the other things to make her feel better until that course is indeed run. (See page 176 for virus-treating tips.)

Prevent Medication Mistakes. While most medication mistakes aren't serious, in a small percentage of cases they can lead to serious harm or death, so it always pays to be vigilant when doing your own dosing (in the case of OTC meds) or following instructions from the doc. Bottom line: *Ignore the ages on the recommended dosing charts on OTC meds;* go by weight and start with the lowest suggested dose. Also, do not redose before the recommended time limit. If you child throws up medicine right after he takes it, consult your doc on guidelines for redosing. Some other things you can do:

⊃ Make sure that the doc uses electronic prescriptions, so no handwriting errors get made and the computer program can check the prescribed dose against the child's reported weight as well as any possible interactions with

THE IDEAL MEDICINE CABINET

When your child is sick or has an accident, the last thing you feel like doing is hopping in the car to find a twenty-four-hour pharmacy. At home, you want to have a well-stocked (and well-locked) cabinet containing items that can help you handle garden-variety health issues that affect kids. Here's how we'd stock it:

MUST HAVE

⊃ **Acetaminophen and ibuprofen (children's Tylenol and Motrin):** for pain relief and reducing fevers (see exceptions for use on page 275).

⊃ **Antihistamines such as Benadryl (diphenhydramine), Claritin (loratadine), and Zyrtec (cetirizine):** for allergic reactions and hives. Always Benadryl; the other two are optional.

⊃ **An antibiotic ointment such as Neosporin or Bacitracin:** for cuts and scrapes.

⊃ **Saline drops:** for stuffy noses.

⊃ **Calamine lotion and hydrocortisone cream:** for stings (no Caladryl or Benadryl cream; it's too easy to overdose the Benadryl component in the topical formulation).

⊃ **Moisturizers such as Cetaphil, Lubriderm, and Aquaphor:** for preventing and relieving dry, itchy skin and chapped lips.

other meds the child might be taking. Everyone can read these, and hopefully the EMR has built in fail-safes, as well as those checks in the pharmacy, to further reduce medicine errors.

⊃ When your doc is prescribing a medicine, ask that your child be weighed in kilograms; that's the unit of measurement used to calculate proper doses for kids. Make sure that you get the weight of your child *that* day, since kids grow faster than weeds.

- ⊃ **Hydrogen peroxide:** for puncture wounds and ear infections. Also dissolves ear wax, which can harbor bacteria and cause pain independently. Mix a small amount half and half with water in the cap, then just pour a few drops into each ear; the wax will soften and fall out. Hydrogen peroxide is also good for cleaning bloodstains from clothing, furniture, and carpeting.

- ⊃ **Band-Aids**

OPTIONAL

These are some of the remedies that the authorship team has used:

- ⊃ **Honey:** works as an effective cough suppressant, but don't it give to children under one because of the risk of infant botulism.

- ⊃ **Rescue remedy:** a Bach flower essence that may work to calm kids. It's unknown whether the effect is biological or psychological, but it seems to work.

- ⊃ **Arnica gel:** to rub on bruises or muscle soreness for topical support.

- ⊃ **Aromatherapy:** ImmuPower from "Young Living Oils" (www.young-living-oils.net/oilblends.html) on the infants' feet comforted the Oz children and might help children's immune systems.

- ⊃ **Elderberry extract syrup:** might help immune function. Starting at age two, children can take a half teaspoon daily for up to three months.

⊃ Get the dosage from the doctor in milliliters, not teaspoons, because milliliters are more precise. One homemade teaspoon can actually contain between 2 and 9 milliliters, so there's lots of variance. And use an accurate, medically labeled syringe or dosing cup instead of the ol' spoon.

⊃ Clarify where the decimal point goes. Half of all dosing errors come from the fact that the parent didn't know whether the dose was, say, 1.0 milligram or 10 milligrams. Always make sure you know the position of that plucky point. For liquid medications, ask the nurse to demonstrate the correct amount using water and a syringe or dosing cup.

◒ Ask the doc to read the prescription aloud to you. Bad handwriting and similarly spelled meds can cause mistakes. Reading it back to you will help you cement in your mind what you're supposed to get, so you can double-check it with the pharmacist.

◒ Ask about any possible interaction with foods, vitamins, or other meds. Does your little guy need to avoid the sun while on this medicine?

◒ Don't fall into the trap of thinking that over-the-counter meds are safer than prescription meds. They can be just as dangerous. For example, one overdose of acetaminophen (Tylenol) can be toxic to the liver. And be aware that marketing claims on packaging are just that: marketing claims. Follow your doc's and our recommendations about using OTC drugs for common self-treatable health issues.

◒ Write down the time whenever you give your child any med, especially if two caregivers are doling out the medicine or if you have multiple sick children at once. That will help you avoid any "uh . . . uh . . . uh . . ." moments when trying to remember the last time you gave the medicine.

◒ Make sure that the dosing instructions are clear to other caregivers (babysitters, day care) and that medicine is properly stored: for instance, refrigerated if required, or kept out of direct sunlight.

◒ Check and follow expiration dates on meds, and do not "share" meds between children, just because you suspect they may have the same illness. Expiration dates are very conservative on meds, and even the YOU docs cheat a little bit on expirations of OTC pills or chewables. But we don't recommend pushing the dates on liquid forms, and please make sure to store them in a cool, dark, and dry place (not the bathroom). The issue of expiration dates really has more to do with potency (does it work?) than toxicity (will it harm?).

- Always complete a course of antibiotics, even if your child appears to be cured after the first few doses. Incomplete dosing invites a recurrence of the infection as well as development of a resistant strain.

- Throw out any extra medicine.

- Be careful about potentially overdosing your child by other means (such as using topical and oral Benadryl simultaneously) or unintentionally causing adverse interactions (using herbal remedies with pharmacologically active ingredients).

Use These Guidelines. You'll see medication recommendations throughout the book, but here are some general principles to keep in mind about specific medications:

- Avoid decongestants because they contain ingredients that can make your child agitated, irritable, or unable to sleep. Try saline drops instead.

- Never give your child aspirin—not even baby aspirin. Aspirin plus a viral infection can cause Reye syndrome, a combination of liver and brain dysfunction that can lead to death.

- Don't give acetaminophen (Tylenol) unless you're sure of the dose, and if you are needing it for five days consistently, it's worth checking in with your doc to see if your child needs to be seen. Persistent fever can occur with illnesses such as influenza, but if that has not been formally diagnosed, consult with the pediatrician to make sure other processes are not going on, such as Kawasaki syndrome, which causes five-plus days of fever, cherry red lips, peeling fingers, toes, and bottoms, often with a more generalized rash, and requires medical treatment as promptly as it is diagnosed.

- Avoid giving combined cough and cold medicines, because they're often made up of a combo of drugs, which can be a lot for small bodies to take. And they tend to treat the parents' symptoms (Mommy and Daddy are tired and need sleep), not the kid's.

Help the Medicine Go Down. Skip the spoonful of sugar, but use these tips to help your little one swallow the icky stuff. With infants, use a dropper to squirt the medicine toward the side and back of the cheek. If your baby doesn't take well to the medicine and refuses to swallow it, try blowing in his face. It sounds cruel, but it makes him swallow—and it's for his own good, right? With toddlers, you can role-play (giving it to a stuffed animal first), distract the child (giving it to him while he's watching TV), or even freeze his taste buds with a pre-medicine Popsicle. After a few doses, even a resistant kid will usually give in. You can also mix it into food or a bottle, as long as you know she's a good eater and will down the whole portion.

Uh-Oh: Navigating the ER

We hope that the closest you get to an ER is watching the popular TV show in syndication, but the simple fact is that almost one-third of children go to the emergency department every year. The cause can be anything: a broken bone, a febrile seizure, a fever that seems way too high, a Lego that decided it wanted to be built inside the intestines. No matter the case, it's a very tense and scary time for parents. We hope that you can avoid emergencies. (See our prevention tips from the previous chapter.) But the fact is that no matter how careful you are, you can't prevent everything, and accidents can't be timed to coincide with your doc's office hours. So it's best to be well versed in how to handle these tough situations *before* they occur. Here's our best advice.

Make a Plan. Discuss with your pediatrician how she likes to handle emergencies. Should you call her before going to the ER? (The answer should be yes; many pediatricians will call ahead or meet you there to help the process along, so it's wise to program your pediatrician's number into your cell phone. The exception is major trauma, when your first call should be to 911; then call the pediatrician while you're en route.) Getting some of these issues straightened out before an emergency happens will speed things up and make sure you get great treatment pronto. One more tip: Make sure you always have your insurance card on hand.

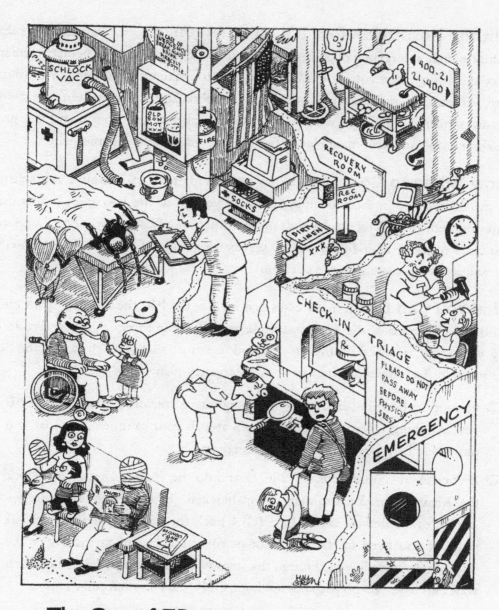

Figure 10.1 **The Cast of ER** The ER is filled not only with lots of anxiety but also with lots of people doing different jobs. To help your child stay calm in what's likely a scary situation for her, it will help for you to stay calm (or at least look like you are!) and be prepared as much as possible by understanding how the process works. It's smart to do homework on the best pediatric ERs in the area, and always remember: Hold her hand. She needs it, even if she doesn't ask for it.

Visit the Hospital Before It's an Emergency. Once you and your doc identify which emergency department you prefer (ideally one with pediatric emergency specialists), then you should take a dry run to make sure you know how to get there, navigate the area, and figure out where to park. You'd be surprised how many ERs are actually hard to find within a hospital complex. A dry run can save you precious minutes—and keep panic levels from rising—during a real emergency.

Know When to Go. Sometimes it's a true judgment call: Should you wait to call the doc's office in the morning, or should you go to the ER or an urgent care center immediately? While it depends on the situation, of course, you can always call your doc's office or after-hours on-call service to get his or her take. The following box will also help you make the decision.

What You Can Do. In many cases that involve the ER, the health of your child will be in the hands of the pros. But there are still some things that you can do to help your child, to speed up the process, and to ensure that your child gets the best care possible. Add these activities to your emergency plan:

➲ Pretend to be calm; anxiety is as contagious as rotavirus. Your child needs your soothing voice, not anxiety. She'll absorb your calmness, and that will ultimately help her manage a scary situation.

➲ If your child is unresponsive, call 911 and do the "ABC" check: (A) Check the **Airway**, to make sure that it's not blocked. (B) Check for **Breathing**—sounds of inhaled or exhaled air. (C) Check for **Circulation**—your child's pulse. If you need to start CPR or perform the Heimlich maneuver, the dispatcher can walk you through the steps while the paramedics are on their way. Better yet, be prepared by taking a CPR class or a refresher course.

➲ Stop any bleeding by applying pressure on the wound. Keep holding the pressure for at least ten minutes and do not cheat by peeking early, since, once the bleeding restarts, you have do it all over again for another ten minutes.

➲ Don't move your child if you suspect a head, neck, or back injury. Cover her with a blanket and wait for the paramedics.

Call 911 and Use Ambulance (Call Doc En Route) No Matter What Age of Child	For Infant: Call/See Pediatrician (and on His Recommendation or When in Doubt, go to ER)	For Age One and Older: Call/See Pediatrician (and on His Recommendation or When in Doubt, go to ER)
• A laceration (wound or cut) that is deep or large or involves the chest, head, or abdomen • A large burn that involves the hands, face, or groin • Evidence that your child has swallowed a poisonous substance or medication • Confusion, headache, vomiting, or loss of consciousness after a head injury • Uncontrollable seizures • Severe respiratory distress and/or skin or lips that look blue, purple, or gray (bright red skin and lips usually aren't a serious problem) • Loss of consciousness	• Inconsolable crying or lethargy • Vomiting and/or diarrhea for twenty-four hours or more • Dry diapers for twelve hours or more • Difficulty breathing • Refusing fluids for twenty-four hours or more • A fever above 100.2 degrees *in infants less than two months old* • Fever with a red or purple rash • Seizurelike jerking movements • Loss of consciousness or syncope—the medical term for fainting • General listlessness, dry mouth, crying with no tears, not urinating or urinating very dark urine (all signs of dehydration)	• Abdominal pain • Difficulty breathing • Severe headache or neck pain • Increasing trouble breathing or chest pain • General listlessness, dry mouth, crying with no tears, not urinating, or urinating very dark urine

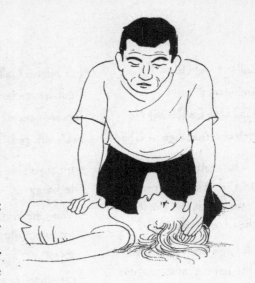

- ⊃ Call your pediatrician on your way to the ER—as long as you're not driving! If your doc talks to the emergency department, there's a good chance that you'll be seen faster.

- ⊃ Be nice. It's simple human nature: Nicer people get treated better than mean, angry, irritated people. You can be assertive, but don't be antagonistic.

- ⊃ Don't give your child food or drink in the waiting room. If he needs surgery, the food won't mix well with anesthesia.

- ⊃ If your child's symptoms have worsened while you've been waiting to be seen, tell the triage nurse, "My child's getting worse." You are your child's advocate and protector. You can be assertive without being rude. If your child needs to be seen, let it be known. Then describe what's changed. It will get some attention from the triage nurse. But don't try to snow the nurse just to get faster attention; that won't help.

Extended Stay: Hanging in the Hospital

There are plenty of heartbreak moments that come for parents: when you have to leave your child for the first time, when he learns that Santa lives in the same house as he does, when he gets rejected at the school dance. But one of the toughest challenges for parents comes when they have to see their child in pain. We've dealt with many levels of pain and sickness throughout the book, and sometimes those issues may warrant more attention than a quick trip to the doc or even the ER. An overnight hospital stay—whether necessary because of an infection that requires IV antibiotics or an operation of some sort—requires a special mind-set and level of parental insight. Consider these steps if you have time to prepare (might not be the case if your child is admitted in an emergency):

Find the Right Place. For something like IV antibiotics, you'll most likely go to the hospital with which your child's doctor is affiliated. But if you're in a situation where you have a choice and some time to find a hospital that fits your needs, check to see that the hospital is accredited by the Joint Commission (www.qualitycheck.org), which helps hospitals and other health care organizations provide a safe and high-quality environment. Of course, you'll also want to talk to your doc to make sure that the hospital matches your needs when it comes to insurance, location, and the procedures or treatments your child requires. Finally, the best question you can ask your doc is this one: Which hospital would she choose if her child were in the same situation?

You definitely want a pediatric hospital, which has specialized docs like pediatric anesthesiologists. Why? Because children are *not* small adults, biologically or emotionally. In a study comparing general hospitals and pediatric centers, the rate of kids' medical complications was a whopping 80 percent lower at the children's facilities, where the staffs were experienced in treating youngsters. The next best thing is a hospital with a full-scale pediatric department. You may find that a center outside of your immediate area might turn out to be a better option for a specific procedure or specialization.

Once you ID the few hospitals that you and your doc like, you should ask the following questions (the hospital's website may have some of the answers, too):

⊃ What percentage of staff docs are board certified? This means that the docs have passed an exam given by a specialty board of the American Board of Specialties. About 85 percent of U.S. docs are board certified.

⊃ Can you see the hospital's patient-satisfaction surveys? If they're doing a good job, they'll be more likely to share them with you. If they're feeding patients leather sandwiches regularly, they may not want to.

⊃ What percentage of the nurses are RNs? Registered nurses have more training than licensed practical nurses (LPNs). On average, about 85 percent

WHO'S THE DOC?

A list of other docs that some children may need to see:

- **Pediatric neurologists:** M.D.s who evaluate children with possible neurological problems to determine whether or not there is a neurological problem and especially look at the causes of problems. Their bread-and-butter diagnoses are seizures and headaches. Some specialize only in epilepsy and its management, while others may concentrate on cerebral palsy or children with other physical challenges. They usually see children of all ages.

- **Child and adolescent psychiatrists:** M.D.s who address psychological disorders such as depression, bipolar, schizophrenia, and ADHD. They focus on the diagnosis, although sometimes they depend on a psychologist to do the diagnosing and counseling while they focus on the medication management. They mostly see children who are school age through adolescence.

- **Developmental-behavioral pediatricians:** M.D.s who evaluate children with developmental and/or behavioral problems and usually focus on children with

of a hospital's nursing staff is made up of RNs. That's not to say there aren't some outstanding LPNs out there, but you want to make sure that the majority of nurses are RNs.

- Does a pharmacist participate in rounds? If so, that will help reduce the risk of medication errors.

- Does the facility have pediatric supplies and equipment, and can you tour the pediatric floor? Or do they keep it more closely guarded than a celebrity A-lister's hotel room?

- Is there a fall-prevention program? Recent studies show that one-third of pediatric patients fall while in the hospital. Good places have systems and behaviors like aggression, ADHD, autism, developmental delays, and learning disabilities. They provide diagnosis and develop a management plan regarding school, behavioral interventions, medication, and therapeutic interventions, which include PT, OT, speech, and home interventions. They work with children under the age of twelve and often younger than six.

⊃ **Pediatric physiatrists (or physical medicine doctors):** M.D.s who work with children and adolescents who have suffered a traumatic brain injury or cerebral palsy. They usually work in a center and manage a team of therapists, including PT, OT, speech pathologists, and psychologists, who develop a plan to maximize function.

⊃ **Clinical or pediatric psychologists:** Ph.D.s who provide counseling for psychological problems. This may include behavioral management of children with disruptive behaviors, social problems, and depression. They frequently focus on a particular problem such as anxiety, a particular age group (teens, for instance), or use a particular technique such as cognitive-behavioral therapy or family therapy.

⊃ **Pediatric neuropsychologists:** Ph.D.s who conduct psychoeducational testing for problems such as learning disabilities and various forms of brain damage.

devices that help reduce the chances of an accident, such as child-sized beds and floor mats in the bathroom.

⊃ How does the medical center ensure the security of its pediatric patients? Some hospitals use an electronic bracelet system that buzzes if the child is outside the area where she should be. Fake handcuffs? Not a good sign.

⊃ What are the rules for visitors and for parents who want to stay overnight?

⊃ For surgeries: How many of that particular surgery does the hospital perform annually, and what is the success rate? The higher the numbers, the better. Is the surgeon a specialist in pediatric surgery, and is there an on-staff (and available) board certified pediatric anesthesiologist? If no, say no to that hospital, unless there is no place that can say yes within 150 miles.

Be Prepared. You'll have several people who will tell you what to bring for a child's hospital stay. Here's our checklist:

- ⊃ A list of any medications, vitamins, and supplements that your child takes. Give a copy to the pediatric nurse in charge.

- ⊃ Slippers to keep germs off your child's feet. Some kids like having their own pajamas, while others like wearing the hospital gown.

- ⊃ Toiletries. Yes, hospitals may provide these, but it can feel "homier" if they are actually from home.

- ⊃ Clothes to go home in, like a loose T-shirt and pants.

- ⊃ A favorite stuffed animal or toy, and other comforting reminders of home.

- ⊃ Your own games or toys to occupy time. Great hospitals have a Child Life Program, or special people whose goal is to make your child's stay more enjoyable, or at least tolerable; they come around with games and videos to help keep your child occupied.

- ⊃ A notebook for you to write down information about tests, procedures, medications, or post-stay instructions.

- ⊃ An overnight bag for you that includes a pillow, toiletries, and your cell phone charger.

- ⊃ Books,* and maybe even a portable DVD player for your child to watch her favorite movies or shows.

- ⊃ iPod with your child's favorite tunes (great for relaxation and distraction).

- ⊃ Photos of family, friends, pets.

- ⊃ Don't forget to clean the items that your child may touch in the hospital—

---

* For yourself, bring a copy of YOU: The Smart Patient, which can help you become a strong advocate for your child during her stay.

like computer keyboards and remote controls—with rubbing alcohol to help prevent infection.

Put Him at Ease. There's no doubt that your child is just as nervous as you are about the upcoming hospital visit. And there's also no doubt that he's looking to you for cues that everything is going to be all right. Even babies can pick up on nonverbal signals, so you need to stay as soothing and relaxed as you can.

You should do the same for toddlers, too, but you can also add in some verbal comfort as well. For example, be up front with your child: Take a few minutes to explain to him what is going to happen and why he's going to the hospital. But avoid using scary words like *needle* and *knife,* and don't compare anesthesia to going to sleep, because he may equate going to sleep with the way that the family dog was "put to sleep." One of the best things you can do is talk about the future—talk about things you're going to do next week, or next summer, anything that helps your child think a little bit past the immediate issue.

Make Little Requests. In scary situations, you can help reduce anxiety with some simple gestures. How can you help him feel more comfortable? For one, you can ask the nurse to apply a numbing gel before your kid gets a shot or has blood drawn. That'll take some of the ouch out. And if your child has to have a surgical mask, have it lined with flavored ChapStick.

Watch the Wash. You have many things to think about while you're with your child in the hospital, but put this one at the top of the list: Make sure that everyone—*everyone*—who touches or treats your child washes his or her hands. The staff needs to use sanitizer or wash with soap and warm water. It's the single most effective way to keep your child from picking up an infection in the hospital. Many staffers fail to wash their hands before seeing a new patient, so it's up to you to make the request. If you don't see staffers wash their hands, ask them to do so. Because they know the importance of it, they will. Don't feel uncomfortable, like you're being the bad cop. You're speaking up to protect your child, and you shouldn't have one iota of guilt for doing so.

YOU: Raising Your Child

The Plan

Okay, folks. Time to get going. You've got quite a ride ahead of you as you guide your child through life. It's a challenging journey, but there are some amazing sights along the way. First steps! Hugging the neighbor's puppy! Dance recital! Above all, your job is to help your child chart a healthy and happy course through life by giving her the tools she needs to maximize her potential socially, intellectually, and biologically. While you're taking the lead on this metaphorical river journey, it's important to remember that the ultimate aim is to hand the paddle over to your child so that she can confidently navigate the currents of life on her own. Until that time, your child will trust in and rely on you—that you love her and care for her, and that you're going to do what you can to protect her while still giving her the opportunity to experience all of life's adventures (within reason and the law).

Quite the responsibility. Amazing levels of potential satisfaction.

While this book is about children's health, it's also as much about you: how you model behavior, how you guide your child toward making healthy choices, and how you create the optimal environment for learning and developing.

We hope that you will use our miniature river (and accompanying map) as your manual: the guide's guide, if you will. In it, we highlight some of the milestones and obstacles you'll encounter along the way, as well as some tips and tricks to make the ride a little smoother. You can always refer to the rest of the book if you'd like more information on a particular subject.

Before we begin, we're going to remind you of our overriding parenting principles, the Super Six—a map of actions. We'd also like you to remember that this timeline is very general: Although there are so-called "typical" ranges for reaching various developmental milestones, not every child follows the same schedule, so don't interpret these as hard-and-fast rules and don't panic if your child is a little off. Do, however, use them as markers to help you figure out if some things don't seem quite right. Our timeline will help you understand your child so you can interpret his behaviors and nudge his progress along with less worry.

When you're on the river, we encourage you to consult the book for advice both practical and philosophical, but oftentimes, instinct is the best compass of all. Since your child is not a blank slate (parental DNA ensures that), your job is to help her become who *she* wants to be, rather than trying to grow the "perfect" child. If your nose is too far in a book, then you may just miss the rocks looming ahead. Good parenting is about being aware of your child and of the environment.

Enjoy the ride.

THE MAP

The Super Six Principles You Need to Remember—and Actions You Should Take

ACTION 1 ➤ GIVE ATTENTION

Early on, kids can't tell you their needs or wants by speaking, so they tell you by crying. Later, they can tell you very well what they need and want, but they opt to do it with text messages (and sometimes crying). In any case, no matter how young or old a child is, the fact is that the thing they want most of all—and the thing that's most crucial to their biological and psychological development—is simply this: your attention. Research shows that giving positive attention to children, in the form of everything from babbling back to them as infants to having regular family dinners, is associated with healthier and better-adjusted kids. And kids who cannot find positive attention will figure out how to use negative attention to get what they need (the toddler banging his head against the floor in the middle of a tantrum to get something sugary in the grocery store, for example). So find the ways to use positive attention to direct behaviors in the way you want, rather than waiting for the negative behaviors to take over. It takes energy, creativity, a bit of humor, and tons of patience to keep that attention positive.

Another key is figuring out how to give attention without spoiling. This can be especially tough for working parents, who may feel they need to find ways to make up for the hours they spend away from their children. Just remember that attention isn't about things, it's about taking a walk in the park and pointing out different kinds of birds rather than taking a walk through the mall and buying the latest toy or gadget. It's about talking to your child rather than plopping him in front of the TV. It's about getting down on the floor to play and having a catch without checking your BlackBerry in between throws. It's about using your eyes and your ears and your hugs, not your credit cards, to make a difference in your child's life. The benefits are immeasurable for them—and for you too.

ACTION 2 ➤ BE A MODEL

Everything you do—and we mean everything—is observed and processed by your child. She's like a human recording device. Your child takes all of that info and figures, "Hey, that's the way I'm supposed to act!" (See our discussion of mirror neurons in chapter 3.) You may also remember from early on in the book that most of the messages that kids receive don't come from what you tell them but from all the *nonverbal* cues that accompany the actual words: your tone of voice, your body language, the gestures you use. If you want your child to eat healthfully, telling her to eat sautéed cauliflower while you order fried onion rings isn't gonna work. If you want her to have healthy friendships, make sure she sees you resolving conflicts in a respectful way. What is that they say about actions speaking louder than words?

ACTION 3 ➤ PLAY TO THEIR STRENGTHS

Back in chapter 2, you read about connections between neurons. Those connections are how we learn, how we form memories, how we develop skills. Connections that we don't cultivate disappear. It's the ol' "use it or lose it" phenomenon in action. This is especially true for kids, because our neural network is most malleable when we're young. But the thing is, young kids are really unaware of the areas in which they have talent or skill, be it art, music, sports, or soufflé making. Our job as parents is to help identify the areas where they have both interest and perhaps natural talent, and when we find those areas, gently nudge them in that direction to allow them to experience the satisfaction and self-esteem that comes from fulfilling their potential. That doesn't mean signing them up for hours of tennis lessons or chaining them to a piano, and it also doesn't mean telling them they shouldn't take art classes because it's clear they're no Picasso. There are benefits to doing things purely for pleasure, too. Follow your youngster's lead and resist imposing your own agenda.

ACTION 4 ➤ MAKE IT AUTOMATIC

Bottom line: Parenting can be darn hard. It's tiring, it's challenging, it's exasperating, and on any given day, you can be filled to your eyeballs with stress. There's no denying it. Part of the trick to effective parenting is to take away some of the struggles by making good, healthy behavior automatic. How do you do that? Through repetition early on. It's easier to get a child to eat healthfully if he's fed good foods right from the start, for example. If you go back to our river analogy, it makes sense: In a river that has several possible branches, the direction the boat will naturally gravitate to is the path where the channel is deeper and the water runs faster; the depth of the channel comes from the repetitive pounding and churning of the water. Just as kids develop muscle memory, they also develop behavioral memory. Establishing good habits early leads to the most benefit later on.

ACTION 5 ➤ FIND THE "YES" POINTS

From the perspective of many kids, parents have a four-word vocabulary: "No!" and "Don't you dare!" And while there's nothing wrong with establishing limits for your child and teaching her that there are boundaries and safety issues, you do need to be thoughtful about how you dole out your allotment of no's. Parenting doesn't have to be all about crisis management. Instead find calm(ish) opportunities where you can talk to your child and explain why it's indeed unsafe to choose the top of the fridge as a hiding place. On an even deeper level, you need to watch your child with a level of anticipation (experts call it anticipatory guidance), where you learn to see potential problems before they happen and steer your child to something else—kind of like keeping a soccer ball in play. This can mean diverting your child from the monkey bars if he's not ready and toward another piece of equipment, or allowing the game of "close the cupboard" to proceed with pinch-free fingers because you already put the safety latch on that door. It's not that "no" doesn't have a place; it's just that "yes" gives your child more opportunities to explore and learn about the world. Redirection and distraction are important skills a parent must learn early on.

ACTION 6 ➤ REMEMBER, LIFE IS A PLAYGROUND

We've spent a lot of time in this book talking about the hallowed middle ground: trying to strike the right balance between too much and not enough, whether it's in the areas of discipline, food, or TV habits. And that's where you should try to live your parenting life, neither overwhelming nor underwhelming your child. That's especially true when it comes to the topic of hyperparenting, or overparenting. While it makes sense to have your child involved in all kinds of activities and to allow her to cultivate new talents, we don't think it makes much sense to have children scheduled like little CEOs. Leave them time to play, to create, to use all of their senses, to bang pots, to see what games they can invent with a couple of pillows and a cardboard box. Unstructured playtime—the time when a child's imagination goes wild and his brain development does the same thing—needs to be sacred time. Remember that, enjoy it, maybe try to catch what you can on video, and reap its joys and rewards.

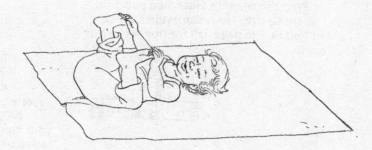

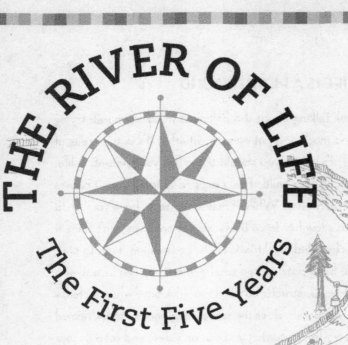

THE RIVER OF LIFE
The First Five Years

BEFORE BIRTH

Find a pediatrician whose principles are aligned with you about such things as vaccinati schedules, complementary medicine, and how to treat infections, and whose style is a good fit in terms of degree of guidance, attitude, and office responsiveness. (See page 258.)

Those outlets covered? It's easier to childproof the house now than in between naps, cries, bottles, and those precious little poops.

Prep the car seat. Make sure it's installed correctly (more than 80 percent aren't; we recommend that you consult a certified technician). She starts out facing back. (See page 257.)

Begin interviewing nannies or researching day care if you plan to return to work soon after birth. (See pages 324–25.)

Prep the nursery. Have Dad paint the room so that Mom can avoid exposure to toxins. See page 319 for tips on buying a crib.

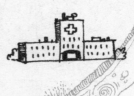

Talk to your baby-to-be and use his name (if you have one picked out); it will help him get used to your voice, just as he gets used to the food you eat.

BIRTH

Lesson from epigenetics: Changes made early can alter the way genes are expressed. Make healthy choices right from the start, and you'll set your kid on a course toward great health.

Give breast feeding a try and stick with it, even if it's tough early on. It's the best nutritional nectar for a baby. Though we realize there are some circumstances that [mak]e it hard to breast-feed, we [enco]urage you to do it if at all [poss]ible.

Make sure to get your own nutrients, including 600 milligrams a day of DHA, which is not only crucial for baby's brain development but can also keep your gray matter firing and stabilize your mood. (See page 112.)

Keep taking your prenatal vitamins for as long as you breast-feed.

THREE DAYS

Sniff, sniff. Babies this old who breast-feed can distinguish their mother's milk from that of other mothers based on smell alone.

To prevent SIDS, put Baby to sleep on his back or side and keep all potentially suffocating objects out of the crib.

TWO WEEKS

First posthospital pediatrician visit. Bring up any concerns you have; write them down beforehand (and leave room to write answers) and get the most pressing ones out quickly. Most times, everything you're going through is perfectly normal. Baby sneezing? He's clearing his nose in the best way he can.

Breast-fed babies tend to poop more than formula-fed ones (two to five per day compared to one or two). The good news? Baby poops smell better while Baby is breast-feeding. Adding formula changes the odor, texture, and color. Either way, at this age, stools should be brown or a seedy yellow green.

The key to a successful burp: Apply counterpressure (hic!) by gently pushing against his belly with your collarbo

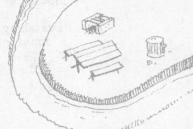

ONE MONTH

Listen up. Your child can't talk, but she may be "pinging" to you by sending nonverbal cue about what she wants and needs. Mimic her sounds and pay attention to how she responds to you, too. She may start making little noises or barks—it's fun to echo them back to her. (See page

High-contrast toys (black-and-white) are great at thi age. Choose them over pastel-colored ones, which will harder for Baby to focus on.

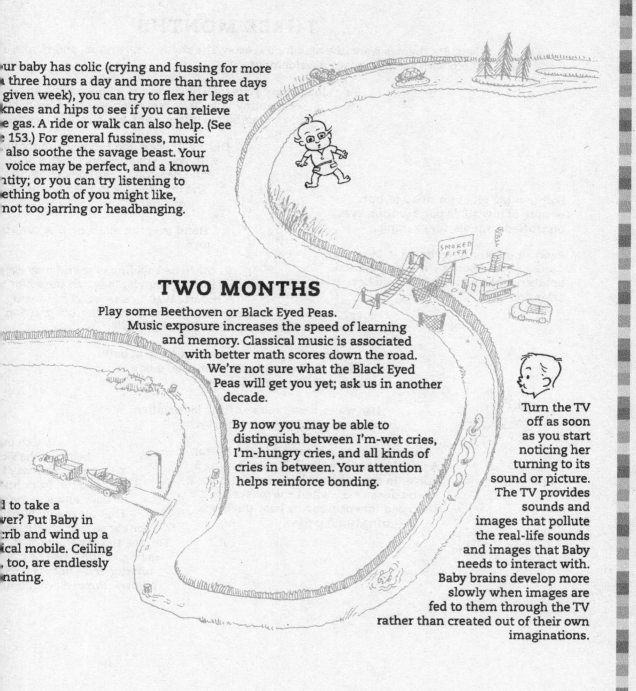

ur baby has colic (crying and fussing for more
a three hours a day and more than three days
given week), you can try to flex her legs at
knees and hips to see if you can relieve
e gas. A ride or walk can also help. (See
e 153.) For general fussiness, music
also soothe the savage beast. Your
voice may be perfect, and a known
ntity; or you can try listening to
ething both of you might like,
not too jarring or headbanging.

TWO MONTHS

Play some Beethoven or Black Eyed Peas.
Music exposure increases the speed of learning
and memory. Classical music is associated
with better math scores down the road.
We're not sure what the Black Eyed
Peas will get you yet; ask us in another
decade.

By now you may be able to
distinguish between I'm-wet cries,
I'm-hungry cries, and all kinds of
cries in between. Your attention
helps reinforce bonding.

Turn the TV
off as soon
as you start
noticing her
turning to its
sound or picture.
The TV provides
sounds and
images that pollute
the real-life sounds
and images that Baby
needs to interact with.
Baby brains develop more
slowly when images are
fed to them through the TV
rather than created out of their own
imaginations.

d to take a
ver? Put Baby in
rib and wind up a
ical mobile. Ceiling
, too, are endlessly
nating.

THREE MONTHS

Nursery rhymes were invented for a reason: The rhythm, repetition, and rhyme a[...] help with early language development.

Talk slowly, vary your tone of voice, and go ahead and speak [...] of mommy talk. Okay, bubsy wubsy? It not only hol[...] your baby's interest but actually helps learnin[...]

During the day, don't forget tummy tim[...] with good supervision. It helps your child develop upper-body strength. She may be able to raise her head a[...] chest now.

Soft toys are great for this age, but beware of ingestible parts (button eyes on stuffed animals, for example).

Hand over the maracas. She can sh[...] toys.

Read aloud. And keep doing it. Every day. Cloth or board books with well-defined, boldly colored pictures will hold her attention best.

She'll be babbling now and may eve[...] imitate sounds, so watch the sailor mouth! Well . . . she won't be making words for a few more months, but you don'[...] want the first one to be "#@#!"

Don't forget to check water temp at bath time. And never leave your child alone or with a sibling around water.

Use water-based moisturizing lotion after baths to keep Baby's skin supersoft.

She may like to see herself in the mirror. A priceless smile indeed. Bonus: Putting a mirror in the crib may keep Baby occupied, so she doesn't cry when she wakes up. It's also good for encouraging baby push-ups during tummy time.

Watch ou[...] because she's o[...] a roll! She may b[...] able to roll from fro[...] to back and vice vers[...] That means no puttin[...] the car seat or bouncy se[...] on the table with her in it. O[...] leaving her on a bed or couc[...] unattended—not even wit[...] pillows propped around he[...]

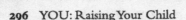

FOUR MONTHS

...is when babies start to get on a schedule; up until now, it may change day to day.

...n now until about six months, you can experiment with starting ...l foods. Baby foods, not rib eye. No need to hurry, and use ...y simple foods. Start with cereals, then puréed ...s and veggies; you can add meats a ...ple of months later. (See page 118.)

...time for naps? For most, it's ... in the morning and two in ...afternoon, but every baby is ...rent, so follow your little ...s clues.

...of massaging, kissing, ...hugging: Touching ...eases levels of ...eel-good and ...ly-bonding ...none ...ocin.

Most of the neurons that a human being has are present at birth; the huge growth in the brain in the first year is the richness of sensory experiences reflected in a proliferation of neural connections. At the end of the first year, the long process of pruning away unnecessary or underutilized connections begins. Expose your baby to lots to give his brain as much to work with as possible. (See page 71.)

To treat eczema (rash of red, scaly patches), wash with water only and bathe her no more than every two or three days. (See page 220–21.) Ask your pediatrician if you need any medicated creams such as hydrocortisone.

➤A ¼ teaspoon (1.25 milliliter) of Karo corn syrup added to breast milk or formula can help ease constipation.

SIX MONTHS

Having another domestic dispute about taking out the trash?
Even if your child can't talk, she gets vibes
about relationships and can feel stress
during arguments. Conflict is okay—
as long as it's controlled and as
long as there's resolution.

Tempting as it is to
plop your baby
in front of a
DVD, she'll
learn more
through
listening to
live words and
watching the
faces that make
them. Hold a convo
with your baby, even
if it's only babble
coming back at you.

Baby
can sit up, but
remember, no walkers.
Use a stationary ExerSaucer
instead. Surround her with toys and
see how long she can entertain herself.

Still reading every night?
You may be sick of green
eggs and ham, but she isn't.

The key to a
good night's
rest a few months
down the line is
establishing good sleep
hygiene now. Create a routine:
warm bath, book, song, and a "Good night,
sweetie." Keep it low-key and simple, so that
she'll be better able to self-soothe and fall
back asleep if she wakes up quietly in
the middle of the night. (For our advice
on crying episodes during the night, see
page 317.)

NINE MONTHS

...member, there's no such thing as perfect parenting.
...e key is to create an environment that allows your
...d to explore and be challenged in a safe
...d loving way.

...s called busy boards, which hang on the
...de of cribs, are terrific for buying you a
...extra minutes of sleep in the morning.

...y is crawling at this point and may
...n be standing and cruising.

...should have your home
...dproofed by now, and make
...e those bookcases are bolted to
...wall.

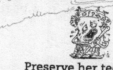

Preserve her teeth:
No bottles in bed. And
feel free to try giving her a
sippy cup for daytime drinking!

The pediatrician will check to see if
she is ready for walking by looking
at her parachute response: The doc
will lift Baby up, then aim her toward
the ground. The baby who is getting
ready to walk will put her arms out
to prepare for touchdown; the baby
who is not ready to walk will still
be angling headfirst toward the
ground. When she is ready to
walk, she will also start standing
flat-footed, instead of perched
up on her toes.

Play lots of
peekaboo.

...Standing up
...ding furniture!

ONE YEAR

Your child should recognize her name and look to you when you say it.

She should have at least one word in addition to Mama and Dada, even though you may be the only one who understands it.

She can pick up Cheerios (as well as stray buttons, dead bugs . . .) with two fingers—and put them in her mouth.

He's doing a good job of developing fine motor skills: banging objects, poking fingers, making marks on paper. No piano concertos just yet, but he's working on it.

She may be able to hold a cup up to her mouth.

She knows "no."

First steps!

Brush his teeth once or twice a day, even if it's just with your finger and baby toothpaste.

Is your child constipated? Try the CRAP diet (cherries, raisins, apricots, prunes). If he's under four years old, purée these fruits, as they don't go down the windpipe so well for babies and toddlers. Bran cereal will also help loosen him up, as will physical activity.

Two naps begin to consolidate into one midday nap around this age.

Your child should be weaned off puréed food around one year; she can eat everything you eat if it is in chewable pieces (except potential allergens, if there's a family history).

wh
milk f.
twelve mo
up until age
Babies need the
for brain developm
After that, your doc
suggest you switch
percent. There's absolu
no need to give your c
soda or even fruit juice, with
exception of calcium-fortified
he doesn't drink milk or prune juic
constipation. (But dilute these with e
parts water, so that your child doesn't
used to overly sweet taste.)

FIFTEEN MONTHS

e yourself: Walking, and perhaps running, will have begun by now.
world as she knows it—and as you know it—has officially changed.
ready to get moving.

your child on a visual leash at all times.
page 242.)

time, playtime, playtime. Get
de and expose her senses
e world. There'll be time
oap and water later.

Remember the mantra
that good foods are just
that: good for you. The more
you give in to marketing tactics
and sugary evil, the harder it will
be to get your kid to eat right.
The more you expose your child
to healthy food, the better the
chances that eating right will
become a habit.

A child's intestines
are about three and a
half times the length of her
height. That's a long way; hope
those smashed peas have frequent-flier
miles.

EIGHTEEN MONTHS

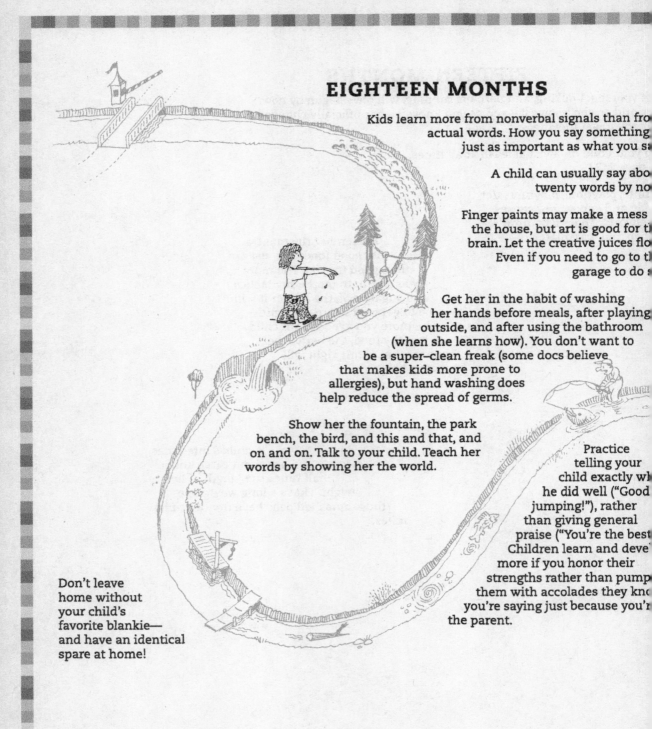

Kids learn more from nonverbal signals than fro[m]
actual words. How you say something [is]
just as important as what you s[ay.]

A child can usually say abo[ut]
twenty words by no[w.]

Finger paints may make a mess [of]
the house, but art is good for t[he]
brain. Let the creative juices flo[w.]
Even if you need to go to t[he]
garage to do s[o.]

Get her in the habit of washing
her hands before meals, after playing
outside, and after using the bathroom
(when she learns how). You don't want to
be a super–clean freak (some docs believe
that makes kids more prone to
allergies), but hand washing does
help reduce the spread of germs.

Show her the fountain, the park
bench, the bird, and this and that, and
on and on. Talk to your child. Teach her
words by showing her the world.

Practice
telling your
child exactly wh[at]
he did well ("Good
jumping!"), rather
than giving general
praise ("You're the best[").]
Children learn and deve[lop]
more if you honor their
strengths rather than pump[ing]
them with accolades they kn[ow]
you're saying just because you'r[e]
the parent.

Don't leave
home without
your child's
favorite blankie—
and have an identical
spare at home!

k for a big smile from Dad about
: She can throw a ball while
ding up.

l daily menu for a toddler: 100
ent whole-grain cereal, whole
, and milk for breakfast; fruit
0 percent whole-grain crackers
water for snack; a half
wich, applesauce, and milk
unch; yogurt for snack;
ein, starch, colored veggie,
, and water for dinner.
can also offer some
before
ime. (Don't
t to brush!)

If you can expose your
child to two (or more)
languages, do it. The brain
structure of children who learn
two languages before age five
changes so much that they have
thicker brains as adults.
Mamma mia!

Get out
the pots
and pans
and let
Junior play
the kitchen
band!

Talk, talk, talk to your child.

She can stoop and pick up objects
and then keep on truckin'. She can also stack
objects, kick a ball, and move backward, forward, up,
down, and sideways.

You should be
omfortable
hoosing
o "agree to
isagree" with
our pediatrician.
ut in some cases,
hoosing a different
oc—one whose
rinciples align more
losely with yours—may
e in order.

TWO YEARS

Spend time with your child as he falls asleep. As children lose their energy, they become more receptive to hearing your words. The last words that they hear should be yours; try "I love you!" or something else that is a major positive. Develop a bedtime routine that brings them comfort.

The best tactic for dealing with a tantrum may be the hardest: Acknowledge your child's anger or frustration but don't get into a power struggle and escalate the emotions. Remember, tantrums usually pass quickly (although it may feel like the longest ten minutes of your life), especially if your child has other ways to communicate. Prevention is best, and you can often predict times when tantrums will take place, such as when a child is hungry or tired. (See page 94.)

Though it's often easier to yell "No!" when Junior tests his physical limits, it's more effective to express other emotions, too. Saying you'd be disappointed if he got hurt can be a better way to teach him about physical safety than forbidding the activity and tempting the gods of rebellion.

Sharing is caring! Now is a good time to teach how to take turns.

She can now do lots of things she couldn't do just a few months ago: Stand on toes, kick a ball, run, jump, and climb up and down your favorite pieces of furniture.

Social skills are at a high. She lov being with others, so a good time to schedule playdates. Bonus: You ca notes (and adult conversa with other parents!

By now, she'll be sleeping about twelve to fourteen hours a day and may be giving up her nap, although so children continue to nap until four or five years old.

Tricycle gassed up and ready to go? Start the heln habit as soon as he's using vehicles other than his feet.

A child can usually say at least fifty words by now. "Ma Dada! SpongeBob!" He can put together two- to three-wo sentences. Don't fret if most of them start with "I want . . ."

Toilet training can happen a little earlier than now, or a little later, but the key is looking for the cues that she's ready. One big one: clutching the crotch or indicating discomfort when wet. (See page 89.) Another is when poops are like a punctual employe on time all the time.

h should be brushed twice a day. Use a soft
h with just a dab of fluoride toothpaste.
h for two minutes.

a thumb sucker? You can use a reward system
stickers) to derail the bad habit. Or try foul-
ng nail polish on the offending thumb(s).
page 102.)

e it a mission to laugh with your child
y day: Make a silly face, read a funny
, wrestle—whatever it takes. Laughter
e best medicine indeed.

t be alarmed. This is the age at which
may start comparing genitals with one
her. Your job is to teach your child
t what's appropriate and what's not,
that private parts are private. (See
68.)

ember:
biotics treat
erial infections,
iruses. Don't push
pediatrician for
ntibiotic if the doc
that your child has
us. That will only
ase the chances that
become infected with
ntibiotic-resistant strain.
page 271.)

Begin researching preschools.

Blocks, dress-up clothes, pretend
kitchens, and other toys that
promote imaginary play are all
appropriate for this age.

SMOKED
FISH

Family dinner = numerous benefits.
Having it just twice a week can yield
improvements in a child's eating
behavior, social skills, and overall
development. Sitting down together
five to seven days a week: priceless!
If you can't do dinner, try family
breakfast.

If you haven't yet,
practice separation:
for instance, leaving her
with a sitter or relative for
the afternoon. It will make the
transition to preschool much easier.

THREE YEARS TO FIVE YEARS

She has a wide range of emotions and can express them all. Sometimes all within nineteen seconds!

It's never too early to make sure that your child is active: getting out, playing tag, doing gymnastics, swimming, and learning to love the fun that comes from moving, stretching, jumping, and running. Activity is one of the greatest ways to combat childhood obesity. Make it a family fun time. (See our plan on page 376.)

Starting at about age four, the number of fat cells a child has begins to increase. That's why it's especially important now to reinforce good eating habits—and to make sure that you're doing so, too. Kids model parental behavior more than they listen to instructions.

Teach your kids some basics about good food and explain why certain foods are better than others. (See pages 124, 137.) Start with observing that foods without food labels are good for you.

Puzzles = good fun and high learning.

Reinforce good manners. There cannot be too many pleases and thank-yous.

No TV in the bedrooms. No TV during meals. No TV as a replacement for real people. Set a daily limit for TV and video games. (We recommend no more than one or two hours a day for children over age two.) Instead of TV and the risk of inappropriate commercial messaging, we recommend child-friendly DVDs such as *Magic School Bus*, *Sesame Street ABCs*.

If your child is interested in computer video games, limit her to a maximum of one or two hours of combined screen time a day (TV, video games, computers). Some great educational websites for kids are www.Funbrain.com and www.pbskids.org. The computer is not a babysitter—it's essential that you supervise your child; in fact, a one-letter typo in the Funbrain site can lead your kid to Vegas—not a trip that's a trip you want your kid to t

fun games that keep your child active, like keeping the
[ball]oon off the floor or throwing socks at each other in the
[living]room. Even a nice game of catch or hide-and-seek
[will] do the trick. If you have a specific game that you
[want] to play, be open to playing it another way.
[Your ch]ild may not be able to play Candy Land
[by th]e rules, but if you sit back and watch
[and] listen, he may choose another way to
[play] that he enjoys just as much.

[Teac]h your child her first and last name,
[your] real names (other than Mommy
[and] Daddy), and her telephone number
[(imp]ortant) and address. A great way to
[help] her memorize your phone number is to
[set i]t to the tune of the first line of "Twinkle
[Twin]kle Little Star."

Keep on reading to your child.
Just because she's started school
doesn't mean that your job as
teacher is over.

Remember,
this may be your
last opportunity to spend
such a high percentage of time
with your child; teachers and peers
get big-time attention starting soon.
Take advantage of it and bask in
the opportunity to have a lasting
impact on your child. Now's
a great time to start talking
about meaningful things: to
communicate your own values
to your child and to teach her
about how she fits into this
great, big, wide world.

[Be care]ful not to
[over]program. Leave
[som]e down time for R &
[R an]d independent play,
[espe]cially with you. This
[is ho]w kids develop social
[skill]s and learn to cope
[with] conflict.

YOU
TOOLS

THE NEWBORN SURVIVAL GUIDE

Coming home with your first baby is a bit like coming home with a new gadget or gizmo. You're excited to start playing with it, but you may have no idea how the heck it works and what to do if something goes wrong. Only now, there's not an instruction manual that came tucked away in the pretty ol' placenta that you can refer to in time of need. For that reason, we offer you our guide to taking care of your newborn. We cover issues ranging from how to feed your baby to how to give him his first bath and everything in between. There's a lot to know, but you can take comfort in the fact that every day, millions of new parents go through exactly what you are going through, and they do just fine. As will you.

You'll also find many more newborn tips throughout the book, such as:

How to find a pediatrician, page 259.

Breast-feeding guidelines, page 110.

How to treat colic, page 153.

Laying the groundwork for good sleep habits, page 82.

Developmental milestones, page 54.

Childproofing your home, and home safety tips, pages 251–55.

Preparing the Home for Baby

Before you deliver, it's a good idea to prepare for your bundle of joy's arrival by readying his room (or area in your room) and making sure that you have all the key supplies you'll need—for him *and* for you. This is a great job for your significant other if you have one conveniently handy.

If your baby will have his or her own room, paint in advance so that fumes have dissipated by the time Baby comes home. Don't be the one to scrape off the old paint, especially if you are pregnant, as the risk of lead toxicity remains high for all homes painted before 1976. While you're at it, cover all outlets, check smoke alarms, and be sure to remove all cleaners and toxins from lower cabinets. (See chapter 9.) Here's a checklist to make sure you've got everything in place before your baby comes home:

For Baby

⊃ Infant car seat—and make sure you've practiced installing it! (See page 257.)

⊃ Extra electric outlet covers.

⊃ Crib, bassinet, or co-sleeper. (See "Crib Guidelines," below.)

⊃ Storage area for clothes and diapers.

⊃ Place to change the baby (changing table, padded foam form that attaches to any bureau top, changing pad if you plan to use the floor or bed).

⊃ Large tote or diaper bag.

⊃ Diapers. Expect to use 350 disposables the first month. If using cloth, contact the delivery company, because you'll need 90 the first week; also buy 6 to 10 diaper wraps or plastic pants and 4 sets of diaper pins, or "snappies."

⊃ Diaper pail or garbage can. A product called Diaper Genie is great for containing bad smells.

- Alcohol-free wipes.

- 10 to 12 extra cloth diapers for burping and other uses.

- 5 to 10 T-shirts or Onesies. Kimono style is easiest; avoid those that slip on over the head.

- 3 to 5 pairs of booties and/or socks.

- 1 or 2 knit hats.

- 1 sun hat (if summer).

- 5 to 7 cotton sleepers or gowns.

- 1 or 2 fleece sleepers, depending on season or temperature of room.

- 1 bunting, a warm Snuggie outfit (if winter).

- 5 to 7 receiving blankets.

- 1 or 2 thermal blankets.

- Waterproof mattress pad for crib.

- 3 or 4 bed pads for crib.

- 3 to 5 soft washcloths.

- 3 to 5 hooded towels.

- Baby nail scissors or clippers.

- Digital thermometer.

- Baby brush and comb.

- Mild soap.

- Baby shampoo.

- Vaseline.

➲ Diaper rash cream (Desitin, Balmex, A+D ointment, Pinxav, or Cleveland Clinic butt paste; see more on diaper rash on page 225).

➲ Q-tips (not for ears!).

➲ Cotton balls.

➲ Rubbing alcohol (for umbilical cord care).

➲ Mobile (high-contrast colors).

➲ Baby monitor.

➲ Baby tub or large sponge to lay baby on in bathtub or kitchen sink.

➲ If bottle-feeding: bottles, nipples, bottle brush, formula.

➲ Perfume- and dye-free laundry detergent.

Note: Wash all of Baby's clothes, sheets, and towels before use. There's no need to wash the baby's things separately from your own or to use special baby detergent; the whole family can use perfume- and dye-free detergent. They're better for you, too. Avoid commercial fabric softeners and dryer sheets, as they contain harsh chemicals. If you must soften clothes, add either ¼ cup baking soda or ¼ cup white vinegar to the wash cycle. The vinegar will also take care of static cling. The companies Seventh Generation and Ecover also make safe fabric softeners and static cling removers based on vegetable products and essential oils.

For Mom

➲ If nursing, at least two cotton nursing bras, nursing pads, and one tube of udder cream or lanolin for treating cracked nipples.

➲ If pumping, either buy a portable pump (good for taking to work) or rent a hospital-grade one (stronger, but not easy to tote around). Also buy glass storage bottles, as well as bottles, bottle brush, and nipples for Baby.

TAKING CARE OF YOURSELF

As we've said several times in the book, your child will model her behavior not necessarily on what you say but on how you act. So taking care of yourself, even at a time when your sole focus is your baby, is vitally important. You can see some of our tips for getting your body back in order and dealing with other postpartum health issues in *YOU: Having a Baby*, but it is important to pay attention to your emotional health as well. Up to 15 percent of women suffer from postpartum depression and many more for the baby blues (and dads can suffer, too; recent research put the number at about 10 percent). The first step, of course, is recognizing (or having your partner recognize and articulate) that something doesn't quite feel right for you. Some symptoms include changes in sleep and energy, significant anxiety, feelings of guilt, and not feeling bonded with your baby. You can also use an official depression scale to gauge whether you fall into the category of having the blues, which will go away by themselves in a matter of weeks, or postpartum depression, which requires treatment. (See www.doctoroz.com or www.realage.com for the test.) If you do suffer from postpartum depression, there are a number of different therapies, including medication. But one of the best treatments is the most simple: talking. Talk to other moms. Talk to friends. Talk to support groups. Talk to a professional counselor. You should also work on relationship issues: trying to spend time together (see our guidelines on choosing a sitter on page 327) and helping each other out (like taking turns sleeping). You can also contact Postpartum Support International (www.postpartum.net; or call 800-944-4773) or the National Women's Health Information Center (www.4woman.gov) for more resources.

⊃ Maxi pads. (Get overnights, the big ones.)

⊃ Tucks medicated pads.

⊃ K-Y Brand Jelly or Astroglide personal lubricant (especially necessary if you're breast-feeding).

⊃ Witch hazel astringent.

○ Plastic bags with ice (good for sore bottom and breasts).

○ Waterproof mattress pad for your bed.

○ Ready-to-eat meals for freezer and pantry.

○ Easy-to-grab, healthful snacks.

Other Useful Items to Add to Your Wish List

○ Stroller. (See page 320.)

○ Sling or baby carrier (BabyBjörn, Snugli, and so on).

○ Bouncy seat.

○ Battery-operated or closed-spring-operated swing.

○ Gymini or similar colorful padded mat with suspended objects that baby can look at or kick while lying on his or her back.

○ Soft toys with varied textures and sounds but no removable parts (like button eyes). Black, white, and red toys are best seen by baby eyes, followed by primary colors. Pastels aren't ideal.

○ Rattles, rings, and toys that Baby can grip.

○ Crib mirror.

○ Fabric books, board books.

○ CDs of nursery rhymes (or Mozart—your choice). Sharon, Lois, and Bram's *Mainly Mother Goose* was a favorite in our homes.

○ A few days' worth of meals delivered to the house.

○ Help from partner and others who will ideally take care of "everything" while you get to know your baby.

Interpreting Cries

It won't take long before you can ID your baby's cries. But to help you early on, here are some tip-offs about what he wants when he's fussing.

IF HE'S CRYING AND ALSO . . .	IT COULD BE . . .
Squirming	He has a dirty diaper.
Turning his head to the side or putting his fist to his mouth	He's hungry.
Pulling his legs up to his chest and has a tense body	He has gas. Burp him.
Sweating and has red ears	He's too warm. Check his temp and loosen his clothing.
Getting goose bumps or has some purplish tones to his hands and feet	He's cold. Go get a blanket or a hat and socks.
Flailing his arms and legs, or turning from the light	He's overstimulated, so take him out of his current environment to a quieter one. Try swaddling him. (See below.)
Blinking and yawning, as well as kicking	He's tired.
Squirming, looking around	He just needs a cuddle.

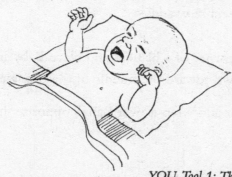

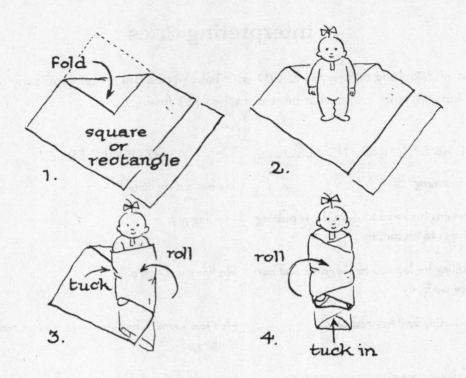

The Proper Swaddle

The major reason that swaddling is so important is that it helps limit the startle reflex, so babies don't wake themselves up. You can swaddle your newborn for much of the day when he's sleeping or resting and loosen the reins as he stays awake longer and seems curious about moving around, starting at about three months. Swaddling is very effective for cranky babies, since the reason they're fussy is often that they actually want to sleep but can't calm themselves down. Follow these step-by-step illustrations for creating a secure swaddle:

- ⊃ Fold down the top corner of a blanket and place Baby in the middle, with her feet pointing down toward the middle of the triangle.

- ⊃ Pick up a side corner and wrap it over Baby's opposite shoulder and tuck it under her back.

⊃ Fold the bottom corner of the blanket up to Baby's stomach or chest.

⊃ Fold the last remaining corner over Baby's other shoulder and tuck it under her back.

How to Change a Diaper

⊃ Lay your baby flat and lift his ankles. For boys, put a wipe over the penis to avoid a spray.

⊃ Slide the diaper underneath so that the top of the diaper is even with his belly button.

⊃ Bring the front of the diaper up between his legs.

⊃ Unfasten the tabs on the side, point his penis down, and close up.

⊃ Make sure it's snug. Diaper leaks can ruin your day—or at least your carpet.

Crib Guidelines

Make sure your crib has:

⊃ A firm, tight-fitting mattress, so Baby can't get trapped.

⊃ No missing, loose, or broken screws or brackets.

⊃ No more than 2⅜ inches between crib slats, so Baby's head and body cannot fit through the slats.

⊃ No corner posts over ¹⁄₁₆ inch high, so clothing can't get caught.

⊃ No cutouts in the headboard or footboard, so Baby's head doesn't get stuck.

How to Choose a Stroller

⤳ If you live in the country or suburbs, get a newborn car seat with a stroller attachment. That way you'll have fewer worries about waking him when you move from car to stroller. If you live in the city or do a lot of errands by foot, a carriage that can be positioned to lie flat with a large basket underneath might be your best bet.

⤳ Jogging strollers and umbrella strollers don't offer back support and are not good for newborns.

⤳ When "test driving" a stroller in the store, consider how heavy it is, how the restraint straps fit, whether it has a removable seat that you can clean, the handle height (and whether it's adjustable), and whether or not you'll be having more than one child in a stroller at any given time.

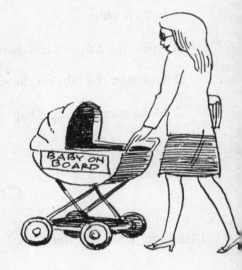

⤳ There is some research to suggest that rear-facing strollers are better for a baby's brain development than forward-facing ones. The rear-facing ones allow better interaction between caregiver and child, while forward-facing strollers expose kids to more white noise, like traffic and wind.

⤳ If you're going to get around using an on-the-body carrier, the baby needs to be seven days and seven pounds before you use it.

Circumcision

Circumcision does reduce certain infections, including HIV and other sexually transmitted diseases, and a circumcised penis reduces transmission of STDs to partners many years hence. But there are no strong data to show that it absolutely must or must not be done; it's an elective procedure, after all. Most parents make the decision based on religious and cultural customs, as well as the simple "what Pop looks like" or "what he'll look like in the locker room" arguments. Management of baby pain during circumcision has improved, and the local anesthetic does appear to soothe the pain, as does sucking on a pacifier after. Sucking on a pacifier with sucrose on it has also been associated with higher comfort and less pain during newborn circumcision.

Siblings

Once you have more than one child, the dynamics of every relationship in the home can change. Here's how to reduce potential conflicts:

➲ Talk to older siblings about what's happening—that is, if they haven't already noticed your growing belly. Discuss potential names you're thinking of, to involve them, and even consider enrolling them in a sibling class, which teaches them how to interact with their new brother or sister. Playdates with friends who have siblings can also help normalize the experience without spending extra dollars on a class.

➲ Have your siblings-to-be pick out (or help pick out) an appropriate welcome gift, and then make sure to get a little surprise gift for the baby to give to the older ones.

➲ If your older kids don't want to be involved, don't force them; they're carving out their own spaces, and the bonding may take a little more time. If they do, give them jobs they can handle.

- Remember, an older child may have gone from a situation in which he was the focus of your world to one in which he has to share your attention, and sometimes it's hard for us to fathom how that truly feels. So be patient.
- Arrange special playdates, visits with relatives, or outings for your older children.
- Leave the baby with a friend, relative, or sitter for a couple of hours and spend one-on-one time with your older children.
- When on outings, if a friend or stranger oohs and ahhs over your new arrival, make sure to emphasize—in front of your older child—how proud you are of him/her for being such a good big brother/big sister, and what a good helper he/she is. This specific praise helps shape the older child's identity as a good big brother or sister.

OTHER CAREGIVERS IN BABY'S LIFE

We've all heard the expression "It takes a village." Part of your job as a parent is to create that special community for your child. Your village will include you, a partner if you have one, as well as grandparents and other family members who will interact with your child regularly. It may also include a nanny, day care professionals, and an assortment of occasional babysitters or mother's helpers. Enlisting qualified, nurturing caregivers is one of the best things you can do for both yourself and your child. For one thing, every parent needs a break now and again—either to revive the romance in your relationship that led you to become a parent in the first place, or simply to recharge your batteries so you can return to diaper duty relaxed and refreshed. For another, it's vitally important for your child to interact with adults other than you in order to learn how to socialize and to separate, skills that she'll need to successfully start school. Unfortunately, not all caregivers are created equal, and it's important to choose carefully and to pay close attention to the signs your child gives you after spending time with each one to know whether or not this is someone you want to trust with your most prized possession.

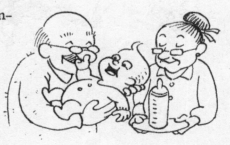

Choosing a Nanny. Many people hire a nanny either because they prefer the convenience and individual attention a nanny can provide or else because, with multiple children, it may end up being more economical than day care. The key thing to remember is that, whether the nanny lives in or out, or works part time or full time, she is someone you are inviting into your home and your family. It's a very intimate relationship, but it must also remain professional.

The most important criterion for a nanny is that she share your ideas and values about child rearing. That is best determined not only in a personal interview but also while watching her interact with your child. Accordingly, we suggest hiring her for a trial day before you seal the deal. Of course, you'll also check all references, and in conversations with her former employers listen for nuances carefully. What is her approach to discipline? Nutrition? Sleep? TV? Is she a homebody or does she like to spend time outdoors? Is she someone who will take the initiative to make playdates for your child, take her to the zoo, the park, or enrichment classes? How are her language skills? Is she comfortable reading to your child and playing number games?

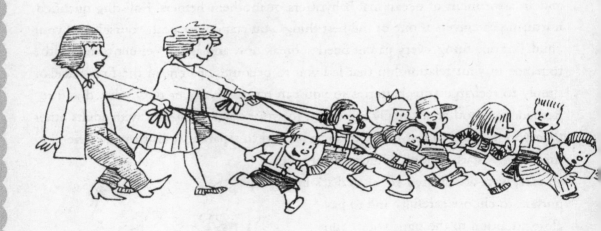

Does she talk or sing to her, or does she spend more time chatting with friends on her cell phone?

As wonderful as a nanny may be with your child, it's also important that you find someone who meets your needs. If you work long hours, can she come early and leave late, or does she have family obligations of her own? How is her health? Is she energetic enough to care for a young child? Does she know CPR? If not, you should arrange for her to take a class. If you need her to travel, is she comfortable doing so? Will you require her to do additional household chores, such as shopping, cooking, cleaning, or laundry? Be up-front about your expectations, as well as about salary, vacation, and sick days. And don't hesitate to run a background check, including of her driving record if she will be driving your child. Finally, when you do reach an agreement, include a trial period of a few weeks; it gives both of you the chance to opt out if it looks like the arrangement isn't working.

By the way, surveillance cameras, or "nanny cams," are legal in all fifty states, but in some states it is not legal to record voices, so check before you do. If your nanny finds out that she has been secretly recorded, it may damage the trust on which your relationship is based; a better alternative is to be up-front about your intention so she knows you're just doing due diligence.

Choosing a Day Care Center. Day care can be an excellent choice for many reasons: It can be more affordable than a nanny. It can be more reliable; you don't have to find coverage when the nanny is out sick or on vacation. And it can be more socially enriching, even if it provides less one-on-one attention. Again, the most important thing is to find a day care center that reflects your philosophies and values in terms of the level of structure, the approach of the providers, and the policies on nutrition, sleep, discipline, and TV. While all day care facilities must be licensed (if it's not, don't even consider it), requirements vary from state to state. In addition, check to see if the facility you're interested in has been accredited by the National Association for the Education of Young Children or the National Early Childhood Accreditation Program, or if it has won any local award or recognition. Other key elements to discuss on the telephone with the director and confirm upon visiting include:

⊃ **Child-to-staff ratio:** The American Academy of Pediatrics recommends the following:

AGE	CHILD-STAFF RATIO	MAXIMUM GROUP SIZE
Birth to 12 months	3:1	6
13 to 30 months	4:1	8
31 to 35 months	5:1	10
3 years old	7:1	14
4 to 5 years old	8:1	16

⊃ **Staff qualifications:** In addition to being cheerful and loving, the staff should have a minimum of two years of college, with training in early childhood education and knowledge of first aid, including CPR. Ask about ongoing faculty development opportunities as well as the average length of tenure or rate of staff turnover.

⊃ **Safety and cleanliness:** Is the facility light and airy? Are there safe indoor and outdoor play spaces? Are the walls, floors, kitchen area, and bathrooms clean? And while you're looking, are there developmentally appropriate pictures on the walls, or is it all signs saying, "Don't Do That," or pictures with a big X on them? Do the decorations stimulate or stifle creativity? Are the toys clean and in good repair? Are there visible first aid kits, fire extinguishers, smoke detectors and carbon monoxide detectors? Is there a child-proof storage area for cleaning materials? Does the staff wash its hands after changing diapers and before preparing meals? How often do the children wash hands?

⊃ **Clear policies:** The center should have clear policies on everything from drop-off and pick-up procedures to fees, health, and vaccination requirements. If your child is sick, can you be reimbursed for missed days? And when is it okay for her to return to day care? Most important, the center should have an open-door policy for you to drop in unannounced to check on your child. Some facilities even have cameras set up so you can watch your child from your computer.

⊃ **Scheduled activities:** The best day care facilities have scheduled times for indoor and outdoor play, snack, meals, and naps or rest. Ideally, preschool-age children should have two hours a day of active play, including two visits a day to an outdoor play space, weather permitting. TV and video watching should not be on the schedule. Rather, there should be plenty of opportunities for creative play, including arts and crafts, music, story time, as well as games involving letters and numbers.

As with any child care arrangement, check references—in this case, current and former parents. Also, in addition to visiting the day care center yourself, visit a second time with your child and gauge her reaction to the staff and environment.

Home-Based or Family Child Care.

Some people prefer family child care to day care because it is less formal, includes fewer children, allows for different-aged siblings to be cared for together, and is in a home environment with a single caregiver. It is also less expensive. Most states require regulation of providers who care for more than four children, including background checks; ongoing training in early childhood development; minimum health, safety, and nutrition standards; and regular or random inspections. Nonetheless, you still have to do your homework, which includes checking references, inspecting the home to make sure it is smoke free and at least as safe and clean as your own, and confirming that there are age-appropriate toys and books and that children are not parked in front of the TV. If there are pets in the home, make sure they are well trained and that your child does not have an allergic reaction. Confirm that the children are never allowed outdoors unsupervised, especially if there is a swimming pool or hot tub. (Watching from the kitchen window doesn't count.) And don't be afraid to drop in for a random spot check to make sure everything is as it should be. Home-based child care providers may be accredited by the National Association for Family Child Care.

Babysitters and Mother's Helpers.

Chances are, even if you are a full-time mom, you'll want to go out to a movie or run an errand sometime in the next five years and will have to hire a babysitter. Or you may find you want someone else to watch Junior for a couple of hours while you clean out your closets in peace. In these cases, babysitters and mother's helpers are ideal. They're not expensive, they don't require a big commitment, and they usually have tons of energy and think it's really fun to take care of kids. Mother's helpers are traditionally preteens who provide an

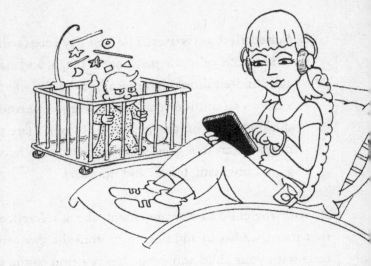

extra pair of hands while you're still in the house. Babysitters are slightly older and more experienced, either from having been mother's helpers themselves, having babysat other children, or having cared for younger siblings.

While there are certification classes for babysitters, an enthusiastic, intelligent, responsible teen doesn't require certification (unless you want her to know CPR). You may have to teach her how to warm a bottle or change a diaper the first time around. Depending on your comfort level, you can allow her to bathe or cook a simple meal for your child or, if she is old enough, to drive Junior to an activity.

And on a very serious note: While there are wonderful male baby sitters out there, we do not recommend them. With boys, there's a 1 in 6 chance that they've been sexually abused as children. With girls, there's a 1 in 4 chance. But here's the difference: Boys who are abused tend to take it out on another victim, while girls tend to be depressed and take it out on themselves. We're not saying that males cannot be good caregivers, but if you're playing the odds with people you don't know (and perhaps even people you do), the evidence simply shows that your child is safer with female sitters.

• • • •

The most important thing is to always leave your sitter with your cell phone number, numbers for a couple of neighbors and relatives, and the numbers for your pediatrician and for Poison Control. By the way, if you're at a movie, put your cell phone on vibrate and instruct the sitter to call only in an emergency.

FAMILY-FRIENDLY RECIPES

In the beginning, feeding your baby can be pretty straightforward. You've basically got three choices: breast milk, formula, or a combination of the two. But once she gets older, starts cutting teeth, and starts deciding that, mmm-hmm, potatoes taste good, then things can get a little more complicated. Please see chapter 4 for our explanation of childhood nutrition (plus how to deal with picky eaters). The big challenge, of course, can be trying to concoct dishes that are tasty, nutritionally powerful, and good for the whole family. That's where these recipes come in. They're quick to make and healthy. And judging from the huge number of kids who tasted them, we can also tell you that they're quite the tongue pleasers as well.

Note: Some of the recipes contain tree nuts, peanut butter, honey, and raisins (which we don't recommend until age three). Those recipes are noted with a special star. ✳

ABOUT LIFESTYLE 180

Lifestyle 180 is one of the disease-reversal programs used at the Cleveland Clinic to help people with such chronic diseases as Type 2 diabetes, coronary artery disease, prostate cancer, etc . . . , learn lifestyle changes that allow them to get rid of their disease or their need for medications. The program has four specific areas including physical activity, stress management, and nutrition and cooking. The recipes have to be quick to cook, inexpensive, and delicious if these individuals are to stick with the program. And they do—so here are a few of the recipes designed for kids (and their moms and dads) to keep healthy and taste great.

Lifestyle 180 **100 Percent**
Whole Wheat Pizza Dough

Yield: 2 pizza crusts

1 package active dry yeast

1¾ cups warm water (110°F), divided

1 teaspoon honey

1 tablespoon plus 2 teaspoons extra-
   virgin olive oil, divided

1 teaspoon salt

3¼ cups whole wheat flour, divided

2 teaspoons cornmeal

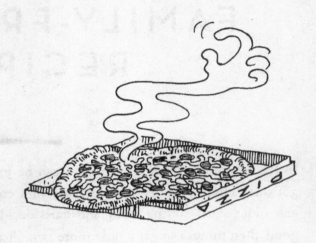

In a small bowl, combine yeast with ½ cup of the warm water and honey; let stand until bubbly, 5 to 10 minutes. In large bowl of electric mixer fitted with dough hook, combine remaining 1¼ cups warm water, 1 tablespoon of the oil, and salt. Add 2 cups of the flour and the yeast mixture. Mix at medium speed until well blended. Add remaining flour in three batches, mixing until flour is incorporated before adding more. Dough should be sticky and hold together.

Oil a large bowl with ½ teaspoon of the oil. Place dough in bowl; brush ½ teaspoon oil over dough. Cover bowl with plastic wrap; place on top rack of an oven that is off. Place a bowl of hot tap water on bottom rack of oven to create humidity. Close oven; let dough rise for 1½ hours.

Remove dough from oven; punch down and divide in half. Oil each of two pizza pans with ½ teaspoon oil; sprinkle 1 teaspoon cornmeal over each pan. Stretch each ball of dough to fit size of pizza pan. Pierce dough with a fork intermittently about six times. Return to oven on top rack with fresh hot water on bottom rack. Close oven and let rise 30 minutes.

Remove dough and water; heat oven to 350°F. Bake dough for 10 minutes. Remove from oven; let cool 10 minutes. Pizza crust is ready to be topped and baked, or refrigerated up to 24 hours before baking, or frozen up to 1 month.

WHAT YOU AND YOURS CAN COUNT ON PER SERVING

Calories (kcal) 99 Fat 2 g Saturated Fat 0.1 g Trans Fatty Acid 0 g Healthy Fats 1.5 g Dietary Fiber 3.1 g
Carbohydrates 18.5 g Total Sugars 0.4 g Protein 3.5 g Sodium 148 mg Calcium 9.5 mg Magnesium 34.7 mg
Potassium 109 mg Iron 1.03 mg

Lifestyle 180 **Any Shape Snack Bars** ✱

Yield: 16 servings

1 cup walnuts, toasted

1½ cups seedless golden raisins

¾ cup sugar-free dried cranberries

5 rice cakes, broken into chunks

2 tablespoons agave nectar

2 tablespoons unsweetened orange juice

1 tablespoon pure vanilla extract

¼ teaspoon cinnamon

Heat oven to 300°F. Place walnuts in a food processor; pulse until finely chopped. Add raisins and cranberries; pulse until mixture is sticky. Add rice cakes; pulse until fine and mixture is loose. Add agave nectar, orange juice, vanilla, and cinnamon; pulse until mixture is sticky and holds together.

Divide mixture into 16 balls. Flatten and shape as desired: round like a circle, rectangle like a bar, or long and narrow like a pencil and then bent into your initials. Place on a nonstick baking sheet; bake 20 to 25 minutes or until firm, or longer to desired crispness.

WHAT YOU AND YOURS CAN COUNT ON PER SERVING

Calories (kcal) 149 Fat 5 g Saturated Fat 0 g Trans Fatty Acid 0 g Healthy Fats 4 g

Dietary Fiber 1.7 g Carbohydrates 25 g Total Sugars 18 g Protein 2 g Sodium 22 mg Calcium 17 mg

Magnesium 12.3 mg Potassium 177 mg Iron 0.70 mg

Lifestyle 180 CMSD Berry-Banana Smoothies

Yield: 5 ½-cup servings

1 ripe banana, peeled, broken into chunks

½ cup fat-free plain yogurt (no sugar added)

½ cup fresh or frozen blueberries

½ cup unsweetened orange juice

½ cup fresh or frozen strawberries or additional
   blueberries

2 teaspoons agave nectar

1 teaspoon chia seeds

½ cup silken extra-firm tofu

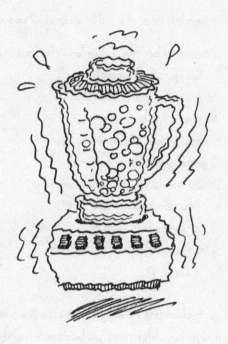

Place all ingredients in a blender container. Cover;
blend until smooth. Serve immediately.

WHAT YOU AND YOURS
CAN COUNT ON PER SERVING

Calories (kcal) 80   Fat 1.5 g   Aging (Saturated) Fat 0.1 g

Trans Fatty Acid 0 g   Healthy Fats 1.4 g

Dietary Fiber 2 g   Carbohydrates 12 g   Total Sugars 10 g

Protein 4 g   Sodium 20 mg   Calcium 70 mg

Magnesium 9.4 mg   Potassium 147 mg   Iron 0.6 mg

Lifestyle 180 "YOU" Chicken Fingers for Dr. Mike

Yield: 6 servings, 3 "fingers" each

Chicken cut into small, thin strips will require much less fat and shorter cooking time.

1 6-ounce boneless, skinless chicken breast half
½ teaspoon ground cumin
½ teaspoon garlic powder
¼ teaspoon kosher salt
½ cup whole wheat flour
2 large egg whites, beaten
1 cup whole wheat panko bread
    crumbs, ground in a food
    processor until fine
1 tablespoon plus 2 teaspoons
    canola oil

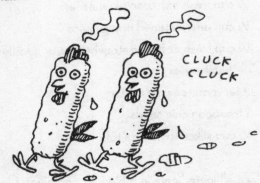

CLUCK
CLUCK

Cut chicken breast lengthwise into 3 equal pieces. Cut each piece crosswise into 6 strips. Season chicken with cumin, garlic powder, and salt. Dredge strips first lightly in flour, then egg whites, letting excess drip off, then in bread crumbs.

Heat oil in a 12-inch nonstick skillet over medium heat until hot. Add chicken; cook until golden brown on bottom. Turn; continue cooking until chicken is golden brown and cooked through. Serve with BBQ Dipping Sauce.

Chef Notes: Tips to Use Less Fat
- Always use a nonstick pan.
- Ensure oil is hot but not smoking. Test by dropping in a pinch of bread crumbs to see if the oil bubbles quickly.
- Oil will bubble up in a nonstick pan when you use small amounts that do not cover the bottom, so place a chicken finger in bubble and drag to a dry spot in the pan. Repeat process until all chicken strips are in the pan.

WHAT YOU AND YOURS CAN COUNT ON PER SERVING
(3 CHICKEN FINGERS AND ¼ CUP DIPPING SAUCE)

Calories (kcal) 300   Fat 11 g   Aging (Saturated) Fat 1.1 g   Trans Fatty Acid 0.02 g   Healthy Fats 3.7 g
Dietary Fiber 4 g   Carbohydrates 20 g   Total Sugars 3 g   Protein 22 g   Sodium 585 mg   Calcium 18 mg
Magnesium 41 mg   Potassium 266 mg   Iron 1.2 mg

Lifestyle 180 BBQ Dipping Sauce
for Chicken Fingers

Yield: 12 ¼-cup servings

This sauce is wonderful to dip crunchy Lifestyle 180 "YOU" Chicken Fingers in. Extra sauce may be refrigerated up to 4 days or frozen up to 3 months.

1 14-ounce bottle organic corn syrup–free and sugar-free ketchup
¼ cup organic reduced-sodium soy sauce
¼ cup red grape juice
¼ cup dark sesame oil
2 tablespoons fresh lemon juice
2 tablespoons agave nectar
1 tablespoon black pepper, coarsely ground
2 teaspoons garlic, minced

Combine all ingredients in a medium saucepan. Bring to a simmer, stirring occasionally. Remove from heat; cool completely.

(Nutritional information is included in the Lifestyle 180 "YOU" Chicken Fingers recipe above.)

Lifestyle 180 Beans and Farro

Yield: 4 ½-cup servings

Farro, also known as emmer, is higher in fiber than common wheat with a wonderful chewy and hearty texture. Loved by our kids. Look for packages of farro in the grain section of natural food stores or some (really good) supermarkets.

2 tablespoons canola oil
½ cup sweet onion, chopped
1 tablespoon garlic, minced
2 cups green beans, blanched and thinly sliced
½ teaspoon kosher salt
¼ teaspoon black pepper, coarsely ground
1 cup cooked farro
2 teaspoons lemon peel, finely shredded

Heat oil in a 12-inch skillet until hot. Add onion; sauté 5 minutes or until translucent. Add garlic; sauté 1 minute. Stir in green beans, salt, and pepper; sauté 1 minute. Add farro and lemon peel; sauté until heated through.

WHAT YOU AND YOURS CAN COUNT ON PER SERVING

Calories (kcal) 131   Fat 4 g   Aging (Saturated) Fat 0.3 g   Trans Fatty Acid 0.01 g   Omega-3 Fatty Acid 0.3 g
Omega-6 Fatty Acid 0.7 g   Healthy Fats 3.1 g   Dietary Fiber 4.8 g   Carbohydrates 20 g   Total Sugars 3.1 g
Protein 4.1 g   Sodium 305 mg   Calcium 40 mg   Magnesium 27 mg   Potassium 116 mg   Iron 1.3 mg

Lifestyle 180
Pumpkin Walnut Muffins ✳

Yield: 14 muffins

Oprah loved this one when we made it for her—your kids will, too.

Chia seeds come from the desert plant *Salvia hispanica*. These high-fiber bundles of nutrition are high in omega-3 fatty acids, absorb up to ten times their weight in water (so the muffins taste moist for a long time) and have been found to help with everything from lowering blood cholesterol and blood pressure to decreasing depression. Including chia seeds and walnuts in your diet is one way to get in those great omega-3 healthy fats!

1 tablespoon chia seed, ground

½ cup orange juice

1½ cups whole wheat flour

2 teaspoons baking soda

2 teaspoons cinnamon

½ teaspoon salt

½ teaspoon nutmeg

1 15-ounce can pumpkin

¾ cup walnuts, chopped and toasted

¼ cup water or unsweetened apple juice

¼ cup canola oil

2 tablespoons agave nectar

1 tablespoon pure vanilla extract

1 cup (packed) fresh apple, peeled and coarsely grated (5.5 ounces by weight)

Heat oven to 350°F. Combine chia seed and orange juice and let it sit for 15 minutes. Add in flour, baking soda, cinnamon, salt, and nutmeg in a small bowl; mix well. In a large bowl, combine remaining ingredients except apple; mix well. Add dry ingredients, stirring until dry ingredients are just moistened. Fold in apple. Spoon into paper-lined muffin cups. Bake 33 to 35 minutes or until wooden pick inserted in center comes out clean. Serve warm or at room temperature. Muffins may be frozen up to 3 months.

WHAT YOU AND YOURS CAN COUNT ON PER SERVING

Calories (kcal) 150   Fat 8.8 g   Aging (Saturated) Fat 0.8 g   Trans Fatty Acid 0.02 g   Healthy Fats 7.5 g
Dietary Fiber 3.5 g   Carbohydrates 16 g   Total Sugars 4.1 g   Protein 3.2 g   Sodium 265 mg   Calcium 30 mg
Magnesium 37 mg   Potassium 164 mg   Iron 1.2 mg

Lifestyle 180 **Better Than Dairy Pudding**

8 ½-cup servings

1 cup natural, no-sugar-added peanut butter

2 ounces 70 percent bittersweet chocolate candy bar, chopped

1 12-ounce package silken extra-firm tofu, drained

2 ripe bananas, peeled, broken into chunks

6 tablespoons unsweetened cocoa powder

1 tablespoon plus 2 teaspoons agave nectar

1 tablespoon pure vanilla extract

Combine peanut butter and bittersweet chocolate in a microwave-safe bowl. Cook in microwave oven at high power in 20-second increments, stirring after each until chocolate is melted and well blended with peanut butter; set aside.

Process tofu in a food processor until smooth, scraping down sides of bowl as needed. Add bananas; process until smooth. Add cocoa powder, agave nectar, and vanilla; process until smooth. Add peanut butter mixture; process until smooth. Spoon into 8 small bowls or one large bowl; refrigerate until chilled.

WHAT YOU AND YOURS CAN COUNT ON PER SERVING

Calories (kcal) 309 Fat 22 g Aging (Saturated) Fat 4 g Trans Fatty Acid 0 g Healthy Fats 0 g

Dietary Fiber 4.4 g Carbohydrates 20.2 g Total Sugars 9 g Protein 11.7 g Sodium 113 mg Calcium 77 mg

Magnesium 8 mg Potassium 158 mg Iron 1.9 mg

Lifestyle 180 Blender Potato Pancakes

Yield: 6 servings of 2 4-inch pancakes

1 tablespoon plus 1 teaspoon extra-virgin olive oil, divided

1 cup chopped onion

½ cup whole wheat flour

1 tablespoon baking powder

½ teaspoon kosher salt

1¼ pounds (about 5 medium) potatoes, peeled, finely diced

3 tablespoons fat-free milk

1 cup zucchini squash, coarsely grated and squeezed to remove excess water

Heat 1 teaspoon of the oil in a large nonstick skillet. Add onion; sauté on medium-low heat until onion is golden and caramelized, 15 to 20 minutes. Remove from heat; set aside.

Combine flour, baking powder, and salt in a large bowl. Combine potatoes and milk in a blender container. Cover; blend until puréed, scraping down sides often. Add potato mixture to flour mixture; mix well. Fold in zucchini and onion.

Heat remaining 1 tablespoon oil in a large nonstick skillet over medium heat until hot. In three batches, drop potato mixture by ¼ cupfuls into hot oil; press with a large spatula to form 4-inch pancakes. Cook until golden brown on each side. Transfer to a baking sheet; keep warm in a 200°F oven. Serve warm.

WHAT YOU AND YOURS CAN COUNT ON PER SERVING

Calories (kcal) 170   Fat 3.5 g   Aging (Saturated) Fat 0.5 g   Trans Fatty Acid 0 g   Healthy Fats 2.8 g

Dietary Fiber 4.2 g   Carbohydrates 33 g   Total Sugars 4.6 g   Protein 5.4 g   Sodium 478 mg   Calcium 94 mg

Magnesium 20 mg   Potassium 142 mg   Iron 1.4 mg

Lifestyle 180 Carrots in Your Cake (or Muffins)

Yield: 16 servings

2 cups carrots, coarsely grated

1 8-ounce can crushed pineapple in juice, drained

½ cup orange juice

¼ cup canola oil

2 tablespoons agave nectar

1 tablespoon orange peel, finely shredded

2½ cups whole wheat pastry flour

¾ cup walnuts, toasted and chopped

2 teaspoons baking soda

2 teaspoons cinnamon

½ teaspoon allspice

Heat oven to 350°F. Combine carrots, pineapple, orange juice, oil, agave nectar, and orange peel in a large bowl. Combine remaining ingredients in a medium bowl; mix well. Add dry mixture in three increments to wet mixture, mixing until dry ingredients are just moistened. Pour batter into a 9-inch square baking dish (lightly oiled with 1 teaspoon canola oil) or 16 paper-lined muffin cups. Bake 45 to 55 minutes for cake or 30 to 32 minutes for muffins or until a wooden pick inserted in center comes out clean. Serve slightly warm or at room temperature. Leftover cake or muffins may be frozen for up to 3 months.

WHAT YOU AND YOURS CAN COUNT ON PER SERVING

Calories (kcal) 135　Fat 4 g　Aging (Saturated) Fat 0.4 g　Trans Fatty Acid 0 g　Healthy Fats 3.1 g

Dietary Fiber 3.7 g　Carbohydrates 22.5 g　Total Sugars 6 g　Protein 3 g　Sodium 169 mg　Calcium 31 mg

Magnesium 14 mg　Potassium 114 mg　Iron 1.2 mg

Lifestyle 180 Chia Gingerbread Cake

Yield 16 servings

1 cup canned pumpkin

⅓ cup canola oil

¼ cup agave nectar

1 tablespoon molasses

2 teaspoons chia seed

1¾ cups whole wheat pastry flour

2½ teaspoons cinnamon

2½ teaspoons ground ginger

2 teaspoons baking powder

2 teaspoons baking soda

¾ teaspoon nutmeg

¼ teaspoon salt

Heat oven to 350°F. Combine pumpkin, oil, agave nectar, molasses, and chia seed in a large bowl. Mix well; set aside for 15 minutes to allow chia seed to swell. Combine remaining ingredients in a medium bowl; mix well. Add mixture to wet ingredients in three parts, mixing until dry ingredients are just moistened. Spread mixture evenly into a sprayed or lightly oiled 9-inch square glass baking dish. Bake 30 minutes or until a wooden pick inserted in center comes out clean. Transfer dish to a wire rack; cool completely.

WHAT YOU AND YOURS CAN COUNT ON PER SERVING

Calories (kcal) 98 Fat 5 g Aging (Saturated) Fat 0.4 g Trans Fatty Acid 0.02 g Healthy Fats 4.3 g
Dietary Fiber 2.2 g Carbohydrates 14 g Total Sugars 4 g Protein 1.2 g Sodium 264 mg Calcium 34 mg
Magnesium 7 mg Potassium 55 mg Iron 0.6 mg

Lifestyle 180 **Chia Guacamole**

Yield: 4 ½-cup servings

½ cup plum tomatoes with juice, diced

½ teaspoon chia seed

1 large ripe avocado, peeled, seeded, diced

1 tablespoon cilantro, finely chopped

2 teaspoons fresh lime juice

½ teaspoon jalapeno pepper (optional), minced

½ teaspoon salt

¼ teaspoon garlic, minced

Combine tomatoes and chia seed in a medium bowl; let stand 10 minutes for chia seed to swell. Add remaining ingredients to bowl; mash to desired consistency. Serve immediately with vegetable sticks or place a sheet of plastic wrap directly on surface of guacamole and refrigerate up to 2 hours before serving.

WHAT YOU AND YOURS CAN COUNT ON PER SERVING

Calories (kcal) 90 Fat 7.6 g Aging (Saturated) Fat 1.1 g Trans Fatty Acid 0 g Healthy Fats 5.6 g
Dietary Fiber 3.9 g Carbohydrates 6.3 g Total Sugars 1.4 g Protein 1.4 g Sodium 367 mg Calcium 16 mg
Magnesium 15 mg Potassium 248 mg Iron 0.6 mg

Lifestyle 180 Chicken Salad of Champions

Yield: 8 ½-cup servings

½ cup Vegenaise nondairy dressing

2 tablespoons Dijon mustard

½ teaspoon salt

¼ teaspoon pepper

1 pound cooked chicken breast, cut into ¼-inch pieces

1 cup seedless red grapes, quartered or halved if small

⅓ cup cooked egg whites, chopped

⅓ cup celery, finely chopped

½ cup walnuts or pecans or half of each, chopped and toasted

1 tablespoon fresh parsley, chopped

Combine dressing, mustard, salt, and pepper in a medium bowl; mix well. Add remaining ingredients; mix well. Cover; refrigerate at least 30 minutes or until serving time. Salad will keep up to 2 days.

WHAT YOU AND YOURS CAN COUNT ON PER SERVING

Calories (kcal) 229   Fat 15.5 g   Aging (Saturated) Fat 2 g   Trans Fatty Acid 0 g   Healthy Fats 2.1 g
Dietary Fiber 0.9 g   Carbohydrates 6.6 g   Total Sugars 3.2 g   Protein 15.2 g   Sodium 567 mg   Calcium 12 mg
Magnesium 9 mg   Potassium 82 mg   Iron 1.1 mg

Lifestyle 180 Chocolate Raisin Pudding ✳

Yield: 6 ½-cup servings

If you're looking for a nondairy option for your cereal in the morning that does not have soy or rice, almond milk is tops! Almond milk is made from ground almonds and contains no lactose. The vitamin D in almond milk will help to keep you younger and to mature your child. If you're worried about not getting your calcium, don't! Most almond milks are fortified with calcium to help keep bones strong.

- 1 cup seedless golden raisins
- ¾ cup almond milk
- 1 ripe avocado, peeled, seeded
- 1 large ripe banana, peeled, broken into chunks
- 3 tablespoons unsweetened cocoa powder
- 1 tablespoon plus 2 teaspoons agave nectar

Place raisins in a food processor; process 20 seconds or until raisins are ground. Add almond milk; process 30 seconds or until well blended. Add avocado, banana, cocoa powder, and agave nectar. Spoon into one large bowl or 6 small serving bowls; cover and refrigerate at least 30 minutes before serving.

WHAT YOU AND YOURS CAN COUNT ON PER SERVING

Calories (kcal) 182 Fat 6.7 g Aging (Saturated) Fat 0.7 g Trans Fatty Acid 0 g Healthy Fats 4 g
Dietary Fiber 4.5 g Carbohydrates 32.7 g Total Sugars 25.5 g Protein 2.1 g Sodium 31 mg Calcium 43 mg
Magnesium 18 mg Potassium 468 mg Iron 1.5 mg

Lifestyle 180 Create Your Own
Chia and Fruit Pancakes ✳

Yield: 6 servings (12 to 14 pancakes total)

Feel free to substitute the same amount of any fruit for the blueberries, apple, pear, and banana.

- 1⅓ cups whole wheat pastry flour
- 1 tablespoon chia seed
- 1 tablespoon baking powder
- ¾ teaspoon salt
- ½ teaspoon cinnamon
- 1⅓ cups water
- 1 tablespoon pure vanilla extract
- 1 ripe banana, peeled, halved, thinly sliced
- 1 apple, unpeeled, coarsely grated
- 1 ripe pear, unpeeled coarsely grated
- ½ cup fresh blueberries
- ½ cup walnuts, toasted and chopped

Combine flour, chia seed, baking powder, salt, and cinnamon in a large bowl; mix well. Add remaining ingredients; mix until dry ingredients are just moistened. If batter seems very thick, add 1 to 2 tablespoons water.

Heat a large nonstick skillet coated with a thin film of oil over medium heat until hot. Drop batter by ¼ cupfuls into hot skillet. Cook several minutes or until pancakes forms bubbles and bottoms are golden brown. Turn; continue cooking until bottoms are golden brown. Pancakes may be kept warm in a 200°F oven as they are made. Serve with fresh assorted berries rather than a sugary syrup.

WHAT YOU AND YOURS CAN COUNT ON PER SERVING

Calories (kcal) 237   Fat 7.89 g   Aging (Saturated) Fat 0.7 g   Trans Fatty Acid 0 g   Healthy Fats 6.3 g
Dietary Fiber 7.6 g   Carbohydrates 39 g   Total Sugars 9.7 g   Protein 5.1 g   Sodium 567 mg   Calcium 100 mg
Magnesium 27 mg   Potassium 191 mg   Iron 2 mg

Lifestyle 180 Different Noodles
with Broccoli and Red Pepper

Yield: 6 1-cup servings

1 pound 100 percent whole wheat spaghetti

3 cups small broccoli florets

4½ tablespoons dark toasted sesame oil*

3½ tablespoons organic reduced-sodium soy sauce

2 tablespoons agave nectar

1½ tablespoons balsamic vinegar

1 teaspoon salt

½ teaspoon garlic, minced

1½ cups red bell pepper, finely diced

⅓ cup green onions, sliced

Cook spaghetti according to package directions. Meanwhile, blanch broccoli in lightly salted boiling water 2 to 3 minutes. Drain; place on plate in refrigerator to stop the cooking.

Combine sesame oil, soy sauce, agave nectar, vinegar, salt, and garlic in a large bowl; mix well. Drain spaghetti; rinse with cold water and drain again. Add to bowl; toss with sesame oil mixture. Add broccoli, red pepper, and green onions; toss well.

WHAT YOU AND YOURS CAN COUNT ON PER SERVING

Calories (kcal) 215   Fat 9.8 g   Aging (Saturated) Fat 1.4 g   Trans Fatty Acid 0 g   Healthy Fats 0.4 g

Dietary Fiber 5.1 g   Carbohydrates 29 g   Total Sugars 4.6 g   Protein 6.6 g   Sodium 550 mg   Calcium 53 mg

Magnesium 46 mg   Potassium 362 mg   Iron 1.7 mg

* For a spicier dish, substitute 1 teaspoon hot chile-toasted sesame oil for 1 teaspoon of the regular sesame oil.

Lifestyle 180 Ever So Easy Turkey and Chia Enchiladas

Yield: 12 servings of ½ an enchilada each

1 tablespoon extra-virgin olive oil

2 cups onion, chopped

1½ cups zucchini squash, diced

1½ cups red bell pepper, diced

1 tablespoon garlic, minced

1 pound 99 percent lean ground turkey breast

2 teaspoons chili powder

1 teaspoon salt

1 teaspoon ground cumin

1 16-ounce can fat-free vegetarian refried beans

1 cup frozen corn kernels, thawed

1 tablespoon chia seed

1 teaspoon canned chipotle pepper in adobo sauce, minced (optional)

6 10-inch whole wheat flour tortillas

3 10-ounce cans enchilada sauce

Heat oven to 375°F. Heat oil in a large nonstick skillet over medium heat. Add onion; sauté until translucent. Add zucchini and red pepper; sauté until just tender. Add garlic; sauté 2 minutes. Transfer mixture to a large bowl. Add turkey, chili powder, salt, and cumin to same skillet; break up turkey with a wooden spoon. Cook until turkey is no longer pink, stirring frequently. Stir in beans, corn, chia seed, and chipotle pepper; mix well. Add to bowl of reserved vegetables; mix well. Spoon about 1 cup filling down the center of each tortilla; roll up. Spoon a small amount of enchilada sauce over bottom of a baking pan large enough to hold enchiladas in one layer. Place enchiladas seam side down in pan. Spoon remaining enchilada sauce over enchiladas. Bake 20 to 25 minutes or until heated through.

WHAT YOU AND YOURS CAN COUNT ON PER SERVING

Calories (kcal) 198   Fat 4.7 g   Aging (Saturated) Fat 0.2 g   Trans Fatty Acid 0 g   Healthy Fats 1.3 g

Dietary Fiber 4.9 g   Carbohydrates 24.8 g   Total Sugars 3.4 g   Protein 14 g   Sodium 583 mg   Calcium 44 mg

Magnesium 8.4 mg   Potassium 121 mg   Iron 0.8 mg

Lifestyle 180 Fiesta Bean Salad

Yield: 14 ½-cup servings

½ cup red wine vinegar

¼ cup canola oil

1 tablespoon plus 2 teaspoons agave nectar

1 teaspoon kosher salt

1 teaspoon dry mustard

1 teaspoon garlic, minced

¼ teaspoon black pepper

¼ teaspoon paprika

1½ cups canned black beans, rinsed and drained

1½ cups canned red kidney beans, rinsed and drained

1½ cups canned cannellini beans, rinsed and drained

1 cup frozen corn kernels, thawed

1 cup celery, finely diced

½ cup onion, finely diced

¼ cup green bell pepper, finely diced

¼ cup red bell pepper, finely diced

¼ cup yellow bell pepper, finely diced

2 tablespoons fresh parsley, chopped

Combine vinegar, oil, agave nectar, salt, mustard, garlic, pepper, and paprika in a large bowl; mix well. Add remaining ingredients; mix well. Chill at least 2 hours before serving. Salad will keep up to 4 days in the refrigerator.

WHAT YOU AND YOURS CAN COUNT ON PER SERVING

Calories (kcal) 311 Fat 24.5 g Aging (Saturated) Fat 1.8 g Trans Fatty Acid 0.09 g Healthy Fats 20.8 g

Dietary Fiber 4.5 g Carbohydrates 17.8 g Total Sugars 3.4 g Protein 5.3 g Sodium 358 mg Calcium 45 mg

Magnesium 2.6 mg Potassium 46 mg Iron 1.33 mg

Lifestyle 180 "Fuji Chips"

Yield: 2 servings

These chips are a great substitute for the sugary fruit roll-ups at the grocery store because they have the same texture but no artificial dyes or corn syrup.

1 cup lemon juice
¼ cup water
2 large Fuji apples, washed, halved, cored, cut into ⅛-inch thick slices
cinnamon to taste

Heat oven to 150°F. Combine lemon juice and water in a medium bowl. Add sliced apples to bowl and toss well. Drain well; place in a single layer on a large nonstick baking sheet. Sprinkle cinnamon from a shaker evenly over apples. Bake 2½ hours. Cool and store in an airtight container at room temperature for up to 2 days.

WHAT YOU AND YOURS CAN COUNT ON PER SERVING

Calories (kcal) 150 Fat 0.4 g Aging (Saturated) Fat 0.1 g Trans Fatty Acid 0 g Healthy Fats 0.1 g
Dietary Fiber 6.5 g Carbohydrates 42.4 g Total Sugars 26 g Protein 1.1 g Sodium 4.8 mg Calcium 36 mg
Magnesium 20 mg Potassium 395 mg Iron 0.4 mg

Lifestyle 180 Banana and Pumpkin Mousse

Yield: 7 ½-cup servings

1 large ripe banana, peeled, broken into chunks

8 ounces extra-firm tofu

1 15-ounce can pumpkin

2½ teaspoons cinnamon

1¼ teaspoon ground ginger

1¼ teaspoon nutmeg

Place banana in a food processor; process until smooth. Add tofu; process until smooth. Add remaining ingredients; process until smooth. Spoon mixture into individual bowls or one large bowl. Freeze until solid. (Alternately, mousse may be refrigerated rather than frozen.)

WHAT YOU AND YOURS CAN COUNT ON PER SERVING

Calories (kcal) 80 Fat 1.9 g Aging (Saturated) Fat 0.13 g Trans Fatty Acid 0 g Healthy Fats 0 g

Dietary Fiber 3.1 g Carbohydrates 13.9 g Total Sugars 7.7 g Protein 3.7 g Sodium 3.2 mg Calcium 86 mg

Magnesium 19 mg Potassium 186 mg Iron 1.5 mg

Lifestyle 180 **Green Soup**

Yield: 8 ½-cup servings

2 ripe avocados, peeled, pitted

2 cups fresh asparagus, trimmed, finely chopped

½ cup fresh spinach, stems removed

½ cup fresh kale, finely chopped

2 tablespoons celery, chopped

4 teaspoons tamari or organic
    reduced-sodium soy sauce

1 tablespoon fresh lime juice

1 tablespoon fresh lemon juice

1 teaspoon green onion, chopped

1 teaspoon garlic, minced

½ teaspoon salt

½ teaspoon fresh tarragon, minced, or
    ¼ teaspoon, dried

¼ teaspoon black pepper

¼ teaspoon dried thyme

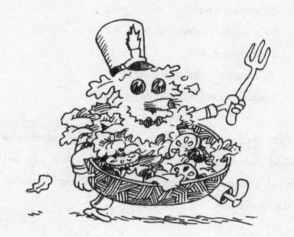

Combine all ingredients in a tall saucepan; purée until smooth with a vertical stick blender. (Or, purée in batches in a food processor or blender.) Serve at room temperature or heat until warm. Soup may be refrigerated up to 2 days before serving.

WHAT YOU AND YOURS CAN COUNT ON PER SERVING

Calories (kcal) 94   Fat 7.5 g   Aging (Saturated) Fat 1.1 g   Trans Fatty Acid 0 g   Healthy Fats 5.6 g

Dietary Fiber 4.5 g   Carbohydrates 6.7 g   Total Sugars 1.1 g   Protein 2.2 g   Sodium 312 mg   Calcium 31 mg

Magnesium 31 mg   Potassium 400 mg   Iron 1.5 mg

Lifestyle 180 Healthy for You Red Pepper Hummus

Yield: 4 ½-cup servings

2 cloves garlic, peeled

1 15-ounce can garbanzo beans, drained

1 4-ounce jar roasted red peppers (packed in water, not oil), drained

3 tablespoons fresh lemon juice

½ teaspoon ground cumin

¼ teaspoon salt

⅛ teaspoon cayenne pepper

1 tablespoon fresh parsley, chopped

With motor running, drop garlic through feed tube of food processor; process until minced. Add remaining ingredients except parsley; process until fairly smooth. Transfer to a serving bowl; cover and refrigerate at least 1 hour. Garnish with parsley just before serving with vegetable dippers.

WHAT YOU AND YOURS CAN COUNT ON PER SERVING

Calories (kcal) 131 Fat 1.29 g Aging (Saturated) Fat 0.01 g Trans Fatty Acid 0 g Healthy Fats 0 g

Dietary Fiber 5.5 g Carbohydrates 23 g Total Sugars 2.1 g Protein 6.5 g Sodium 282 mg Calcium 69 mg

Magnesium 34 mg Potassium 229 mg Iron 1.7 mg

Lifestyle 180 Less Than 30 Minutes
Roasted Red Pepper Tomato Sauce

Yield: 8 ½-cup servings

1 tablespoon extra-virgin olive oil

½ cup onion, chopped

1 tablespoon garlic, minced

1 28-ounce can crushed tomatoes, no sugar added, undrained

1 8-ounce jar roasted red peppers (packed in water), drained, puréed in a food processor

½ teaspoon salt

¼ teaspoon black pepper

1 tablespoon dried basil

1 teaspoon dried oregano

Heat oil in a large saucepan over medium heat. Add onion; sauté until translucent. Add garlic; sauté 2 minutes. Add tomatoes, puréed peppers, salt, and pepper; bring to a boil over high heat. Reduce heat; stir in basil and oregano. Simmer 20 minutes, stirring occasionally. Serve over whole wheat pasta. Sauce will keep refrigerated up to 4 days.

WHAT YOU AND YOURS CAN COUNT ON PER SERVING

Calories (kcal) 70   Fat 2 g   Aging (Saturated) Fat 0.3 g   Trans Fatty Acid 0 g   Healthy Fats 1.5 g

Dietary Fiber 2.2 g   Carbohydrates 10.1 g   Total Sugars 5.1 g   Protein 2.8 g   Sodium 414 mg   Calcium 51 mg

Magnesium 3 mg   Potassium 41 mg   Iron 1 mg

Lifestyle 180 **Grrreat Meatballs**

Yield: 10 servings (4 meatballs)

1 cup nonalcoholic red wine, divided

2 tablespoons garlic, minced

2 tablespoons chia seed

1 cup whole wheat panko bread crumbs

2 egg whites

¼ cup fresh parsley, chopped

1 tablespoon fennel seed

2 teaspoons seasoned salt

½ teaspoon crushed red pepper flakes

½ teaspoon dried basil

¼ teaspoon dried oregano

¼ teaspoon dried thyme

¼ teaspoon black pepper

2 pounds 99 percent lean ground turkey breast

Heat oven to 375°F. In a large bowl, combine ½ cup of the wine with the garlic and chia seed; let stand 10 minutes for chia seed to swell. Add remaining ingredients except turkey to bowl; mix well. Add turkey; mix well. Roll mixture into 40 1-ounce meatballs; place in a 15-x-10-inch jelly roll pan or shallow baking pan. Bake 18 to 20 minutes or until internal temperature of meatballs

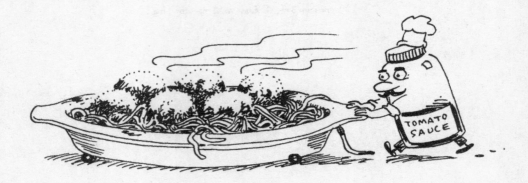

reaches 165°F. Serve immediately with Less Than 30 Minutes Roasted Red Pepper Tomato Sauce (see page 355) and whole wheat pasta, or cool and refrigerate up to 4 days or freeze up to 3 months. Note: Do not reheat meatballs in pasta sauce; they will become tough.

WHAT YOU AND YOURS CAN COUNT ON PER SERVING

Calories (kcal) 180   Fat 2.8 g   Aging (Saturated) Fat 0.1 g   Trans Fatty Acid 0 g   Healthy Fats 0.8 g
Dietary Fiber 2.5 g   Carbohydrates 9.3 g   Total Sugars 0.5 g   Protein 25.8 g   Sodium 370 mg   Calcium 44 mg
Magnesium 9.4 mg   Potassium 70 mg   Iron 2.3 mg

Lifestyle 180 **No Potato, No Fryer French Fries**

Yield: 8 ½-cup servings

1 tablespoon canola or extra-virgin olive oil

2 teaspoons garlic, minced

1 teaspoon ground cumin

1 teaspoon chili powder

1 teaspoon salt

½ teaspoon black pepper

2 pounds butternut squash, peeled, seeded, and cut into strips (3" x ½" x ½")

Heat oven to 375°F. Combine oil and remaining ingredients except squash in a large bowl, and mix. Add squash; toss until well coated with oil mixture. Arrange in a single layer on a nonstick baking sheet or shallow pan. (You may need more than one.) Bake 35 minutes or until tender.

WHAT YOU AND YOURS CAN COUNT ON PER SERVING

Calories (kcal) 73 Fat 2 g Aging (Saturated) Fat 0.2 g Trans Fatty Acid 0.01 g Healthy Fats 1.7 g

Dietary Fiber 2.5 g Carbohydrates 13.9 g Total Sugars 2.5 g Protein 1.2 g Sodium 299 mg Calcium 58 mg

Magnesium 39 mg Potassium 407 mg Iron 1 mg

Lifestyle 180 **Nut and Broccoli Sizzle**

Yield: 8 ½-cup servings

1 tablespoon sesame oil, toasted

½ cup walnuts, chopped

1 teaspoon garlic, minced

4 cups broccoli florets

½ cup red bell pepper, finely diced

2 tablespoons tamari or organic reduced-sodium soy sauce

1 teaspoon sesame seed, toasted

Heat oil in a large nonstick skillet or wok over medium heat. Add walnuts; stir-fry 1 minute. Add garlic; stir-fry 1 minute. Add broccoli and red pepper; stir-fry 5 minutes or until broccoli is crisp-tender. Add tamari and sesame seed; stir-fry 1 minute.

WHAT YOU AND YOURS CAN COUNT ON PER SERVING

Calories (kcal) 79 Fat 6.9 g Aging (Saturated) Fat 0.7 g Trans Fatty Acid 0 g Healthy Fats 4.2 g
Dietary Fiber 1.8 g Carbohydrates 3.6 g Total Sugars 0.6 g Protein 2.4 g Sodium 235 mg Calcium 26 mg
Magnesium 22 mg Potassium 169 mg Iron 1 mg

Lifestyle 180 **Walnut Pecan Pesto** with Green Beans ✳

Yield: 8 ½-cup servings

1 clove garlic, peeled
¼ cup fresh basil leaves
¼ cup fresh parsley leaves
¼ cup fresh spinach leaves
¼ cup chopped fresh kale leaves, ribs removed
3 tablespoons pecans, chopped and toasted
3 tablespoons walnuts, chopped and toasted
¼ teaspoon salt
3 tablespoons extra-virgin olive oil
4 cups hot cooked green beans, drained and cut

With motor running, drop garlic through feed tube of food processor; process until minced. Add basil, parsley, spinach, kale, pecans, walnuts, and salt; process to a coarse purée. Add oil; process until well combined. Toss with green beans. Serve warm or at room temperature. Leftover bean mixture will keep refrigerated up to 4 days.

Note: Pesto is also good tossed with hot cooked whole wheat spaghetti. Or toss with cubes of extra-firm tofu, roast, and serve over brown rice.

WHAT YOU AND YOURS CAN COUNT ON PER SERVING

Calories (kcal) 114   Fat 9.1 g   Aging (Saturated) Fat 1.1 g   Trans Fatty Acid 0 g   Healthy Fats 6.0 g
Dietary Fiber 2.7 g   Carbohydrates 5.3 g   Total Sugars 2.2 g   Protein 2 g   Sodium 85 mg   Calcium 41 mg
Magnesium 10 mg   Potassium 51 mg   Iron 0.8 mg

Lifestyle 180 Nutty Fruity Vegetable Salad

Yield: 6 ½-cup servings

This Nutty Fruity Vegetable Salad is a great way to showcase jicama, a crunchy vegetable that tastes like water chestnut. The salad makes a wonderful lunch-box treat that keeps at room temperature for several hours.

2 cups unsweetened pineapple juice
1 Fuji apple, unpeeled, diced (½-inch pieces)
1 Bartlett pear, unpeeled, diced (½-inch pieces)
¼ pound jicama, peeled, diced (½-inch pieces)
½ cup seedless red grapes, halved (or cut smaller)
¼ cup walnuts, chopped and toasted
½ cup Vegenaise nondairy dressing
1 tablespoon sesame seed, lightly toasted

Combine pineapple juice, apple, pear, and jicama in a large bowl; let stand 5 minutes. Drain; reserving pineapple juice for another use. Combine drained fruit, grapes, and walnuts in same bowl. Add dressing and sesame seed; toss well. Serve immediately or chill up to 1 hour before serving.

WHAT YOU AND YOURS CAN COUNT ON PER SERVING

Calories (kcal) 232   Fat 16 g   Aging (Saturated) Fat 2.3 g   Trans Fatty Acid 0 g   Healthy Fats 2.9 g
Dietary Fiber 3.4 g   Carbohydrates 20.3 g   Total Sugars 13.7 g   Protein 1.6 g   Sodium 113 mg   Calcium 22 mg
Magnesium 14 mg   Potassium 198 mg   Iron 0.7 mg

Lifestyle 180 **Orange Mashers**

Yield: 6 ½-cup servings

1 large (12-ounce) rutabaga, peeled, diced (½-inch pieces)

4 cups vegetable broth

8 ounces carrots, peeled, diced (½-inch pieces)

4 ounces potato, peeled, diced (½-inch pieces)

½ teaspoon kosher salt

¼ teaspoon black pepper

Combine rutabaga and broth in a large saucepan. Bring to a boil over high heat; reduce heat, simmer 15 minutes. Add carrots and potato; simmer 15 minutes or until vegetables are very tender.

Drain vegetables, reserving broth in saucepan. Simmer broth until reduced to ½ cup. Return vegetables to saucepan; add salt and pepper. Use a potato masher to mash vegetables to desired consistency.

WHAT YOU AND YOURS CAN COUNT ON PER SERVING

Calories (kcal) 51 Fat 0.2 g Aging (Saturated) Fat 0.03 g Trans Fatty Acid 0 g Healthy Fats 0 g

Omega-3 Fatty Acid 0.03 g Omega-6 Fatty Acid 0.07 g Dietary Fiber 2.7 g Carbohydrates 11.7 g

Total Sugars 5.1 g Protein 1.5 g Sodium 232 mg Calcium 42 mg Magnesium 22 mg

Potassium 39 mg Iron 0.6 mg

Lifestyle 180 **Popeye Would Be Proud Smoothie**

Yield: 4 ¾-cup servings

½ cup firmly packed spinach leaves

½ cup firmly packed kale leaves, chopped, with large ribs removed

½ cup seedless green grapes, frozen

½ ripe banana, peeled, sliced, and then frozen (takes 1–2 hours)

½ Fuji apple, diced

½ fresh orange, peeled

½ cup water

½ teaspoon chia seed

1 cup crushed ice

Place all ingredients except ice in a blender container. Cover; blend on low speed 1 minute. Add ice; cover and blend on medium-high speed until smooth.

WHAT YOU AND YOURS CAN COUNT ON PER SERVING

Calories (kcal) 48 Fat 0.4 g Aging (Saturated) Fat 0.1 g Trans Fatty Acid 0 g Healthy Fats 0.3 g

Dietary Fiber 1.9 g Carbohydrates 11.8 g Total Sugars 7.9 g Protein 0.8 g Sodium 7 mg Calcium 27 mg

Magnesium 10 mg Potassium 160 mg Iron 0.4 mg

Lifestyle 180 **Orange Tapioca Pudding**

Yield: 6 ½-cup servings

1 cup unsweetened pineapple juice

1 cup orange juice

¼ cup tapioca

½ cup canned mandarin oranges, drained

1 tablespoon agave nectar

Combine pineapple juice, orange juice, and tapioca in a 1½-quart saucepan; let stand 5 minutes. Bring to a boil over high heat, stirring once. Remove from heat; stir in mandarin oranges and agave nectar. Pour into an 8-inch square glass dish or 6 individual serving bowls. Refrigerate until set.

WHAT YOU AND YOURS CAN COUNT ON PER SERVING

Calories (kcal) 79 Fat 0.1 g Aging (Saturated) Fat 0 g Trans Fatty Acid 0 g Healthy Fats 0 g

Dietary Fiber 0.3 g Carbohydrates 19.4 g Total Sugars 12.8 g Protein 0.4 g Sodium 2 mg Calcium 14 mg

Magnesium 6 mg Potassium 160 mg Iron 0.3 mg

Lifestyle 180 Chilled Red Soup

Yield: 4 1-cup servings

1 cup tomato juice

1 cup cucumber, peeled, diced, and seeded (¼-inch pieces)

1 cup red bell pepper, diced (¼-inch pieces)

1 cup ripe tomatoes, seeded and diced (¼-inch pieces)

2 tablespoons cilantro or parsley, chopped

1 tablespoon red wine vinegar

1 tablespoon fresh lime juice

1 tablespoon garlic, minced

1 tablespoon extra-virgin olive oil

¼ teaspoon salt

2 dashes hot sauce (optional, or more to taste)

Combine all ingredients in a large bowl. Transfer half of the mixture to a food processor or blender. Blend until smooth; return to bowl and mix well. Refrigerate at least 2 hours before serving.

WHAT YOU AND YOURS CAN COUNT ON PER SERVING

Calories (kcal) 88 Fat 4.1 g Aging (Saturated) Fat 0.5 g Trans Fatty Acid 0 g Healthy Fats 3 g
Dietary Fiber 1.9 g Carbohydrates 9.8 g Total Sugars 6.3 g Protein 1.5 g Sodium 332 mg Calcium 45 mg
Magnesium 15 mg Potassium 243 mg Iron 0.9 mg

Lifestyle 180 **Yellow Spaghetti**

Yield: 6 ½-cup servings

1 2-pound spaghetti squash

6 cups vegetable stock or broth

½ teaspoon lemon peel, finely shredded

½ teaspoon salt

¼ teaspoon black pepper

Cut the top and bottom off squash. Stand squash upright and cut off the cream-colored rind. Cut squash lengthwise in half; scoop out and discard seeds. Slice each trimmed half crosswise into ¼-inch thick slices.

Bring stock to a simmer in a 12-inch sauté pan. Add squash; cook 7 to 9 minutes or until squash is tender. Use a slotted spoon to transfer squash to a shallow dish or pan. Reserve stock for another use. While squash is still warm, use two forks to pull squash into strands. Season with lemon peel, salt, and pepper.

WHAT YOU AND YOURS CAN COUNT ON PER SERVING

Calories (kcal) 35 Fat 0.34 g Aging (Saturated) Fat 0.1 g Trans Fatty Acid 0 g Healthy Fats 0.2 g

Dietary Fiber 1.8 g Carbohydrates 8.4 g Total Sugars 3.3 g Protein 0.9 Sodium 217 mg Calcium 28 mg

Magnesium 14 mg Potassium 152 mg Iron 0.5 mg

Lifestyle 180 Salsa Bean Salad

Yield: 8 ½-cup servings

1½ cups no-sugar-added salsa

1 teaspoon fresh lemon juice

1 teaspoon fresh lime juice

1 teaspoon cilantro, minced

¼ teaspoon ground cumin

¼ teaspoon garlic powder

1½ cups canned black beans, rinsed and drained

1 cup frozen corn kernels, thawed

½ cup green bell pepper, finely diced

½ cup red bell pepper, finely diced

¼ cup sweet onion, finely diced

Combine salsa, lemon juice, lime juice, cilantro, cumin, and garlic powder in a large bowl; mix well. Add remaining ingredients; mix well. Cover; refrigerate at least 30 minutes before serving.

WHAT YOU AND YOURS CAN COUNT ON PER SERVING

Calories (kcal) 71 Fat 0.4 g Aging (Saturated) Fat 0.01 g Trans Fatty Acid 0 g Healthy Fats 0 g

Dietary Fiber 2.7 g Carbohydrates 15 g Total Sugars 2.4 g Protein 3.1 g Sodium 457 mg Calcium 19 mg

Magnesium 3 mg Potassium 48 mg Iron 0.7 mg

Lifestyle 180 **Sloppy Jims**

Yield: 8 ½-cup servings

Serve this tasty meat sauce over a toasted whole wheat bun. Or make a version of chili-mac by serving it over whole wheat macaroni. Or use any leftovers to make an egg white breakfast frittata.

 1 tablespoon canola oil
 ½ cup sweet onion, finely diced
 1 tablespoon garlic, minced
 ½ cup red bell pepper, finely diced
 ½ cup green bell pepper, finely diced
 1 pound 99 percent lean ground turkey breast
 ½ teaspoon salt
 ½ teaspoon black pepper
 ¼ teaspoon dried thyme leaves
 1 cup ketchup, made with organic corn syrup
 1 tablespoon Dijon mustard
 1 teaspoon rice vinegar
 1 teaspoon agave nectar

Heat oil in a large nonstick skillet over medium heat. Add onion; sauté 5 minutes or until golden brown. Add garlic; sauté 1 minute. Add bell peppers; sauté 5 minutes or until tender. Crumble turkey into skillet; cook until turkey is no longer pink, stirring frequently with a wooden spoon. Add ketchup, mustard, vinegar, and agave nectar; sauté 5 minutes or until heated through.

WHAT YOU AND YOURS CAN COUNT ON PER SERVING

Calories (kcal) 101 Fat 2.6 g Aging (Saturated) Fat 0.1 g Trans Fatty Acid 0.01 g Healthy Fats 1.6 g
Dietary Fiber 0.6 g Carbohydrates 5.5 g Total Sugars 2.2 g Protein 14.4 g Sodium 325 mg Calcium 8.5 mg
Magnesium 4.3 mg Potassium 64 mg Iron 0.9 mg

Lifestyle 180 "Squished Squash" ✳

Yield: 8 ½-cup servings

1½ pounds butternut squash, peeled, seeded, diced

1 large Fuji apple, peeled, diced

½ cup orange juice

2 tablespoons golden raisins

Heat oven to 375°F. Combine all ingredients in a large bowl; mix well. Transfer to a 9-inch square baking dish; cover with foil. Bake 45 minutes or until squash is very tender; use a potato masher to mash to desired consistency.

WHAT YOU AND YOURS CAN COUNT ON PER SERVING

Calories (kcal) 65 Fat 0.2 g Aging (Saturated) Fat 0.03 g Trans Fatty Acid 0 g Healthy Fats 0 g

Dietary Fiber 2.4 g Carbohydrates 16.6 g Total Sugars 7.4 g Protein 1.1 g Sodium 4 mg Calcium 45 mg

Magnesium 32 mg Potassium 374 mg Iron 0.7 mg

Lifestyle 180 These Banana Pops Are Tops

Yield: 6 servings

½ cup walnuts, toasted

¼ cup pecans or additional walnuts, toasted

¾ cup seedless golden raisins

3 brown rice cakes, broken into pieces

1 teaspoon cinnamon

6 ripe bananas

6 Popsicle sticks

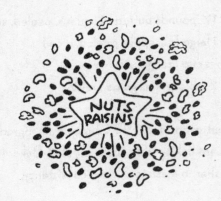

Pulse nuts in a food processor until finely chopped.
Add raisins; pulse until raisins are finely chopped.
Add rice cakes and cinnamon; pulse until mixture is
loose and well combined. Transfer mixture to a single layer in a shallow dish or baking pan. Peel
bananas, roll in nut mixture until evenly coated. Insert a Popsicle stick into each banana. Wrap in
plastic wrap; freeze until firm.

WHAT YOU AND YOURS CAN COUNT ON PER SERVING

Calories (kcal) 307   Fat 10.5 g   Aging (Saturated) Fat 1.1 g   Trans Fatty Acid 0 g   Healthy Fats 5.6 g

Dietary Fiber 5.5 g   Carbohydrates 53 g   Total Sugars 29.4 g   Protein 4.5 g   Sodium 35 mg   Calcium 32 mg

Magnesium 48 mg   Potassium 656 mg   Iron 1 mg

Lifestyle 180 Watermelon Freeze

Yield: 2 ½-cup servings

1 cup seedless watermelon, diced

½ cup ice, crushed

1 tablespoon fresh lime juice

1 teaspoon agave nectar

Combine all ingredients in blender container. Cover; blend until smooth. Transfer to a bowl; freeze until slushy.

WHAT YOU AND YOURS CAN COUNT ON PER SERVING

Calories (kcal) 32   Fat 0.01 g   Aging (Saturated) Fat 0.0 g   Trans Fatty Acid 0 g   Healthy Fats 0 g

Dietary Fiber 0.5 g   Carbohydrates 10.1 g   Total Sugars 9 g   Protein 0.3 g   Sodium 5 mg   Calcium 8 mg

Magnesium 1 mg   Potassium 9 mg   Iron 0.2 mg

Lifestyle 180 Whole Wheat Brownie Bites

Yield: 16 servings

¾ cup whole wheat pastry flour

¼ cup unsweetened cocoa powder

½ teaspoon baking soda

⅛ teaspoon salt

½ cup soy milk

¼ cup agave nectar

1 teaspoon pure vanilla extract

½ cup 72 percent bittersweet chocolate, broken into chunks

1 large ripe banana, peeled, mashed

¼ teaspoon canola oil

Heat oven to 350°F. Combine flour, cocoa powder, baking soda, and salt in a small bowl. Mix well; set aside. Combine soy milk, agave nectar, and vanilla in a small saucepan. Heat over medium heat until warm. Add chocolate; cook and stir until melted. Stir in banana; whisk until well blended. Remove from heat; whisk in dry ingredients. Grease a 9-inch square glass baking dish with the canola oil. Spread mixture into dish. Bake 20 minutes or until set. Transfer dish to a wire rack; cook completely. Cut into squares.

WHAT YOU AND YOURS CAN COUNT ON PER SERVING

Calories (kcal) 122 Fat 8.4 g Aging (Saturated) Fat 1.9 g Trans Fatty Acid 0.02 g Healthy Fats 4.2 g
Dietary Fiber 1.8 g Carbohydrates 12.1 g Total Sugars 5.1 g Protein 1.7 g Sodium 62 mg Calcium 14 mg
Magnesium 3 mg Potassium 80 mg Iron 0.7 mg

Lifestyle 180 **Veggie Rice**

Yield: 6 ½-cup servings

2 tablespoons canola oil

½ cup sweet onion, finely diced

1 tablespoon garlic, minced

¾ cup zucchini squash, finely diced

¾ cup green beans blanched and finely diced

½ cup red bell pepper, finely diced

½ cup yellow bell pepper, finely diced

1 cup cooked brown rice

½ teaspoon kosher salt

¼ teaspoon black pepper

2 teaspoons lemon peel, finely shredded

Heat oil in a 12-inch sauté pan over medium heat. Add onion; sauté 5 minutes or until golden brown. Add garlic; sauté 1 minute. Add zucchini, green beans, bell peppers; sauté 5 minutes or until vegetables are crisp-tender. Add rice, salt, and pepper; sauté until heated through. Stir in lemon peel.

WHAT YOU AND YOURS CAN COUNT ON PER SERVING

Calories (kcal) 108   Fat 5.3 g   Aging (Saturated) Fat 0.4 g   Trans Fatty Acid 0.02 g   Healthy Fats 4.4 g

Dietary Fiber 2.2 g   Carbohydrates 12.1 g   Total Sugars 2.5 g   Protein 1.8 g   Sodium 168 mg   Calcium 19 mg

Magnesium 21 mg   Potassium 125 mg   Iron 0.5 mg

Lifestyle 180 Sweeter Than Sour Chicken, Vegetables and Brown Rice

Yield: 6 1-cup servings

This recipe is a great way for your children to enjoy increasing their intake of plant-based foods and fiber, and it is low in fat. Refrigerate the leftover Ginger Sweet n Sour sauce to serve as a dipping sauce for cooked seafood, chicken, and vegetables.

2 cups cooked broccoli florets

12 ounces cooked chicken breast, cut into 1-inch pieces

1 cup Ginger Sweet n Sour Sauce*

1 cup cooked zucchini squash, sliced

1 cup cooked lima beans

1 cup cooked carrots, sliced

1 cup diced cooked red and/or yellow bell peppers, diced

1 cup hot cooked brown rice

Combine all ingredients except rice in a medium saucepan; cook over medium heat until hot, stirring frequently. Serve over rice.

*Ginger Sweet n Sour Sauce

14 ounces unsweetened pineapple juice

¼ cup agave nectar

¼ cup organic corn-syrup and sugar-free ketchup

2 tablespoons light soy sauce

2 tablespoons white wine vinegar

½ teaspoon fresh ginger root, minced

½ teaspoon jalapeno chili pepper, minced (optional)

1 tablespoon arrowroot or cornstarch

Combine all ingredients except arrowroot in a medium saucepan. Bring to a boil over high heat. Reduce heat; simmer 1 minute. Whisk together arrowroot with 3 tablespoons water; add to saucepan. Whisk constantly until sauce thickens.

WHAT YOU AND YOURS CAN COUNT ON PER SERVING

Calories (kcal) 225   Fat 2.1 g   Aging (Saturated) Fat 0.2 g   Trans Fatty Acid 0 g   Healthy Fats 0.4 g
Dietary Fiber 7.3 g   Carbohydrates 32.7 g   Total Sugars 7.2 g   Protein 19.7 g   Sodium 441 mg   Calcium 48 mg
Magnesium 61 mg   Potassium 536 mg   Iron 2.8 mg

FITNESS FOR FAMILY

One of the many great things about kids is this: Instinctually, they know how to move their bodies. Once they can run, they run everywhere, they climb, they're active. Simply, they play. But sometimes we can stifle that instinct if we're not careful. The downside of having a child who's physically inactive is a higher risk of developing obesity and obesity-related health issues. Right from the start, it's important to make sure your kid moves her body.

Even early on, working out with your child can be a great way to spend quality time together while learning how to improve his focus, memory, muscle growth, and balance. But keep it simple so as to engage all the senses. These workouts need no equipment, but you are more than welcome to use whatever costumes or toys are available to stimulate your child's imagination. This "workout" is designed for both of you to do together, so *you* get a nice total-body workout too.* (We know that it can be tough to squeeze in workouts as a parent, so we made it easy for you to combine fun and fitness.)

Enjoy, and let the child guide you in play. (And be sure there's no glass, pointed edges, or breakable objects nearby.)

* Created by Joel Harper. You can find his workout DVDs at www.joelharperfitness.com.

On Floor

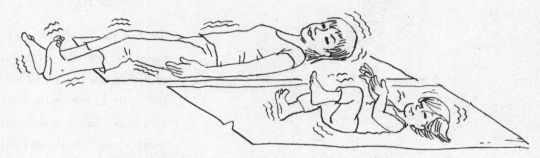

JELLO (Loosens Entire Body)

Try to relax completely and wiggle every single muscle. You can do this while you both lie on your backs. Keep jiggling while naming five things to eat that are red. Change the color each time.

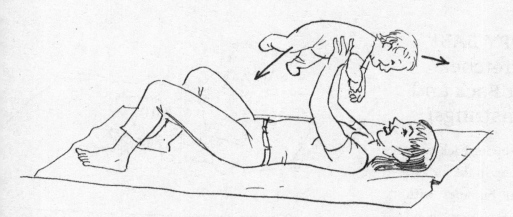

BIRD (Strengthens Arms and Core)

Lie on your back with your knees up and feet flat. Hold your child above you, so that you face each other. Have her stretch out and flap her arms and legs. You can lift and lower your child toward you to simulate flying. Tilt her side to side as your own arm strength builds; make bird or airplane noises and vibrate your lips for variety. Keep going for a few minutes. This is great for face-to-face interaction.

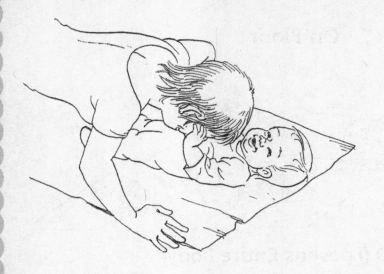

RASPBERRY (Warms Up Body)

Switch places: Now your child is on the ground, and you are above. While on your knees, lean over and make horse noises on your child's belly, trying to get him to wiggle and squirm. Do for a few min-utes, and then you can tickle him or play peekaboo. Most kids love to be tickled. Use a variety of noises to engage your child. Be aware that he may be more sensitive to sounds from one day to the next.

HAPPY BABY (Stretches Lower Back and Hamstrings)

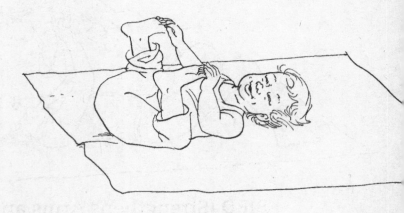

Lie flat on your back with your feet up in the air and grab your big toes with two fingers. Now bend your legs at right angles, bring your heels above your knees, and gently pull your elbows down toward the mat while simultaneously pressing your lower back into the mat. Now giggle, even if you are not feeling it; see if you can giggle until it is real.

SPOTLIGHT
(Great Cardio)

Stand up and leave your child on all fours. Shine a flashlight on the floor and have her crawl to the light. As soon as she gets to it, reward her (with words) and aim the beam somewhere else. Repeat five times, then give her the flashlight and switch places.

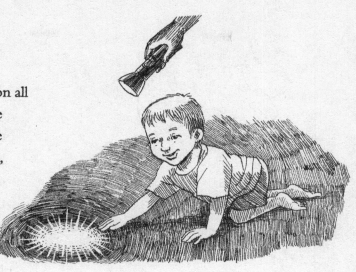

WAG YOUR TAIL
(Loosens Spine and Strengthens Entire Body)

Get onto all fours with your knees below your hips and your hands below your shoulders. Now act like you have a tail and wag it. Really get into it, by moving your shoulders and head, and bark like a dog; see how many different *ruffs!* you can belt out. Crawl around the room chasing each other. Whoever gets caught gets tickled.

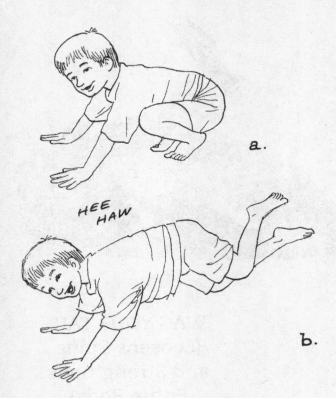

HEE
HAW

DONKEY (Works Quads and Improves Balance)

Stay on all fours facing child. Come onto your toes and kick both feet up like you were a donkey; try to float up and down. Barely hear your feet land. Keep your elbows bent and use your knees as springs. Make donkey noises as you kick up. Do five times. (Make sure coffee tables and other items are out of range before kicking.)

a.

b.

LION (Works Legs and Core)

While on all fours (hands and knees), lift up your upper body and lean back so that you are on your knees. Bring your paws up and roar like a lion, facial expression and all. Do five times. Keep your stomach taut.

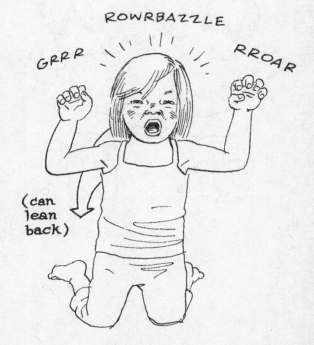

ROWRBAZZLE

GRRR

RROAR

(can lean back)

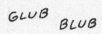

GLUB BLUB

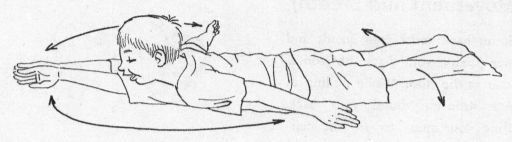

FISH (Strengthens Back)

Lie flat on your stomach and reach your hands out above your head. Bring the back of your hands together and apart and do the same with your heels, as if you were a goldfish swimming around. Pucker your lips and pull your stomach in. Lift your knees as high as you can. Talk as if you were a goldfish and describe what you see in the tank. Don't forget to talk to your fish friends.

LIMBO (Helps Children Learn Body Awareness)

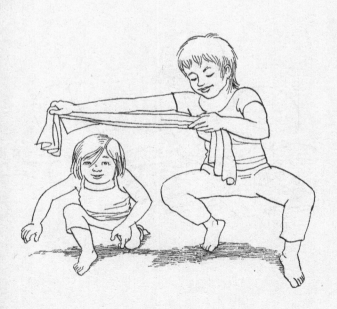

Take a towel and, holding it at both ends, squat down with a straight spine, using your leg strength. Have your child crawl under the towel without touching it. Have him try five times, always coming under a different way (back, side, and so on). Pretend that you are in the circus.

CAT (Coordinates Movement and Breath)

Come back onto your hands and knees, with your back horizontal. Gaze at the floor. While pulling in your stomach, round your back, lifting your spine toward the ceiling. Gently squeezing your butt, look down at the area between your knees. Meow and purr or hiss like a cat. Go back and forth three times. Next, extend an arm out in front of you and the opposite leg behind you; switch and do the opposite arm and leg. Repeat three times on each side.

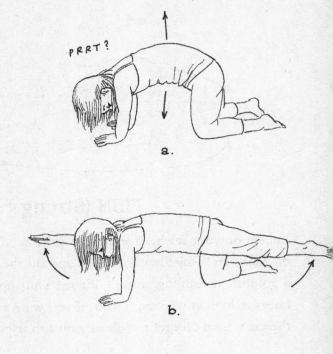

ROLLING PIN (Loosens Entire Body)

Place pillows across the floor and have your child lie on her back with a straight body. Roll her over the pillows like you are rolling out dough. Go back and forth five times. Kids love to experiment with gravity from different angles.

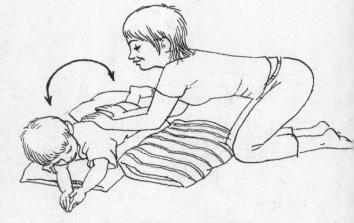

Standing

AIRPLANE (Lower Back, Arms, and Legs)

Place a pillow in the center of the room and reach your arms out to your sides with your palms down, fingers spread. Bend your knees and, with a straight back, lean forward to two o'clock. Circle around the pillows as if you are an airplane flying around a mountain while you are tilting your arms side to side. Circle five times in each direction. Make the sound of a motor while you chase each other. Bend your knees up and down so that your wings reach different altitudes.

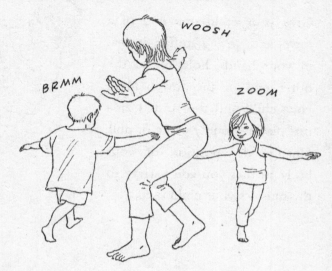

SEAWEED (Arms and Shoulders)

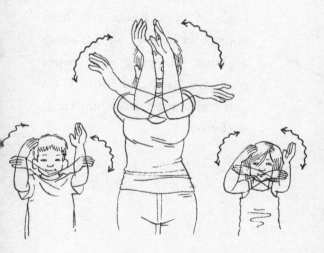

Bring your elbows up to shoulder height, with your fingers above your elbows. Now pretend that the area from your elbows to your fingertips is seaweed at the bottom of the ocean, and sway your forearms from side to side as you tap your elbows and then spread them apart. Stand up straight and name ten things you can find in the ocean (whales, starfish, boats . . .)

TUG OF WAR
(Builds Arm Strength)

Give your child one end of a towel and, with a stuffed animal in your hands, hold on to the other end of the towel. Have your child and the stuffed animal play a friendly game of pull. Change the position of your body so that you add variety to the muscles your child uses.

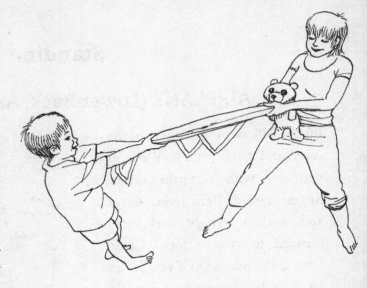

TIGHT ROPE
(Helps with Balance and Concentration)

Place a shoestring straight across the floor. Place a paper plate on both of your heads and have your child walk along the string without dropping the paper plate. Go back and forth. If he gets really good, have him try it backward.

KANGAROO (Legs and Cardio)

Place a shoestring straight across the floor. Hold your arms in front of your chest. Now hop over the string, trying to jump as far as you can each time without touching it. Do it five times in each direction. Take turns. Show your child how to observe and then participate.

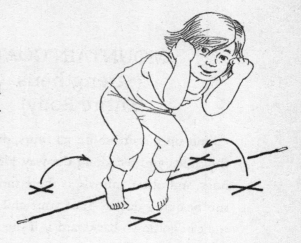

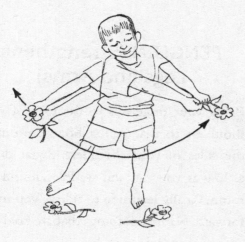

ELEPHANT (Works Your Core)

Interweave your hands together in front of you with straight arms. Lean forward and sway your arms and upper body side to side as you follow each other with a wide stance around the room. Name five wild animals. Lead and then follow. You can stop along the way and grab hay from the floor with your trunk.

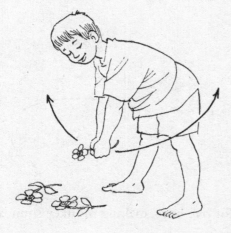

MOUNTAIN GOAT
(Strengthens Entire Body)

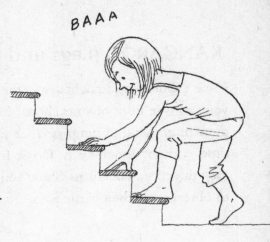

BAAA

Climb up a staircase on all fours, discussing all the sights you see along the way. Flowers, trees, bugs, and other animals. Is there snow, or is the sun beaming down? Spot your child and see if she can go down backward as if she were trying to sneak away without being heard.

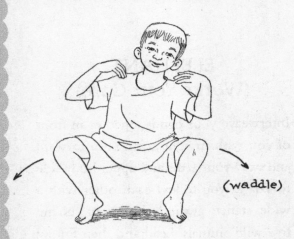

(waddle)

PENGUIN (Strengthens Legs and Arms)

Bring your fingertips to the tops of your shoulders so that your elbows are out to the sides of your shoulders. Squat down as low as you can and waddle around the room. Really lean side to side as you move forward. Name ten things that are cold (ice cream, snow, igloos . . .)

MONKEY
(Works Legs and Arms)

Remain on all fours. Come onto your toes, push off the floor with your hands, and reach forward as far as you can with both arms simultaneously, then plant your hands and hop both

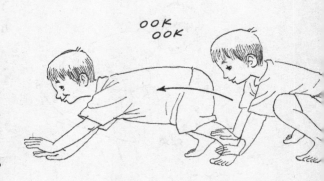

OOK OOK

feet forward. Keep going forward this way for five hops, making monkey sounds and discovering things in the forest.

TREE
(Improves Balance)

Reach your arms out to the side as if they were crooked branches. Spread your fingers. Now lift your left foot off the ground and balance. Hold for ten seconds and switch sides. Name five things you can find in a tree (leaves, birds, apples) or make the sounds of different birds. Kids love the sounds of talking parrots. You can also both rip up old newspapers and make leaves, and as your child is trying to balance, you can toss them over your heads.

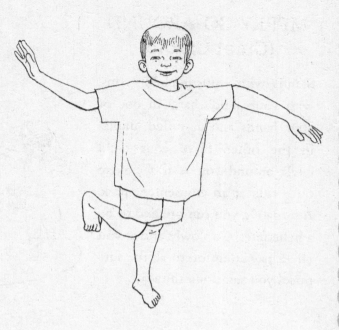

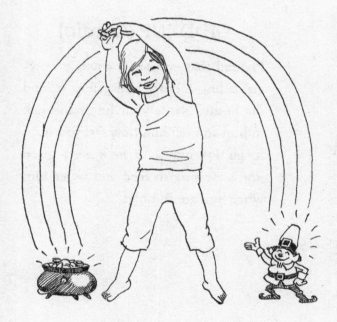

RAINBOW (Stretches Legs and Arms)

With a very wide stance, slowly hang down and walk your hands to your left foot. Now starting there, come up and reach your arms high above your head, making a rainbow until you get to your right foot. Go back and forth, naming the colors of the rainbow.

MERRY-GO-AROUND
(Great Cardio)

Stand with outstretched arms, with your child's hand in one of your hands and a stuffed animal in the other. Have your child circle around you as if she were on a ride at an amusement park. Alternately, you can pretend to be a helicopter. Go slowly, and as you circle, pay attention to all the surprises you see along the way.

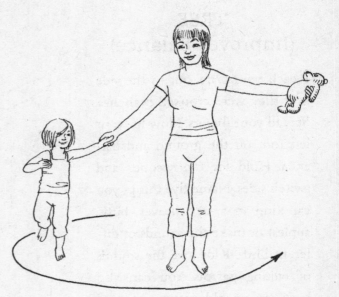

HI YO SILVER... AWAYY!

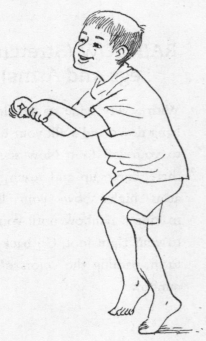

GIDDYUP (Cardio)

Pretend that you are a cowboy/cowgirl riding a horse and gallop around the house. Name your horse and talk to him and tell him how fast you want to go. Pet him as if he were a good horse. Be sure to feed and water him when you are finished.

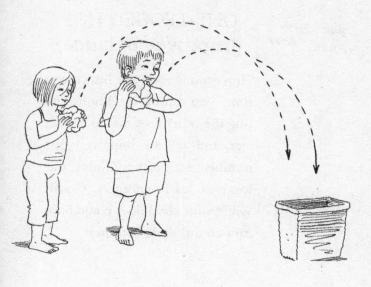

SOCK TOSS
(Increases Focus and Spatial Relationships)

Gather some old socks or ball up some newspaper pages and play toss into a short trash can or a bucket. Start close so you help build confidence and gradually go back. Start with 5 socks each and alternate hands every other time.

WALL CHAIR
(Strengthens Legs)

Put your back flat against a sturdy wall, making sure that your heels are below your knees and your legs are at right angles. Play patty-cake with your child. Then switch places.

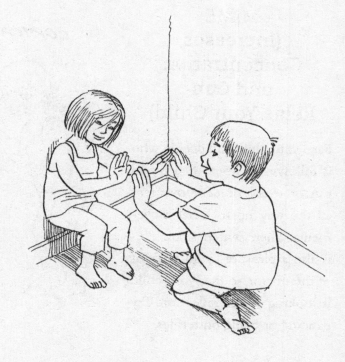

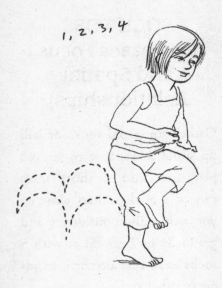

1, 2, 3, 4

ONE, TWO,
THREE, FOUR

ONE-LEGGED HOP
(Improves Balance)

Hop on one foot. See how many times you can do it without setting the other foot down. Switch legs and try to improve your number each time. Count out loud to learn numbers. Count while your child does it and have him count while you do it.

MIME
(Increases Concentration and Can Relax Your Child)

Face your child and decide who is following whom, then try to mirror every single movement all the way up to facial movements. Then switch sides. This is also a pleasure to do in front of the mirror, so that your child is looking at her reflection. Try dancing or being butterflies.

COPYCAT!

MIME!

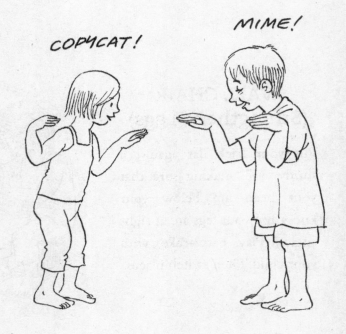

FUN AND GAMES FOR BIGGER KIDS

As your child gets older and more nimble, the world is full of fun fitness possibilities. While one of the goals of being active is to help prevent childhood weight issues, there's also another good reason: High-impact exercises, like jumping, stimulate bone growth and strengthen bone, too. Some ideas to get your older ones hopping to it:

➲ **Create Obstacle Courses:** Use a park, backyard—anywhere—to create a safe course where your child has to run, jump, and hop.

➲ **Play Hop Scotch:** You can use good old-fashioned sidewalk chalk.

➲ **Create Your Own Jumping Game:** Cut out a piece of cardboard and write the numbers on it as pictured below. There are all kinds of jumping and hopping games your child can do from here (going in order, or hopping to numbers that you call out, or doing all even numbers, and so on).

11   12

10

9   8   7

5   6

4

1   2   3

VACCINES

Most of us believe we make important decisions from our heads, rationally weighing the available information. But the truth is that when it comes to the most important decisions, we rely on our hearts and our gut instincts far more than we want to acknowledge. Perhaps nowhere does that become more apparent than it does with the issue of vaccination. It's a hotly debated topic among parents, doctors, and researchers. While there are many viewpoints, all the sides have one thing in common: We care first and foremost about the health of our children. As you make this decision, you will largely be guided by your emotion and instinct, but we also hope to provide some information, especially about prevention and risks, that can help shape your opinions and ultimately help you decide what to do.

In *YOU: Having a Baby*, we dissected the argument from all sides and provided our take. So if you have that book, and here, for those of you who don't, we outline the debate again—complete with updated information and material.

When it comes to vaccines, we are not going to adamantly tell you what to do one way or the other, since even the authorship team has varying opinions on the subject. What we hope is that you will explore both the pros and cons about vaccines (which we outline here), even do additional research, and make a thoughtful decision about what makes sense to you even before Baby arrives, if possible.

In a nutshell, here's the debate: There are surely enough data to show that vaccines do save lives and protect against illness. The extent of that benefit may be debatable, but we consider it significant. There are also safety concerns, as with any medication, in that there are not—and never can be—enough data to guarantee the safety of vaccines in any given individual, especially as they interact with other vaccines, viruses, drugs, foods, and that person's specific internal environment.

So what are we left with? In one corner, we have a group of people who examine the data and believe the advice of the American Academy of Pediatrics, the majority of pediatricians worldwide, and the Centers for Disease Control and Prevention. They conclude that vaccines are much more likely to benefit their children than harm them and are helpful to the long-term health not only of children but of the population at large. They and the American Academy of Pediatrics and the Centers for Disease Control and Prevention cite studies showing that vaccines prevent disease and infant deaths every year. When problems such as epilepsy, delayed development, and impaired communication arise in close proximity to vaccine administration, they are often categorized as "side effects of vaccine"—but close appearance does not indicate cause and effect. Indeed, since studies have shown that more unimmunized kids have these problems than kids who have received shots, blaming the vaccines may not be justified.

In the other corner are those who do not believe that vaccines are safe enough for the long-term health of their children. From their perspective, no studies absolutely demonstrate a vaccine's safety, and the full range of serious consequences caused by vaccines is being minimized and ignored.

The great news is that there is some common ground: Both sides acknowledge that the debate has forced vaccines to become safer, and that's a good thing. Beyond that, your decision may ultimately come down to (1) what kind of person you are at heart (trusting of the medical profession or skeptical of it), (2) how tolerant you are of risk, and (3) your family medical history. One thing is clear: Not vaccinating your child greatly increases his/her risk of getting one of the vaccine-preventable diseases described below (see page 410).

To help you make an informed choice, we questioned over a hundred experts on all sides of the vaccine issue to get their data and understand their points of view. Here's a summary of some of their major arguments for and against vaccination, and at the end of each section is the YOU Docs' take on the issue after considering all the information:

THE ISSUE	ARE VACCINES SAFE AND EFFECTIVE?
Support Vaccines	Vaccines prevent 20,500 infant deaths a year in the United States (compared to the prevaccine era) and innumerable other disorders such as brain dysfunction, paralysis, and even cancer in children and adults. Vaccines are credited with huge decreases in medical illnesses; the polio vaccine prevents polio and alone saves some $100 billion a year that would be spent in caring for polio victims, not to mention preventing suffering of the polio victims themselves. By reducing the prevalence of these infections in the population through vaccination, we can reduce the risk to those not able to be vaccinated or for whom vaccines may not work: to cite a few examples, those with immune deficiencies, those who are receiving treatments that hinder immunization, and those who are too young. If immunization rates were to decrease, the risk of infection would increase for all children, and especially for the most vulnerable members of society. There's no doubt that vaccination can cause some injuries. For example, we believe (based on the studies) that the original polio vaccine, which prevented polio in 1 out of every 245 children immunized, caused polio in 1 out of every 1 to 2 million children back when the vaccine was made from a live weakened virus. The rate is even less for the inactivated vaccine currently used. Measles vaccine causes about 4 cases of serious brain dysfunction a year in the United States, but it prevents 2,000 to 4,000 cases of such brain dysfunction and several hundred deaths from the actual disease. The rotavirus vaccine, before it was reformulated, used to cause intussusception—a serious condition often requiring surgery or a radiologic procedure—in 1 out of every 10,000 to 14,000 kids immunized. This spurred development of a new vaccine that has not been associated with intussusception risk. However, rotavirus vaccine prevents hospitalization for diarrhea in about 1 out of every 200 kids who receive it. (These statistics come from the "Vaccine Injury Table" of the National Vaccine Injury Compensation Program, which lists side effects acknowledged by the government or courts.) Anecdotal information (examples from individuals), even when disproved by large studies, can feel emotionally wrenching, but it is important to remember that when two things happen at the same time in a population, this does not prove that one causes the other.
Against Vaccines	Large European studies showing no adverse effects from vaccines in more than 2.5 million kids were epidemiological, meaning that they examined patterns in the population rather than biological cause and effect in the individual. Large studies also ignore the significant number of anecdotal stories by parents who have witnessed sudden declines in the health of their children after vaccination.
The YOU Docs' Take	"Safe" does not mean without risk. It means that the benefit of a vaccine, or any medical procedure, is greater than the risk involved for the general population. Vaccines save lives and prevent disease, but all seventeen childhood vaccines combined may carry serious risks for anywhere from 1 child in 2,000 to 1 child in 10,000. The chance that childhood vaccines benefit the typical child are at least twenty times greater than the chance of serious injury. Some of us think that it is not just the vaccine but its interaction with another factor—specifically, with a gene turned on by a virus, for instance—that underlies many a bad reaction. One way for parents to "play it safe" is not to immunize their child while he or any family member is sick but to wait a week until he's healthy. In other words, we agree with vaccinating, just not when your child is sick. This is the recommendation of the American Academy of Pediatrics and the federal government as well, so make sure that your child is healthy when vaccines are given. Bottom line for us, immunizing your healthy child against the diseases preventable by currently licensed vaccines is one of the best ways of keeping your child healthy.

THE ISSUE	DO VACCINES CAUSE AUTISM?
Support Vaccines	Large-scale epidemiologic studies in a number of countries, including Finland, the Netherlands, the United Kingdom, Japan, and the United States, clearly demonstrate that vaccines are not responsible for the epidemic of autism. Vaccines *might* trigger autism in a small number of genetically primed individuals with a very rare preexisting disease of the mitochondria (see page 173); and these people most probably would have developed autism even if they hadn't received the vaccine. In this situation, a virus or another environmental insult can just as easily be the straw that breaks the camel's back.
Against Vaccines	The stories of parents describing the transformation of their previously healthy children into children with autism spectrum disorder soon after and in immediate relationship to vaccination are too strong and too common to avoid the conclusion that vaccines can cause autism.
The YOU Docs' Take	There is no known association between vaccination and autism, or, to state it another way, vaccination is not the cause of the autism epidemic. However, environmental circumstances such as another viral infection causing a high fever, or a high fever plus a vaccine may bring out autism in genetically susceptible children. We cannot currently identify such vulnerable children prior to vaccination. As genetic triggers become better known, and as testing becomes safer, less expensive, and more available, we may be able to identify all individuals at risk for virus-plus-vaccine-triggered diseases and avoid vaccinating them, or avoid vaccinating them while they're exposed to a particular infection. For all who choose vaccination, make sure that your child is in good health, is well hydrated before getting the shot, and is not receiving antibiotics. If your child or another family member is sick, schedule his vaccines for another time. Treat any postvaccine fever and irritability aggressively, and hydrate the young patient: with breast milk or formula for children not yet one year old; with water, milk, or Pedialyte for toddlers; and with water, milk, or 100 percent juice for older children. Then proceed according to your pediatrician's instructions.

THE ISSUE	ARE VACCINES EVEN NECESSARY?
Support Vaccines	If we had vaccines for more pathogens (disease-causing agents such as viruses and bacteria), we could decrease the incidence of more diseases. Imagine if there were vaccines against Alzheimer's disease, AIDS, breast cancer, and bacterial infections such as MRSA, a potentially fatal staph bacteria that is alarmingly resistant to antibiotics. Many docs believe it is life threatening *not* to immunize. Children continue to die of pertussis (whooping cough) in parts of the world where this vaccine is not utilized by enough of the population.
Against Vaccines	There are hundreds of pathogens for which there are no vaccines, and the CDC makes very good recommendations for staying healthy while being exposed to those pathogens. The same recommendations should hold true for those diseases for which we have vaccines.

(continued on next page)

THE ISSUE	ARE VACCINES EVEN NECESSARY? (cont.)
The YOU Docs' Take	Our grandparents and their parents didn't get vaccinated, and a number of us didn't get many of the current vaccines. We missed seven to fourteen days or so of school for chicken pox (varicella), and some of us will suffer shingles when that virus resurfaces in us later in life. Our caregivers suffered with us and stayed home from work, too. We weren't allowed to play outside, go to the movies, or go to camp in the summer until the polio vaccine was deployed. Many of us older docs know folks killed or harmed for life with mental dysfunction by a virus for which there is now a vaccine. One in a thousand of our parents' generation who got measles developed brain dysfunction, German measles led to deafness, blindness, and brain dysfunction if infection was contracted in utero, and more kids died in previous eras due to other vaccine-preventable diseases. Vaccination has promoted a better quality of life and has allowed more of us to survive and have children of our own. We're for 'em.

THE ISSUE	WHAT ARE WE EXPOSING OUR KIDS TO?
Support Vaccines	Kids and even adults are exposed to many more than 113 new antigens every *hour* in a new environment such as a zoo or museum. Plus, the smallpox vaccine alone contained 203 antigens. The great news? By wiping out smallpox through mass vaccinations in the past, no one currently gets those 203 antigens.
Against Vaccines	If children receive the entire panel of vaccines recommended by the American Academy of Pediatrics, they get 32 vaccinations (well, 17 vaccines, but some are given more than once to achieve adequate protection) over six years and are injected with 113 vaccine antigens. That's a lot of unnecessary chemicals to put into a child's body and three times as many as was recommended two decades ago. This is also more than what many European countries recommend.
The YOU Docs' Take	The safety of vaccines has improved and the track record for vaccine additives has improved. We are more comfortable with vaccine safety based on scientific study and years of experience. The recent H1N1 (swine flu) vaccination campaign for high-risk individuals demonstrated the ability to contain an epidemic predicted to kill over 40,000 in the United States. By the end of the 2009–10 flu season, only 12,000 people had died of H1N1 (many before the vaccine became available). And 50 million doses of the vaccine were administered with few to no reported long-term side effects, and no deaths in vaccinated people. Of course, more can always be done to improve the quality and delivery speed of vaccines, and the current debate is pushing that research forward.

THE ISSUE	HOW IMPORTANT ARE VACCINES IN A GLOBAL AND UNPREDICTABLE WORLD?
Support Vaccines	Vaccines are necessary because we live and travel in a world where we come into unexpected contact with people who have been exposed to disease or may be asymptomatic carriers. A recent outbreak of measles in unvaccinated teens and adults after a plane ride with a child with measles demonstrates this hazard of lack of vaccination.

Against Vaccines	Children who are not known to be high risk do not need to be exposed to vaccines.
The YOU Docs' Take	If you can identify your child as low-risk for certain diseases, you can be more flexible in terms of timing those vaccines. However, that may not be so easy to do, unless you and your child live without much contact with the outside world. The current schedule is based on getting the most protection when babies are particularly vulnerable. For example, pertussis is most deadly during the earliest months of life. On the other hand, if you, your partner, and your child's caregivers are not carriers of hepatitis B, we recommend waiting to give this vaccination until two months of age or later (if your child has not already started to receive this series of shots). Do note that varying from the recommended schedule places the burden of record keeping on you, but if you're up to the task, it may work well (and may even be safer) for Junior.
THE ISSUE	**CAN WE WIPE OUT DISEASES WITH VACCINES?**
Support Vaccines	Through vaccines, we can achieve what's referred to as herd immunity, making diseases so uncommon in the environment (the herd) that some are eventually eradicated. (And we no longer need the vaccine.) The best example is the global elimination of smallpox. We were very close to eliminating polio until a few countries declined immunization for several years, allowing it to resurface in their populations and then spread to others. Until those outbreaks can be eliminated, polio vaccination is still a necessity.
Against Vaccines	Modern medical advances such as sanitation systems and personal hygiene have also played a major role in wiping out diseases, and children do not need to be vaccinated for diseases that they're at little risk of contracting or suffering life-threatening complications from.
The YOU Docs' Take	We love the smallpox story but think it is unlikely to be repeated for many diseases. And vaccination against some organisms always will be needed. For example, vaccination against tetanus will always be needed, as this tetanus-causing organism is universally present in the soil. Until the smallpox story can be repeated for other diseases preventable by vaccines, we urge parents to protect their children according to current standards set by the American Academy of Pediatrics. These schedules have considerable flexibility, and we urge you to discuss them with your pediatrician.
THE ISSUE	**SHOULD WE USE VACCINES TO PROTECT OTHERS?**
Support Vaccines	Vaccinating your child helps protect others who might be particularly vulnerable to these life-threatening diseases, such as grandparents, infant siblings, pregnant women, or children and adults who suffer from disorders that compromise their defenses against disease or who are undergoing immune-suppressing therapies.
Against Vaccines	People who are vulnerable need to take preventive measures against contracting diseases. And disease risk has gone down substantially as many others are getting vaccinated. My child need not bear the responsibility for other people's health by being vaccinated.

(continued on next page)

THE ISSUE	SHOULD WE USE VACCINES TO PROTECT OTHERS? (cont.)
The YOU Docs' Take	Herd immunity is a wonderful thing. If you're concerned about the health of other people, your choice is clear; if you're concerned solely for the health of your child, your choice may be more difficult. However, since our society recognizes its responsibility to protect all children, laws and regulations may exclude unvaccinated children from public programs such as schools, day care, and camps.

THE ISSUE	WHO SHOULD MAKE DECISIONS ABOUT VACCINATION?
Support Vaccines	The issues around research and ethics are too complex for those not scientifically trained to understand. Complicating the issue is the fact that many believe a gold-standard study would be unethical: How could you carry out what's called a double-blind study of a large group of children—randomly assigning half to be immunized and half not, leaving the second group of kids vulnerable to serious and often deadly diseases? The law says that the community has a say that goes beyond the rights of the individual when it comes to communicable disease, so expect not to be able to send your child to school when there's a chicken pox outbreak and you haven't vaccinated your child.
Against Vaccines	Individuals need to customize their own programs with willing physicians as advisers. The one-size-fits-all schedule is dangerous for too many kids.
The YOU Docs' Take	We think that you are smart enough to digest the arguments in this toolbox and make rational decisions for your children. Most readers will follow the official guidelines established by the American Academy of Pediatrics, which offer the least chance of missing important vaccinations and the best chance of avoiding severe disease or death for your child. Others will follow alternative schedules to reduce to the smallest degree possible the potential perceived complications, while still ensuring that all appropriate vaccinations get in. All of the docs on the authorship team have vaccinated their children, though not always according to the official schedule.

THE ISSUE	HAVE THE YOU DOCS PRESENTED THE ISSUE FAIRLY?
Support Vaccines	You could have done a better job. Giving equal space to those against vaccines makes it seem as though they have a valid argument. You try to be too nice, and maybe you guys don't understand the science well enough.
Against Vaccines	You guys seem to ignore the personal stories of parents whose children suffered real illness and injury right after vaccination. You do not tell the story of how the establishment is hiding data concerning side effects or misleading themselves about the robustness of weak studies.
The YOU Docs' Take	If both sides think that we are giving the other side too much credit, we've probably hit the sweet spot in this argument. But we also believe that we need a new way of presenting the information to help mothers and fathers discuss the options with well-meaning but busy pediatricians who are understandably frustrated addressing the same concerns dozens of times weekly. That's why we introduced in *YOU: Having a Baby* a new way of understanding the issue, called the Number Needed to Treat.

The Number Needed to Treat

To help you understand the risk–benefit relationship with regard to immunization, we calculated for each vaccine a number called the Number Needed to Treat: that is, how many kids have to be inoculated to save a life or prevent a case of that particular disease. (For more information on how we calculated these numbers, please see our explanation on www.realage.com and www.doctoroz.com.) The advantage of this number is that it gives you some perspective on how effective a vaccine can be. How to read it: The smaller the number, the better the figure. For example, when the number needed to treat is 2, that means that for every two children vaccinated, one death or illness is prevented. When the number is high, it's the opposite: For every, say, five thousand children vaccinated, one death or illness is prevented. If you're not comfortable with numbers and statistics (and even if you are), we strongly encourage you to copy this chart and discuss it with your pediatrician to help you understand the numbers as well as you can.

Because vaccination has made many of these diseases uncommon, you may not be familiar with the possible outcomes of contracting them. We encourage you to read our summary of the risks of each disease at the end of this toolbox. The major points that you can take away from these numbers:

In most cases, vaccines prevent high-impact ailments for which there is currently a low probability of contraction. It's up to you to decide where the balance point lies between risk and benefit, according to your own sensitivities. Remember, if there were a simple answer, we wouldn't even be having this debate. Focus also on the Number Needed to Vaccinate to Prevent a Case, not only the Number Needed to Vaccinate to Prevent a Death, because infection often leads to hospitalization and potentially a host of other exposures and lifelong complications, not to mention that infections put others around you at risk as well. These numbers are calculated by comparing the number of cases of a disease before vaccines became available versus after they were used. And they lead to a fundamental question: Is the risk of getting the infection great enough to warrant vaccination, or is it small enough that the risk of the vaccine isn't worth it? Only you can answer that, because we each have our own philosophical take on where to draw that line.

	NUMBER NEEDED TO VACCINATE TO PREVENT A CASE	NUMBER NEEDED TO VACCINATE TO PREVENT A DEATH
Varicella	2	46,512
Rotavirus	2	104,167
Measles	8	9,091
Newborn influenza	13	50,000
Pertussis (whooping cough)	22	998
Mumps	26	102,564
Hepatitis A	39	33,613
Hepatitis B	75	21,053
Rubella	84	235,294
Strep pneumococcus	186	2,424
Diphtheria	200	2,195
Haemophilus influenzae type b (Hib)	201	4,020
Polio	245	2,129
Influenza in pregnant women	952	63,492
Meningococcus (cerebrospinal meningococcal meningitis)	2,689	22,409
Tetanus	7,421	8,547

YOUR VACCINATION OPTIONS

The bottom line is that you can educate yourself to make informed, conscious, and customized choices based on your family's beliefs and values. Essentially, you have three options.

THE OPTION	VACCINATE ACCORDING TO THE CDC AND AMERICAN ACADEMY OF PEDIATRICS' APPROVED GUIDELINES
Support This Approach	The American Academy of Pediatrics and the U.S. Centers for Disease Control and Prevention have assembled the most knowledgeable experts in the world to come up with a vaccination schedule that makes the most sense for the public health. The schedule is based on the knowledge of diverse experts who are best able to synthesize what is known about human developmental biology, the epidemiology and clinical characteristics of the disease, and the characteristics of the particular vaccine.
Against This Approach	Some of these experts earn income by administering or researching vaccines or consulting with pharmaceutical manufacturers. While they are concerned about the health of the general public, few value your individual child's health as greatly as you do. And some recommendations are clearly designed for society in general even if you as an individual might not benefit. For example, the recommendation to immunize against hepatitis B at birth is illogical if you, your partner, and your caregivers are all low risk. But the advice is wise for the U.S. population as a whole, if you consider it unlikely that the parents at high risk for hepatitis B (like IV drug abusers) will bring their children back to the pediatrician in a timely fashion.
The YOU Docs' Take	The advantage of the standard plan is that it represents a broadly based scientific consensus on how to maximize protection of each child. In addition, most docs follow it, making it easier to avoid mistakes, especially if you're moving or switching pediatricians at any point. Combining injections saves money (since many insurers won't pay for alternative plans) and avoids traumatizing the child with multiple injections at every doctor's visit. The downside, some believe, is that some of the early vaccines (like hepatitis B at birth) are unnecessary to be given at that early time for low-risk babies.

(continued on next page)

THE OPTION	VACCINATE ACCORDING TO A POPULAR PEDIATRICIAN'S GUIDELINES OR YOUR OWN PLAN
Support This Approach	Spreading out vaccines reduces the stimulation of your child's immune system caused by administering multiple antigens and toxins at once. Delaying the vaccines allows the infant's immune system to develop so that she can cope more effectively. And when she has completed the schedule, she still gets all the protection offered by the standard approach.
Against This Approach	If you do follow an alternative program, you have to be diligent in your record keeping to help out the doc's office, since the staff there might not be used to the alternative schedule, and it's essential to complete each series for full immunity. Further, no study has been conducted to randomly compare kids who receive vaccinations according to an alternative schedule versus the standard schedule, so we do not know if it is as safe and as protective as the standard schedule. If you are going to use an alternative schedule, check with your insurance company to make sure that the vaccines are covered, as some companies cover only the traditional schedule. If you need to pay for the visits yourself, you may want to consider using the public health department services at a lower cost.
The YOU Docs' Take	With the alternative schedule, you'd still get the recommended vaccines, but they're spaced apart a little more, thus exposing your child to fewer foreign substances at once and spreading out that exposure over a longer period of time. The downside is that it means more doctor visits, more exposure to sick kids at those doctors' offices, more money, more periods of postshot grumpiness, and a greater risk of your child contracting a disease during infancy from either the delayed or missed shots or the extra visits' exposure to sick kids. Plus there are no studies to show that this alternate approach is any safer. We now favor the American Academy of Pediatrics schedule.

THE OPTION	NOT TO VACCINATE YOUR CHILD
Support This Approach	Some believe that all vaccines are unnecessary, especially for people with few risk factors. They also believe that some health benefits are achieved if a child overcomes an illness, such as less asthma and gains in lifelong immunity. If you believe that health is an "inside-out" phenomenon—meaning that if you have a strong immune system, it will prevent you from getting sick—you may decide that you and your children can stay healthy without vaccines. When deciding whether or not to vaccinate, many parents may not know that vaccines are not always mandatory for entering the public school system. Every state has its own rules, but nineteen states have what is called a philosophical exemption, meaning that you have a very simple right to refuse. The other two types of exemptions, religious and medical, are beyond the scope of what we want to discuss here. But it's important for you to know that you don't always have to vaccinate simply to get your kids into school.
Against This Approach	You never know when your child might be exposed to certain diseases, whether through traveling on airplanes or public transportation, visiting foreign countries, going to day care or school, or being taken care of by a babysitter or relative who may be an unknowing carrier. Choosing not to vaccinate puts both your child and your community at risk via loss of herd immunity or protection. If this individual decision makes you or your child contagious, that can set up a larger outbreak of a significant or life-threatening infection.
The YOU Docs' Take	Children deserve our protection, living in today's mobile world. All children are at risk from vaccine-preventable diseases. Some children are at higher risk. That includes children living in cities who take public transportation, whose parents work in health care, who travel (or whose parents travel), and who live in communities with immigrants. We also recommend immunization for kids who live around people at high risk for contracting diseases, such as grandparents and those whose immune systems may be compromised; those who spend time in settings with other children, such as in day care; and children with caregivers who may be exposed through any of these means.

Vaccine Schedule Options

Below you'll find both the official AAP schedule and an alternate one. We include the alternate one because you may have heard of it, so it is here for you to review with your pediatrician. No matter what you decide, we do want to offer some basic guidelines and principles for vaccines and immunity.

⊃ Pregnant women should avoid getting the live influenza vaccine, but the inactivated vaccine is safe and effective. Talk to your doctor about it and always make sure that the vaccine is free of the mercury-based preservative thimerosal. (Single-dose vials are thimerosal free; current vaccines that have thimerosal contain a dose of mercury equal to that ingested in two pieces of tuna sushi or a small tuna sandwich.) We believe that all pregnant women should seriously consider it since they are at extra-high risk of severe, or even fatal, flu. If you choose not to get the flu shot, you can boost your immune system during the winter by taking 2,000 IU of vitamin D_3 daily.

⊃ If your child is at risk of contracting influenza either because you or his caregivers are at risk or because he is exposed to crowds or in day care, he should receive his first flu vaccine at six months and then annually thereafter. One of the reasons you don't want your baby to catch the flu is that antiviral medications such as Tamiflu (oseltamivir) are either contraindicated due to side effects in those under one year of age or have not been tested for safety in that population, and flu is a more serious disease for those not yet in first grade.

⊃ We strongly support breast feeding, as it does offer some immunity to babies, but it is far from foolproof, especially since most mothers who breast-feed discontinue the practice by six months after delivery, and their breast feeding can be sporadic at times.

⊃ We recommend priming your child for a successful immunization by making sure of the following:

1. He has a good night's sleep. Toddlers typically need twelve to fourteen hours of total sleep a night plus naps.

2. He is not showing symptoms of any illness, nor has he been around anyone with an infectious illness for a week before the vaccination.

3. He is well hydrated. Cajole, bribe—do whatever it takes to get him to drink beforehand. Children younger than one year old should have breast milk or formula; those between one and two, a glass of milk or water; and kids three to five years old, one to two glasses of milk, juice, or water.

4. He has had adequate amounts of vitamins A, C, and E for at least a week prior to the appointment. Breast milk provides these vitamins, but we recommend that you supplement with a baby multivitamin such as Tri-Vi-Sol or Poly-Vi-Sol drops—1 milliliter a day starting at age two months. (See page 116.) Older children should also be taking a daily multivitamin. (See page 125.)

· · ·

Here are two user-friendly forms that you can use to help track either the standard vaccination schedule or an alternative devised by Dr. Bob Sears. We are not endorsing the Sears method, just providing the schedule for the families that choose that path, to help those families avoid missed immunizations:

American Academy of Pediatrics Schedule

	Diphtheria Tetanus Acellular Pertussis (DTaP)	Rotavirus	Pneumococcal	Haemophilus influenzae type b	Polio	Measles Mumps Rubella (MMR)	Varicella	Hepatitis A	Hepatitis B
2 months	*	*	*	*	*				*
3 months									
4 months	*	*	*	*	*				*
5 months									
6 months	*	*	*	*					
7 months									
9 months									
12 months						*	*	*	

	Diphtheria Tetanus Acellular Pertussis (DTaP)	Rotavirus	Pneumococcal	Haemophilus influenzae type b	Polio	Measles Mumps Rubella (MMR)	Varicella	Hepatitis A	Hepatitis B
15 months	*		*	*	*				*
18 months								*	
2 years									
2½ years									
3 years									
3½ years									
5 years	*				*	*	*		

★ Influenza: yearly beginning at 6 months.

★ Meningococcal: given before age 11.

★ The last dose of polio, MMR, varicella, and DTaP can be given anytime between 4 and 6 years.

Alternative Schedule by Dr. Bob Sears

	Diphtheria Tetanus Acellular Pertussis (DTaP)	Rotavirus	Pneumococcal	Haemophilus influenzae type b	Polio	Mumps	Measles	Rubella	Varicella	Hepatitis A	Hepatitis B
2 months	*	*									
3 months			*	*							
4 months	*	*									
5 months			*	*							
6 months	*	*									
7 months			*	*							
9 months					*						
12 months					*	*					

	Diphtheria Tetanus Acellular Pertussis (DTaP)	Rotavirus	Pneumococcal	Haemophilus influenzae type b	Polio	Mumps	Measles	Rubella	Varicella	Hepatitis A	Hepatitis B
15 months			*	*							
18 months	*							*			
2 years					*			*			
2½ years											*
3 years							*				
3½ years											*

Risk of Disease

Before making your decision, take a moment to read through the following information. We provide it not to scare you but to let you know the risks of contracting the various ailments against which pediatricians vaccinate.

- ⊃ Diphtheria—attacks the throat and heart; can lead to heart failure and death. The infection is thought to respond to antibiotics. There are fewer than four cases a year in the United States. (Advocates would say, "Thanks to vaccines!")

- ⊃ Pertussis (whooping cough)—causes severe coughing that makes it hard to breathe, eat, or drink; can lead to pneumonia, convulsions, brain damage, and death. Most serious for kids under three because secretions are thick and windpipes are tiny. Older children develop a cough and typically recover uneventfully. Immunity wanes as kids get older, with pertussis outbreaks common and often starting with a coughing adult. This can lead to more potentially fatal cases in unimmunized children and incompletely immunized infants. The booster dosing helps with waning immunity in those over eleven years old.

- ⊃ Tetanus (lockjaw)—a serious infection that can lead to severe muscle spasm and death.

- ⊃ Polio—can cause muscle pain and paralysis; it paralyzes muscles used to breathe and swallow and can lead to death. Most exposed to polio have mild symptoms, but a small percentage get paralysis or debilitating motor impairment.

- ⊃ Measles—causes fever, rash, cough, runny nose, watery eyes; can lead to ear infections, pneumonia, brain swelling, and death. Individuals who are against vaccination contend that if there is an outbreak of measles in your area, give your child approximately 10,000 IU of Mycel vitamin A drops in juice for five days (or a single dose of 200,000 IU of vitamin A orally for children over one year of age, and 100,000 IU in a single dose for children six months to one year of age). That way, if he contracts measles, it will likely be a milder case, and he will have lifetime immunity. But supporters of vaccination ask, Why play Russian roulette with your child's life? In a recent U.S. outbreak among unvaccinated children, several died, and several suffered permanent brain dysfunction.

⊃ Mumps—causes fever, headache, painfully swollen salivary glands; can lead to meningitis and brain swelling. In very rare cases, mumps can cause testicles to swell, which can lead to infertility. Much more common: a parent's spending seven days with the child at home while she recovers.

⊃ Rubella (German measles)—causes fever, rash, and swelling of glands in the neck; can cause brain swelling or bleeding. If a pregnant woman contracts rubella, it can cause miscarriage or put her baby at high risk for neurological problems that resemble autism or life-threatening birth defects involving brain damage, hearing loss, cardiac malformations, and endocrine dysfunction. If you were not immunized earlier in life, get immunized as soon as possible.

⊃ Haemophilus influenzae type b—can cause meningitis, pneumonia, and epiglottitis (a severe throat infection that can lead to choking and death). This infection is less frequent in babies who are exclusively breast-fed, but it is an issue after six months, especially when breast feeding wanes or stops. This infection remains more common than diphtheria, tetanus, and polio. Just a few years back before this immunization was widely used, we saw many more kids with meningitis and severe bacterial infections from the flu.

⊃ Hepatitis B—can cause infection of the liver that can eventually lead to liver cancer and death. Unless you, your partner, or any other caregiver is high risk, the vaccine doesn't need to be given at birth and can be delayed until two months; some argue that any time before age ten is also fine. The Hep B vaccine doubles as a hedge against liver cancer.

⊃ Pneumococcal conjugate vaccine—protects against bacteria that commonly cause ear infections as well as potentially fatal illnesses such as meningitis, pneumonia, and bacteremia (infection of the bloodstream). Those children most at risk are those with predisposing factors, such as certain upper respiratory tract infections, asthma, and other conditions.

⊃ Meningococcal conjugate vaccine—protects against four types of bacterial meningitis (infections and inflammation of the fluid and membrane around the brain and spinal cord) that can cause high fever, headache, stiff neck, confusion, brain damage, hearing loss or blindness, and death. While this infection is unquestioningly severe when it happens, it is sporadic.

⊃ Rotavirus—causes severe acute gastroenteritis (vomiting and diarrhea) that can lead to hospitalization and death. By the time children are two years of age, the vast majority have had a rotavirus infection, and if so, are protected from this virus family going forward.

⊃ Hepatitis A—a liver disease that can cause mild flulike symptoms, jaundice, severe stomach pains, diarrhea, and in rare cases, death.

⊃ Varicella (chicken pox)—a highly contagious, common disease that can cause low-grade fever, rash, complications such as pneumonia and encephalitis, and in severe cases, death. Fetuses of women who contract varicella during the first two trimesters of their pregnancy can acquire congenital varicella syndrome; if a woman is infected between five days before giving birth and two days after, the baby will acquire the virus, which can be fatal. In addition to preventing chicken pox, the vaccine can also protect adults from contracting shingles, a very painful condition that affects more than 30 percent of unvaccinated adults.

⊃ Influenza—a highly common and contagious disease that can cause fever, aches and pains, cough, congestion, and lead to pneumonia, and, in rare cases, death. The vast majority of cases are an inconvenience, not deadly.

Out of four hundred thousand pregnant women in the United States who contract influenza each year, four hundred die of it, and an equal number are believed to have children with some significant abnormality because of it. Keeping the immune system strong with vitamin D_3 during the winter, along with obsessive hand washing and great sleep, helps avoid the flu.

Vaccine Requirements by Schools, Day Cares, Head Start, and Camps

HIGHLY RECOMMENDED (REQUIRED BY VIRTUALLY ALL SCHOOL SYSTEMS NATIONWIDE)	RECOMMENDED (SOMETIMES REQUIRED FOR SCHOOL OR DAY CARE—CHECK YOUR STATE)	OPTIONAL (NOT COMMONLY REQUIRED)
DTaP (the *a* means that it's a less reactive form of the pertussis vaccine) Polio MMR (or separate measles, mumps, and rubella) Hepatitis B (but does not need to be given at birth) Varicella Hib	Hepatitis A Meningococcal conjugate Pneumococcal conjugate especially important if you have depressed immunity (spleen removed), diabetes, asthma, or other heart or lung diseases	Rotavirus (unless your child is in day care, in which case it is highly recommended) Influenza (ditto for this one, and highly recommended for all children with asthma, congenital heart disease, and other risk factors—see page 415)

Our Recommendations on Specific Vaccines

⊃ If you, your partner, or a caregiver is a carrier of hepatitis B, request the first dose of the vaccine at birth. For everybody else, we recommend waiting until two months of age. At this time, it can also be given as part of a combination vaccine.

⊃ Hepatitis A is relatively common in the United States and far more common in other parts of the world. The Centers for Disease Control and Prevention has recommended this vaccine to all children ages one and older since 2006, in part because of increased travel and immigration, but also in an attempt to eliminate indigenous hepatitis A from the United States. Consider it optional if (1) your school system does not require it, (2) your child will not be in day care, (3) you do not live in a high-risk community, (4) everyone who prepares food for your child washes well, and (5) you do not travel to countries with a high incidence.

⊃ The rotavirus vaccine is a live oral vaccine, so one of the side effects is vomiting and diarrhea—exactly the symptoms it is supposed to protect against but exponentially milder than the disease itself. A prior version of this vaccine was withdrawn from the market in 1999 because it was linked to a severe condition known as intussusception, a blockage or telescoping of the intestine that may require surgery or a radiologic procedure and rarely can be fatal. The new vaccine, released in 2006, has not been associated with intussusception, but a version of it has had a forced recall due to the FDA's concern about virus contamination. The vaccine now on the market seems to have been tested sufficiently for us to say that it has much more benefit than risk and that it prevented hospitalization in 1 out of every 200 children. If your child is in day care or exposed to other high-risk circumstances, we recommend that she receive it. If you plan on using babysitting services, even sporadically, we can now recommend this vaccine as well.

⊃ Because influenza is so common and affects young children so severely (20,000 U.S. children under age five are hospitalized with complications of the flu each year), and because children under one year of age cannot be given antiviral therapy, the recommendation of yearly flu shots beginning at six months of age is not unreasonable. (Children ages two and above can take the nasal spray as long as they don't have asthma and are not immuno-compromised and have no one immunocompromised in the household.) Just make sure that the preparation is thimerosal free (from a single-dose package; all flu vaccines for infant use in the USA are as of 2010 thimerosal free). Children at high risk for complications from the flu who should get vaccinated include those with asthma, immune suppression, chronic kidney disease, heart disease, HIV-AIDS, diabetes, sickle-cell anemia, long-term as-pirin therapy, and any condition that can reduce lung function.

⊃ If your child is in day care or a member of your household is elderly or at high risk for flu, we also recommend vaccination. If the flu vaccine is not required for school and you would like to opt out, take precautions to avoid transmission, including frequent hand washing, not sharing cups and uten-sils, and avoiding even small crowds during flu season. This is not foolproof, but does reduce risk of infection.

Further Reading

Because this topic is so complicated and conflicted, we recommend that you explore it further. These are some of the resources that we found extremely helpful when thinking about the issue:

Red Book: 2009 Report of the Committee on Infectious Disease, by The American Academy of Pediatrics (www.aapredbook.aappublications.org)

Saying No to Vaccines: A Resource Guide for All Ages, by Sherri Tenpenny

Vaccinated: One Man's Quest to Defeat the World's Deadliest Diseases and *Autism's False Prophets: Bad Science, Risky Medicine, and the Search for a Cure,* by Paul A. Offit

Vaccine Safety Manual for Concerned Families and Health Practitioners:
   Guide to Immunization Risks and Protection, by Neil Z. Miller

Do Vaccines Cause That? by Martin Meyers and Diego Pineda

The Vaccine Book: Making the Right Decision for Your Child,
   by Robert W. Sears

THE FINE ART OF DISCIPLINE

As parents, we straddle the line between enthusiastic praise for good behavior (fist bump: "You pooped in the bowl!") and consequences for not-so-good behavior ("No playground until you apologize to your sister!").

Part of the issue of discipline—which is different from making and breaking habits but more about incentives and consequences—revolves around your parenting style. Here's how we recommend approaching the tough area of discipline.

As a parent, you need to come up with systems of encouragement and consequences that will help you educate your child and help her establish healthy habits along the way. If you go out on either of the extreme ends of this spectrum (rewarding your child for everything he's expected to do so that he comes to expect rewards for merely existing; or disciplining your child all the time so that he comes to fear you), you're setting up your child for a lot of stress, anxiety, and problems down the road. Your goal should be to function in the middle by saying no when the situation calls for it and dispensing TLC when your child craves it.

Consequences Philosophy. We know that there are several different camps when it comes to punishment. There's the spank camp ("My dad wumped me on the backside, and I turned out fine"), the extreme-threat camp ("No TV for you until you're in college—maybe even graduate school!"), the lecture camp, the time-out camp, the do-nothing camp, the pull-your-ear camp, and many, many more. First and foremost, we don't believe in spanking—because it hasn't been shown to be effective in changing behavior, because it's more about allowing the parent to vent his or her stress, and because it teaches your child to be more aggressive to others (mirror neurons, people!). That's not even mentioning the fact that some research shows that spanking is associated with lower IQs in children. But that doesn't mean we don't think there's sometimes a place for physical reactions from parents. (See our tip about wrestling on page 105.) If you do think you have the tendency to be a spanker, then we ask you one question: Is that how you deal with the people you love when you're angry? By hitting them? (Actually, that's two questions.) Before you react in an uncontrolled way, you need to give *yourself* a time-out.

Fact is, we've found, and data supports, that a time-out is the most effective approach for discipline. It gives both the child and parent a chance to decompress from a stressful event and think about actions that fit the situation. It also allows you the space to explain what's wrong with the behavior and reinforce that said behavior is not acceptable, so that your child learns from it. "If I throw forks down the toilet, I'll be sitting in a chair looking at the wall." The concept is that the time-out habituates the child to being sepa-

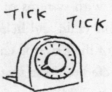

TICK TICK

rated when he misbehaves or loses control so that he can eventually learn to separate himself from the compelling-but-clearly-not-the-right-thing-to-do or from a tough situation in which he may react emotionally. We actually know of kids who will announce they're putting themselves in time-out *before* they overreact; that's the kind of behavior that can eventually lead to an older child learning to take five deep breaths or count to ten when he feels angry, frustrated, or on the verge of an outburst.

Reward Philosophy. The most effective way to form a healthy habit is by giving positive reinforcement when your child does the right thing. Now, of course, there's a fine line between healthy positive reinforcement and indiscriminant rewarding that ultimately harms the child by spoiling him and teaching him to manipulate situations to *get* something. This is how we draw the line:

⊃ Don't reward every behavior with a *thing*. Instead use words and compliments to reinforce actions. If your child goes above and beyond expectations or handles a real tough challenge (Hello, toilet!), a tangible reward may be appropriate. Just make it the exception, not the rule.

⊃ But be careful: After a while, indiscriminate praise loses meaning to a child. So give praise when it's earned, but don't overpraise every little thing.

⊃ It's better to compliment specific things as opposed to giving general or exaggerated praise. Telling a child that you liked the way she drew the lines on the picture is much better than "You're a Monet in the making!" if indeed she's not. Why? Kids know when they're being lied to, and repeated offenses of false praise send the message that, well, you're not to be trusted.

⊃ Choose words wisely. As we mentioned in a previous chapter, even telling a child he's smart can be somewhat damaging. That's because being "smart" becomes the child's self-image, so when he does fail at something, he sees himself as a failure. Down the line, fear of failure may even limit his risk taking (and, thus, his opportunities for success). It's far better to praise a child for working hard or showing a lot of effort—something he feels like he controls, as opposed to his intelligence, which, even at a young age, he feels like he doesn't necessarily control.

⊃ Praise actions rather than characteristics. If your daughter always gets told she is beautiful when you have her at the mall, answer with, "And you should see what a great big sister she is!"

Be careful about ignoring behaviors, in general. In households where no reaction is the norm, *any* reaction can be desirable; if bad behaviors get all the attention, the child will learn to keep doing them rather than risk getting *no* attention.

APPENDIXES

Appendix 1: More Medical Issues

Throughout the book, we've covered a wide range of health and medical issues that affect many children. As an added bonus, we'd like to touch upon some issues that may affect more select groups of children as well. If you know or think your child has one of these conditions, you will need to educate yourself and discuss options with your doctor, but this guide can help you get started, especially when it comes to symptoms and diagnosis.

ADHD
(Attention Deficit/Hyperactivity Disorder)

What It Is: A misfiring of neurotransmitters, which play an important role in orienting attention and regulating alertness. Other conditions may affect brain development and result in ADHD-like symptoms or increase the risk in genetically predisposed children. These include prenatal exposures to cigarette smoking, certain pesticides, lead, alcohol, and possibly cocaine, as well as prematurity, intrauterine growth restriction, brain infections, and inborn errors of metabolism. ADHD is found in at least 3 percent to 5 percent of children, with the most common cause being heredity. (Siblings are five to seven times as likely to be diagnosed as the general population.) If you have ADHD and your partner does not, each of your children has a 25 percent chance of having ADHD.

Identification: Your preschooler has high activity level, impulsivity, and short attention span even for a child his age and developmental level. This is an issue in more than one setting, such as in preschool and at home. Or maybe things are more serious. Other behaviors seen in preschoolers with ADHD include unbuckling seat belts and threatening to open the car door, jumping or falling out of windows, and ingesting toxic chemicals. Frequently, these children need to be supervised closely for their safety and the safety of those around them. As you look back, was Junior an infant who ran as soon as he walked, was hard to please, and had problems sleeping?

Diagnosis: Although ADHD is difficult to convincingly and precisely diagnose in the preschool years, evaluation and associated intervention can dramatically improve the prognosis of the behaviors of concern. You should start with an evaluation by your primary care health provider. There needs to be a diagnostic formulation, and this may require further evaluation by a subspecialist such as a developmental-behavioral pediatrician, pediatric neurologist, pediatric psychologist, or child psychiatrist. (Notice the word *pediatric* or *child* is in the title of each of these because not all specialists have experience with children in this age group.) ADHD more frequently than not coexists with other disorders such as anxiety disorder, disruptive behavior disorders, and learning disorders.

What to Do: Behavior therapy is the type of counseling intervention that has been shown to work best in the youngest age group. In the preschool and early school-age child, parents, caregivers, and teachers need to act in unison to tweak the environment and reward appropriate behavior. The idea is that the likelihood of a specific behavior occurring is determined by the Antecedents (what takes place prior to the behavior), the Behavior, and the Consequences (what takes place immediately afterward), or ABC. Medicating preschoolers with stimulants can be helpful and called for if there are serious safety issues. Treatment with medication at this age tends to be associated with more side effects and less effectiveness than in the older population of school-age children. While not first-line treatments, nonconventional options for ADHD include dietary changes such as eliminating additives and/or gluten or supplementing with essential fatty acids.

Autism

What It Is: A developmental problem that hinders communication and social interaction and is associated with repetitive motor movements and obsessive behaviors.

About 1 in 110 kids have autism spectrum disorder. Experts generally believe we've seen an increase because we've broadened the definition and more children are being identified at earlier ages as having ASD because of early intervention programs, as well as possible genetic-environmental interactions that have yet to be identified.

Risk Factors: Some of the risk factors are having male children, older parents, family history, and a host of syndromes.

Identification: Each child on the spectrum is unique, so every child cannot be expected to be exactly like your sample child that you know from down the street. Nevertheless, parents commonly notice that their child does not make eye contact or may not respond to his name. In ASD, social and language skills are usually more delayed or "out of sync" with motor, self-help, and cognitive or problem-solving skills. Experts can often pick up signs before a year, but many parents don't notice a problem until after that one-year milestone, when delays in language and other skills might become more apparent or the child might begin to regress in these areas. Other children may not show signs of certain ASD processes until later. Any child with suspected ASD needs an evaluation.

A professional who has experience in evaluating children to determine whether they have ASD, such as a child psychologist, child psychiatrist, pediatric neurologist, developmental-behavioral pediatrician, or neurodevelopmental disabilities pediatrician, should evaluate the child. Generally, there should also be an evaluation of the intellectual function, speech-language, and hearing function, as well as a behavioral history and observation.

What to Do: Early, specialized educational-behavioral interventions are generally recommended with one-on-one therapies for twenty-five hours per week and sometimes more. The best-studied intervention is a very structured, repetitive, and intensive behavioral approach, applied behavioral analysis (ABA), which rewards the child for responding to behavioral goals such as looking toward where their name is being called. Another commonly used intervention is "floor time," which focuses on engaging young children in social interactions. In addition, children with ASD receive speech therapy, which focuses on speech development and conversational language skills; and occupational therapy which often focuses on sensory processing issues. Medication is often used for associated inattention and hyperactivity, aggression and disruptive behavior, anxiety, and sleep disturbances that interfere with function and learning.

Developmental Delays

What They Are: Development refers to changes over time, and in children it refers to changes in thought, behavior, and function. With children, we talk about age-appropriate neurodevelopmental milestones in broad areas of language, motor, and social-adaptive development. (See chapter 2.) When an infant, toddler, or young child is not meeting some or all milestones within the window of expected age, we say that they have a developmental delay. This is really a temporary diagnosis or placeholder identifying a child as being at risk for a developmental disability.

Signs: In the first few months of life, signs include a lack of visual or auditory response, an inadequate suck, or increased resistance to moving limbs (spastic muscle tone) or floppiness (decreased muscle tone). Later in the first year, delays in attaining motor milestones of sitting and walking, or language milestones of babbling and words, suggest developmental delays. Between six and fifteen months of age, motor delay is the most common concern, while language and behavior problems are the common concerns after eighteen months. In general, the earlier the identification of developmental delays, the more severe the impairment. Although developmental delay is the most common presenting concern in children who later are diagnosed with intellectual disability, learning disability, autism spectrum disorder, and cerebral palsy, it does not always turn out to be a developmental disability. Isolated mild delays, especially in expressive language, may resolve by the preschool years but may be an early sign of academic or behavioral difficulties that become evident by school age.

Treatment: Parents should voice their concerns and observations to their child's physician when they first cross their minds, and docs should use developmental surveillance as part of routine pediatric care. This includes taking a careful history of the concerns, recording developmental milestones, and using standardized developmental screening tests. If there is evidence of a developmental lag, the child needs an evaluation by a physician experienced in early childhood development such as a pediatrician, neurodevelopmental pediatrician, developmental-behavioral pediatrician, child psychiatrist, or pediatric neurologist, who will refer for further medical testing to identify any associated deficits such as hearing and vision problems. This should be done in tandem with a referral to the state early intervention system so that a clinician experienced in evaluating developmental strengths and weaknesses of young children can develop an educational-developmental intervention plan. Services might include speech therapy, occupational therapy (for fine motor and/or feeding and sensory modulation problems), and/or physical therapy (for gross motor problems such as sitting and walking). The child may also be referred to an infant development specialist (for play and cognitive development) and/or behavioral specialist if he demonstrates aggression toward others and himself.

Hearing Issues

The Hearing System: When we hear a sound, we are actually processing and interpreting a pattern of vibrating air molecules. An initial vibration sets successive rows of air molecules into motion in oscillating concentric circles or waves. The hearing system is divided into a peripheral auditory mechanism, which goes from the external ear and ends in the auditory nerve, and the central auditory system, which extends from the auditory nerve to the brain. A disorder of the peripheral system results in a hearing loss, whereas a disorder of the central auditory system interferes with the *interpretation* of what is heard.

The peripheral system includes the external ear (auricle and ear canal), the tympanic membrane, or eardrum, the middle ear (three small and connected bones: malleus, incus, and stapes), the oval window boundary, and the inner ear (vestibular system and cochlea). The Eustachian tube is a part of the middle ear and runs from the front wall of the middle-ear space down to the back of the throat. The Eustachian tube is usually closed but opens during a swallow or yawn, allowing air to pass between the nose and throat and middle ear to equalize its air pressure with that in the external canal. This is what you do to unpop your ears when the plane goes up and down. When the Eustachian tube is blocked with inflammation or large tonsils, the likelihood of the bacteria causing infection in the middle ear increases.

When sound waves travel down the ear canal, they strike the eardrum (what your pediatrician is looking at to see if there is an ear infection), which vibrates and sets the small bones in the middle ear into motion. The middle-ear bones, through a lever system, amplify the incoming sound pressure by thirty decibels. The cochlea houses the actual end organ of hearing, the organ of Corti, which consists of multiple rows of delicate hair cells that are the receptors for the auditory nerve. The organ of Corti converts the mechanical energy arriving from the middle ear into electrical energy. The hair cells release neurotransmitters that generate impulses that go up the auditory pathway to the brain. Also, when stimulated, the outer hair cells produce very soft sounds called otoacoustic emissions (OAEs), which are used for newborn hearing screening.

Childhood Hearing: From the very beginning, you want to make the world of words and voice and sound and music available to your baby. Chatting to your child about what is going on around her, using statements ("It sounds like someone is at the front door!") and rhetorical questions ("Do you think it is Grandma?"), is extremely important. The first words that children say, they have heard thousands of times. Kids who live in a language-rich environment have bigger vocabularies and consequently higher intellectual function than those in a language-poor home. Reading to your child should be as natural as breathing and a daily activity or habit just like brushing your teeth. It should continue far beyond the time that he can read for himself, as you're able to read at a higher level and share the ideas and thoughts. In these early years, when boys and girls cannot sort out TV voices and household voices, the background noise of TV, CDs, and radio should be kept to a minimum. The natural sounds of a household and life should be available to them.

Diagnosing Issues: With the advent of universal newborn hearing screening, all children should have their hearing screened before they leave the hospital. Make sure that your baby was screened and that the results were normal. If the hearing screen is not passed, then you need to get a definitive evaluation by three months of age. If this evaluation shows that your child has a hearing loss, then it's important to move fast. You need to get to treatment in the form of a hearing aid (amplification) and educational intervention (speech therapist, audiologist, or infant educator who has experience with young children with hearing loss) by six months of age, or her present and future language potential may be greatly compromised. Children with a severe or profound hearing loss (deafness) can be treated surgically with a cochlear implant, which electronically stimulates the auditory nerve. Recent research suggests that children with these implants rate their quality of life as high as children with regular hearing levels.

For older children, any child whose language is not developing properly or shows signs that he is not hearing well needs another hearing evaluation. The question is not whether he hears but whether he hears well enough to develop good speech.

Treatment: The folks who diagnosed your child's hearing loss are very likely the same people who can provide evaluation for amplification. Ask them a lot of questions, including: Where do I go for amplification (hearing aid)? Do you think he will need a cochlear implant, and, if so, where do they have a lot of experience with children? Which pediatric ear specialist (otolaryngologist, or ENT doc) do you recommend and why? What is the contact number for early intervention (specialists with experience with hearing loss) and what can I expect from the system?

Before a cochlear implant can be considered, your child will need to have a trial amplification of three to six months. If your child has hearing loss, she should also be tested for vision issues. (See below.)

How to Protect a Child's Hearing: Since hearing loss can come about because of environmental influences, it's smart to get children in the habit of protecting their ears. Teach them to plug their ears when in the presence of sirens, subway trains, jackhammers, and so on. And, please, don't take them to loud concerts or football games, although if you must, protect their ears with noise-reducing earmuffs. And you should also monitor volume levels on earphones for music and video players.

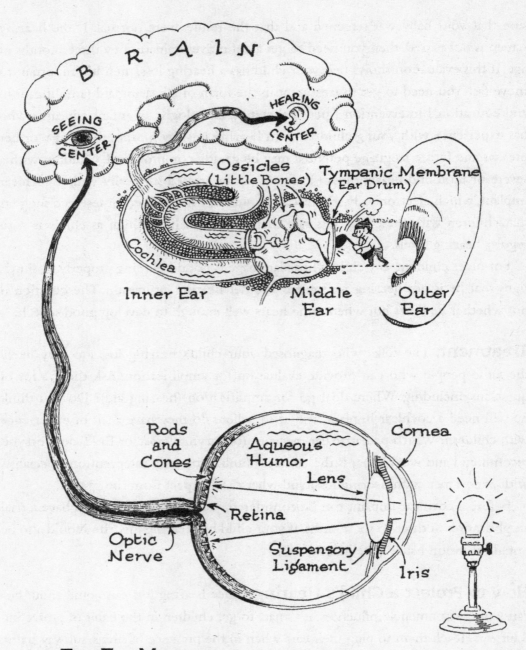

Figure A.1 **Eye Ear You** The brain works as the major processing center for all senses. The eye works as a camera as the brain interprets the snapshot. The brain uses tiny vibrations from sound waves to allow you to hear sounds.

Vision Issues

How the Eye Works: The eye is the most amazing of traditional cameras. The parts include the following: eyelids (the cover on the lens), cornea (the first layer of glass protection), iris (the aperture), lens (the lens—what else?), retina (the film), brain (the photographer's brain). For vision to develop normally, these focusing components of the system must be properly formed and aligned and functioning well. In addition, that brain behind the camera has an important sensitive and dynamic period of development in the first few months of life. The visual system does a lot of maturing in the first year. This is the time of myelination of the optic parts of the brain: the formation of fatty deposits that help speed up brain connections. Most dramatic and important is the brain's ability to make the eyes work together.

Infant Vision: Healthy infants display a wide range of visual behaviors. Some newborns are awake, alert, and following the movement of a face from the first day of life, while others may appear disinterested in their visual world for several weeks. By two months, most infants can visually fix on a face and follow it horizontally. Infants find the human face the most interesting thing to track, followed by a toy and then a light. Some toy companies take advantage of these preferences as well as the preference for patterns to get the attention of infants. For the first months of life, infants focus best at about twelve to fifteen inches from their face. This fixing and tracking behavior is most easily elicited if Baby is awake, alert, and on her back. Being able to elicit this fixing and following, as well as reciprocal smiling, behavior by two months of age offers reassurance for development of good visual acuity.

Most newborns are unable to distinguish colors because the cones, which are responsible for detecting color as well as fine detail, are stubby and widely spaced. As they grow longer and pack more closely together in the retina during the first few months, they become much more efficient at capturing light. By eight weeks, babies can discriminate between large and bright colors, especially reds, oranges, and greens; colors that depend on blue cones, such as purples and yellow greens, are still hard to make out. By three months of age, the blue-yellow system catches up with the red-green system, and babies can make nearly all the same color distinctions as adults.

OTHER EYE-RELATED ISSUES

ISSUE	TREATMENT
Blocked tear duct	In the first months of life, tear ducts can get blocked with normal secretions. You can massage the duct by pressing your clean index finger next to the inside corner of the affected eye and, rubbing from the nose side outward, get the goop out of the duct and help to unblock it. If the tear duct becomes infected, the area will get puffy and swollen (and ooze green goo). An antibiotic can treat the infection. If daily massaging does not open the tear duct, surgery may be called for.
Conjunctivitis (pinkeye)	Eye is red, itchy, and goopy. Need to see a doc to determine whether it's bacterial (which an antibiotic can treat) or viral (which has to run its highly contagious course but will resolve itself in five to ten days). Wash all pillowcases and hand towels that your child uses, so as not to infect the whole household.
Styes	Come from blocked eyelashes or hair follicles with inflammation, making the area around the eyelash follicle red and puffy. Use a hot compress (without scalding your child) on the sty and reapply to help draw the inflammation out.
Sand in eye	Don't rub. Flush with water or saline generously. If still hurting or tearing, see a doc to make sure there's no cornea tear and to make sure everything's out.
Ball to the eye	Check for blurred vision or double vision and to see if eyes are moving together. If vision is blurry or double, call a doc. If you see any blood, go to the ER.

Problems: For the first few weeks of life, often the eyes do not move together. Sometimes one or both eyes will turn intermittently outward or inward. Other times, you may think that they are not quite in sync. A way to tell is to see if the reflection of light falls on the same area of the iris on both eyes. If it does, the eyes are probably moving together. If by six to twelve weeks of age your baby's eyes are still turning out, in, or not together, you should bring it to the attention of your doc. Strabismus—when one or both eyes are clearly misaligned—occurs in about 4 percent of children younger than six years of age. More commonly, if the eye or eyes look toward the nose (cross-eyed) or look toward the side (walleyed), a pediatric ophthalmologist (not an optometrist) needs to evaluate the problem. Early treatment to make sure that there is a well-focused retinal image is extremely important so that the visual cortex mentioned above is stimulated by both eyes. Some treatments include patching the good eye to make the straying eye work harder and eventually correct itself. Special glasses can also help. The earlier the intervention, the less time it takes to fix the problem, and the better the outcome will be. Surgery is also an option to repair the muscle that controls eye movement.

In preschoolers, mild vision loss is usually not suspected or detected until a doc screens them at about age three. Signs include squinting, sitting too close to the TV, or having trouble with tasks that require visual acuity. More serious vision loss may be associated with body rocking and gazing at fingers and hands, as your child moves them quickly in front of her face. If you suspect a problem, you need to get an evaluation as soon as possible. Vision issues aren't just about sight, but they're also associated with developmental issues as well. Treatment can correct or improve not only sight but also many developing skills.

Intellectual Disability

What It Is: The definition of an intellectual disability (previously known as mental retardation) is controversial. But there is general agreement that it is significantly subaverage intellectual function (individually administered IQ test of approximately 70 or below) associated with other deficits or impairments in such areas as communication, self-care, and social skills. In infants and children up through three years of age, infant psychological tests are poor predictors of later IQs. However, children with very low scores (less than 50) will likely have an intellectual disability. Intellectual disabilities are found in about 2 percent to 3 percent of the population.

What to Do: You will go through the same type of evaluation as discussed under "Developmental Delays" on page 426.

Orthopedic Issues

Many orthopedic problems occur because of how the baby is formed in utero in the third trimester, when space is at a premium. (Docs call them packaging or molding abnormalities.) Firstborn children, where that space has not been stretched before, are often most at risk, as are twins (shared space). Some of the more common ones include:

- ⊃ A muscle contraction of the neck with the head tilting away from the affected side; more common in big, firstborn babies with long labor. It usually goes away with gentle manipulation over the first few months.

- ⊃ A dislocation of the shoulder from a too-big baby trying to get through a too-small space. Called shoulder dystocia, this is easily treated after birth.

- ⊃ A clavicle (collarbone) fracture, which is rare but heals well.

Other childhood orthopedic problems:

Duplicated Digits (extra fingers or toes): Being born with a sixth digit is not uncommon. Extra digits can be tied off (and they'll automatically fall off on their own) or surgically removed.

Syndactyly: This is a congenital connection or fusion between digits. Most are repaired when the child is over one year old under anesthesia.

If you have a child with a chronic illness, the internet is a wonderful resource to find not only medical information but also support groups of other parents who are going through the same thing. Their emotional support—as well as even medical suggestions—can be important tools to help you deal with your own situation. To find a support group, we recommend MedlinePlus (www.medlineplus.gov), an information service of the National Institutes of Health. Just use the search tool for the specific condition, and you'll see a link to "organizations" that can help set you in the right direction.

Toeing In: In utero, most babies are stuck with their feet internally rotated or toeing in. Parents don't necessarily see it until the kid starts trying to walk. In 95 percent of children, this torsion resolves itself by twelve to eighteen months, after they start walking. Numerous studies have shown that bracing does not speed up the process. Very rarely, a child will have clinically significant toeing in and torsion leading to ongoing falls by age four years; that child can benefit from a referral to a pediatric orthopedic surgeon to see if he needs corrective surgery.

Rickets: Extreme bowleggedness caused by a body's resistance to vitamin D or prolonged insufficient intake of vitamin D_3. (Mild bowleggedness is common in most kids and resolves itself.) Rickets is often seen in kids who are also short. These kids don't need to be braced, but need nutritional support.

Clubfoot: This is a true congenital deformity involving all bones in the foot. These babies get put in casts for the first year or so of life to help turn the foot and improve long-term flexibility.

Hip Dysplasia: One out of a hundred babies will have a little hip instability, but only one out of a thousand will have true hip dislocation. We catch this in the newborn nursery: When the child is relaxed, and not fighting the examination, we place our thumbs in the hip joint and rotate the leg and hip outward. If we feel a clunk, that is the femoral head (the top of the thigh bone) returning to the hip socket. This does not hurt the babies, and often they're not crying or fussing while we are doing this (especially if we have good timing). Another way we look is to flip the baby on her tummy and see if her butt cheeks have symmetrical folds. Those with congenital hip dysplasia are put into a harness to keep the hips flexed and prevent complete dislocation. This allows the capsular structures to tighten and maintain hip stability. It works 95 percent of the time. If reduced early, there is a great chance that it will be entirely normal at two years and thereafter.

Seizures

Identification: The sudden onset of unusual movements, behaviors, or spells sometime referred to as a paroxysmal disorder may catch your attention or even be brought to your attention. Some of these may be seizures, and some may not. Seizures in newborns are seemingly random and difficult to distinguish from normal activity. Movements that resemble neonatal seizures can be just jitteriness, breath holding, arching, jerking, or startling. Movement patterns in the newborn that are more likely to be seizures would be breath holding with body stiffening, local jerky movements of one limb or both on one side, many focuses of jerky movements, shocklike contractions, deviations of the eyes upward or to the side, and even laughing.

Diagnosis: From one month to two years, "spells," which include seizures (especially febrile seizures), as well as apnea and breath-holding spells with loss of consciousness, are relatively common. When an infant has a seizure, it often occurs at the time of fever. It can be an infection of the nervous system; an underlying seizure disorder in which the stress of fever triggers the seizure; or a simple febrile seizure. A simple febrile seizure is a genetic age-limited form of epilepsy in which seizures occur only with fever. About 4 percent of children experience them. Of the children whose first seizure is associated with fever, only 2 percent have a nonfebrile seizure (epilepsy) by age seven. Apnea is cessation of breathing for fifteen seconds or longer or less than fifteen seconds if accompanied by a slow heart rate. The frequency of apnea is inversely related to age, so it is more often seen in newborns than infants, and is rarely seen in children. Apnea is rarely a manifestation of a seizure and more frequently related to reflux.

Risk Factors: The causes of nonfebrile seizures in infancy are not substantially different from those in childhood. The factors that place a child at risk for nonfebrile seizures are congenital malformations, neonatal seizures, and a family history of epilepsy. In children younger than two, the seizures are more frequently associated with another disorder. Approximately 25 percent of children who have recurrent seizures during the first year are developmental or neurologically abnormal at the time of the seizure. Intellectual disability is associated with seizures that are persistent and difficult to control.

What to Do: If you are seeing unusual movements that occur as "spells," being able to produce a good description of these spells is extremely important, since that's the main clue that the physician uses to determine what is going on. It's important to note what the baby was doing just before the seizure. Eating? Sleeping? Falling? Which parts of the body were moving or stiffening? How long did it last? (This is difficult to judge, as it seems like forever to a parent. So glance at your watch early and then at the end.) Then it's important to note what the child did afterward, such as sleep or resume her activities. Sometimes you are talking about an isolated incident, but other times it repeats. Being able to capture them on a video is extremely helpful. Bring that to your doctor's visit, or email it to him beforehand, to help with assessment.

Cancer

While childhood cancers are rare in children under five, there are a few that can strike. You should let your parental instincts rule. If something doesn't seem right, then get it checked out. Some of them include:

⊃ Acute lymphocytic leukemia (a blood cancer): Occurs mainly in one- to four-year-olds. Signs will be excess fatigue, irritability, pale complexion, and the tendency to bruise more easily than the normal toddler.

⊃ Retinoblastoma (an eye cancer): Kids with retinoblastoma have no red reflex in the affected eye (the red you see in flash photos). The child with retinoblastoma may have one red pupil, but the affected side will look white. That's called leukocoria.

⊃ Neuroblastoma (a nerve tissue cancer): Here a child may develop a new, wobbly gait (after walking well previously), or eyes that seem occasionally to really scramble.

If your child shows a combination of these signs, take him in to his pediatrician ASAP.

Appendix 2: Family Situations

One of the assumptions that tends to be made about families is that most of us live in so-called traditional family units, made up of Mom, Dad, kids, and a leg-licking dog who lives for the moment that a cracker crumb falls from the table. We all know, though, that so-called nontraditional families are really pretty traditional nowadays: In fact, more than 75 percent of American children are being raised in families other than the traditional makeup of two married heterosexual parents. There's no such thing as typical, because there are all kinds of household units and all kinds of ways to get there. We hope that we've done a good job throughout the book of not assuming too much about you and your family. That said, we do think it's worth spending a little bit of time on a few familial situations that may affect some, but not all, of you.

Adoption

About 2 percent of the U.S. population is adopted, with half by nonrelatives and half by relatives. Some issues that you will want to address with your adopted son or daughter:

When to tell the child he is adopted. This issue is somewhat controversial. While many recommend that the child is said to be (and be told he was) adopted from the beginning, many families choose to tell a child at age three or four. If parents wait until the child is older, they need to make sure it comes from them, as opposed to from a sibling, other relative, neighbor, or classmate.

How to tell the child. Certainly this depends a bit on age, but the key thing to remember is to tailor your explanation to the child's developmental level. When you explain that he is adopted (some say "born in my heart, not born in my tummy"), make sure to include your motive (for example, you couldn't conceive a baby yourself), the fact that he was born like any other child, that the decision by the birth parents wasn't your child's fault, and how happy you are that he is part of your family.

How to deal with outsiders. Experts recommend that you don't hide the fact that your child was adopted, but that you also respect the child's privacy about such things as the birth parents' motives and situations. Explain to anyone who asks that you believe it will be your child's choice to reveal that information or not talk about it.

Health issues: Children who are adopted both internationally and from within the United States are two to three times as likely to have developmental problems as nonadopted children. The children are also more likely to have behavior problems and attachment issues. Internationally adopted children often do not come with completely accurate records including date of birth and often have infectious disease issues like intestinal parasites or nutritional issues like anemia. They need careful, thoughtful evaluation and monitoring. There are pediatricians who specialize in international adoptions and who are knowledgeable about specific health issues; it's worth seeking one out in your area.

Cultural issues: It's important to acknowledge and celebrate a child's culture of origin. For international adoptions, there are often support groups where you can meet families who have adopted from the same country. Celebrate holidays of the child's culture of origin, read books about her country of origin or ethnic group, and look for as many ways as possible to positively reinforce her cultural self-image.

Open versus Closed: Open adoption refers to the continuum of options that enables birth parents and adoptive parents to have information about and communication with one another before and/or after the child is placed. One advantage is the ready source of information available as the child feels a need for it. The practice of open adoptions has not been well researched, and the long-term effects on the child are not known. Initial data indicate that open adoption is associated with positive attitudes on the part of the adoptive mother toward the biological mother.

Blended Families

There's some evidence to suggest that blended families, or stepfamilies, are now the most common type of American family. When parts of two families join to make one, that can bring on many emotions for a child who may very well not understand

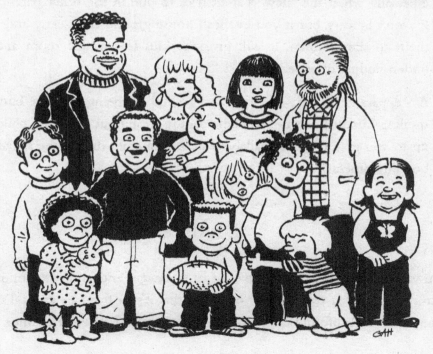

exactly what's happening. With all the changes going on—moving to a new home or having new people moving in to his home, or changing schools, for example—a child has not only had his routine disrupted but also is more likely to question things like loyalty and trust because of all those changes to the family infrastructure. Very often that can bring about feelings of stress, insecurity, anger, even depression. Some things you can do if you're in that situation:

⊃ Do not have unrealistically high expectations of what the new family will be like.

⊃ Do not get stuck on what everyone wants to be called. To force a child to call your new husband "Dad" when she already has a dad will not sit well.

⊃ Be patient. It's going to take some time to get the new family feeling like a family. So don't try to overparent the new kids in your life. Instead focus on building positive experiences that can be the foundation for good memories.

⊃ Establish rules in private. Discipline can be a huge source of tension, especially when the "new" parent tries to punish the other parent's child. It won't be easy, but if you establish house ground rules early and explain them to the children, it will give the kids less wiggle room and more understanding of expectations.

⊃ A stepparent may try to win over a child by being his best buddy and spoiling him. It's best not to come on too strong but to let the child warm up to you gradually. Be available, but let the child dictate the speed of the bonding process.

Divorce

When you consider the fact that half of all marriages end in divorce (most of them within the first seven years), then you know that it's far from an atypical situation—and one that has profound effects on the kids involved. A lot of changes take place for both parents and kids during the divorce process, not only in terms of logistics but also of emotions. Research tells us that many factors can affect how a child reacts to a divorce: everything from his temperament to the stress levels that he faced in the household beforehand. And it's clear that different children react in different ways. Some regress in development, some become more aggressive, and some experience high levels of stress because their habitual worlds have been turned upside down. There are many ways to address this with your ex-partner as you split into two households, such as mutually agreeing to try to establish as much routine as possible (for instance, consistent bedtimes) and providing endless emotional support. Other things that divorced parents should consider:

⊃ Reassure the child that he is not responsible for the divorce.

⊃ Emphasize that the child is a worthwhile, special person no matter what decisions parents have made concerning their own lives.

⊃ Encourage the child to put feelings into words rather than into negative behaviors.

⊃ When conflicts are observed or heard without resolution, the kids begin to feel that it is their fault, which lowers self-esteem.

⊃ Keep any dating invisible at least until a ring on the finger is an eventual possibility. Each breakup from dating is another "divorce" experienced by the child.

⊃ Keep your promises, especially regarding visitation.

⊃ Don't use your child as a messenger to communicate with your ex.

⊃ Refrain from speaking ill of your ex in front of your child. After all, your child is half that person as well. How will she feel about herself knowing that half of her comes from someone you detest (especially if she resembles your ex in some way)?

Appendix 3:
Prematurity and Multiples

While it's true that not all multiples are premature and that not all premature infants are multiples, it is true that prematurity and multiple births go hand in hand like Onesies and spit-up stains. If you're pregnant, we discuss ways to reduce the risk of prematurity in *YOU: Having a Baby.* But for any number of reasons, babies (whether multiple or not) and doctors may decide that it's a safer environment for the baby on the outside than on the inside, and labor begins. Here we'll outline a few things to consider if your baby is born prematurely, as well as some tips for those parents of multiples.

Prematurity

Definitions: Infants born before thirty-seven completed weeks of gestation are premature. Low-birth-weight babies are less than 5 pounds, 8 ounces (8 percent of births) and very-low-birth-weight babies are less than 3 pounds, 4 ounces (fewer than 2 percent of births). The preterm birth rate is about 13 percent in the United States, having risen for the last two decades, mostly because of multiple births due to assisted reproduction.

Implications: Although the prematurity rate increased significantly in the 1980s and 1990s, the complications and mortality associated with prematurity have declined dramatically as more and more hospitals are able to offer neonatal intensive care. Nevertheless, premature infants are at increased risk for chronic problems like asthma, obesity, and developmental delays. The shorter the gestation and the lower the birth weight, the more susceptible the baby is to medical complications. Health problems more common in premature infants include:

- Ophthalmologic: strabismus (crossed eyes), myopia (nearsightedness), retinopathy of prematurity (a complex disease of the blood vessels serving the retina; can result in blinding retinal detachment)

- Neurologic problems such as seizures

- Growth and feeding problems

- Respiratory problems, including chronic lung disease from being ventilated

Prognosis: Fortunately, most premature infants do well, but they are particularly at risk for the "vulnerable child syndrome." This is a child with an imagined or real illness early in life, resulting in the parents developing a long-term sense of the child being particularly susceptible to illness or injury. That means that the child is viewed as incapable of being independent or of performing certain tasks. This leads to ongoing stress, odd dynamics between the child and the parents, and confusion for both parent and child.

Many neonatal intensive care units offer help and instruction for transitioning between their units and home. If the complications of prematurity are caught early, therapy and other interventions can help lessen the effect. Often, preschool programs also can help in many developmental areas. As with most issues, early detection is key, so an active parent serves as the first and best line of defense. (We also recommend additional info about home care for premature babies at www.marchofdimes.org.)

Multiples

The mantra for many parents of twins: two of everything. Yes, that can be the case for some things, like cribs. But perhaps the trickier part about raising twins and higher-order multiples is not the logistical side of the equation but the developmental and emotional side—the side in which you really work hard to treat your same-aged kids as individuals and not as a unit. When you consider that twins account for more than 3 percent of births (an increase we've seen largely because of older adults giving

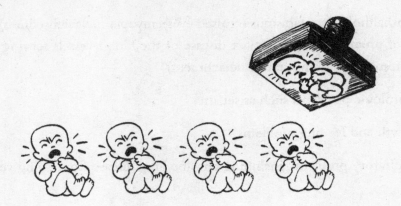

birth and fertility therapies), then it's clear that raising twins is a big issue for a lot of folks. Though much of the advice we give throughout this book can be applied to your kids, because they are, in fact, individuals, we do recommend the National Organization of Mothers of Twins Clubs (www.nomotc.org) for parents raising multiples to address specific issues and concerns and to find a local chapter. Here, a few pointers to get you started:

Stay on Task. In terms of logistics, the big trick is staying organized. As tired as you may be at times, it's imperative (for your own sanity) to stay organized—and to get help from your partner and other family members. You'll always need to be equipped with the right amount of diapers, bottles, etc., and staying prepared will make life easier all around.

Figure out a Feeding Routine. Feeding two infants is tricky no matter how you cut it. And your situation (breast or bottle or both) will dictate how you can manage it. We recommend that you feed both at the same time (or one right after another), so that they can stay on similar feeding and sleeping schedules. While it may be more efficient to feed them in car seats at the same time as they get older, do keep in mind that babies prefer being held when fed.

Think Solo. Even though you can have a lot of fun and enjoy "cute" moments with twins doing things together (and dressing alike), you should really do what you can to make sure that they're treated as individuals as much as possible. That means doing things like:

- ⊃ choosing different-sounding names;

- ⊃ dressing them in different colors;

- ⊃ not calling them "the twins," but by name;

- ⊃ taking time out to spend private time with each individually;

- ⊃ buying different toys, books, etc., based on their personal interests, not focusing so much on trying to be "equal";

- ⊃ having them in different preschool classrooms, if possible;

- ⊃ encouraging cooperation rather than competition between the two.

Appendix 4: Growth Charts

At each visit with your pediatrician, you should ask for the height (called length) and weight of your child as well as the head circumference for children younger than three years of age. You may want to bring your own gender-specific chart and plot the numbers yourself; the nurse can help you if you are unsure how to do it. If a number does not make sense—for example, your seemingly wiry three-year-old is plotting as overweight—check to see that you have not mixed up pounds for kilograms or if Junior needs to be remeasured.

You will note that the charts we show list age on the horizontal axis (sideways). So, find your child's age in months for the birth-to-thirty-six-months growth chart and draw a vertical line up through the weight and length lines. On the vertical axis (up and down), on the left side of the chart, length is listed in both inches and centimeters; weight, in both pounds and kilograms, is listed on the right side. Follow the age line up and mark dark dots where the age line hits the child's weight and then length. These numbers give you your youngster's percentage weight and length compared to other boys or girls of the same age.

Normal growth is when the child's weight and length are between the 3rd and 97th percentiles. The relationship between length and weight is most important, and ideally both are roughly the same percentile for their height and weight. In children younger than two years old, we use the weight for length chart. On this chart, you look for your child's length on the horizontal axis and trace up along that line until you hit the line of your child's weight coming across the page. This tells you what percentage of children of the same length as your child weigh more than your child: for instance, let's say that your child is at the 75th percentile, then 25 percent of children who are the same height as your child weigh more and 75 percent weigh less. These charts are available at www.cdc.gov/growthcharts.

For children younger than three, also keep a head-circumference chart. This also has age on the horizontal axis and head circumference (usually measured in centimeters) on the vertical axis. At birth, children have a large head in relation to their

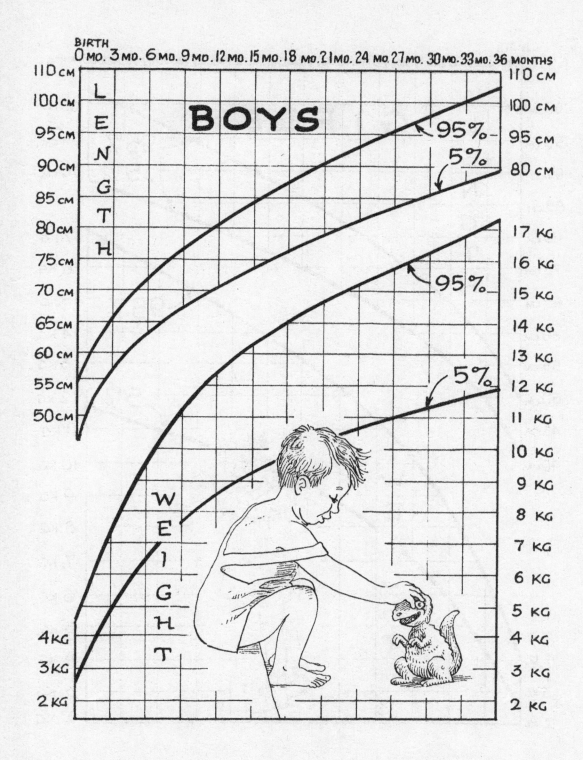

BOYS

BIRTH
0 MO. 3 MO. 6 MO. 9 MO. 12 MO. 15 MO. 18 MO. 21 MO. 24 MO. 27 MO. 30 MO. 33 MO. 36 MONTHS

LENGTH

95% — 5%

WEIGHT

95%

5%

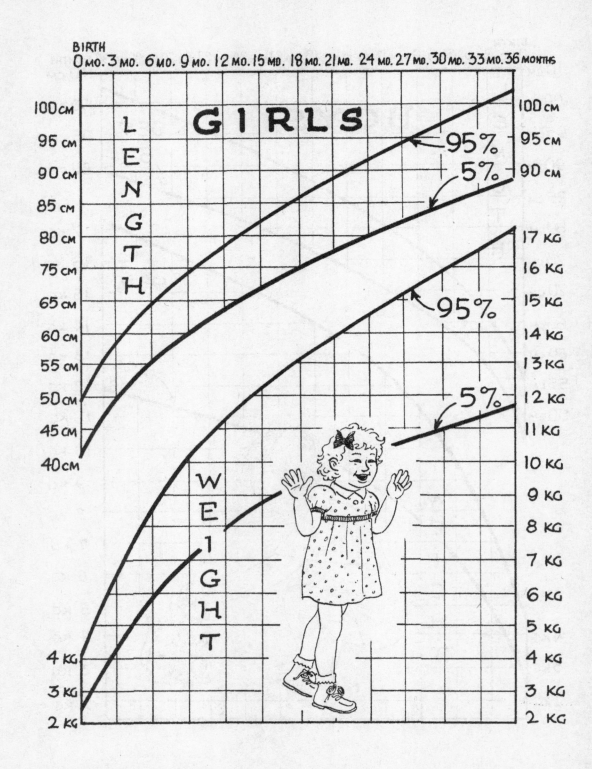

BIRTH
0 MO. 3 MO. 6 MO. 9 MO. 12 MO. 15 MO. 18 MO. 21 MO. 24 MO. 27 MO. 30 MO. 33 MO. 36 MONTHS

GIRLS

LENGTH

100 cm
95 cm
90 cm
85 cm
80 cm
75 cm
65 cm
60 cm
55 cm
50 cm
45 cm
40 cm

95%
5%

100 cm
95 cm
90 cm

17 KG
16 KG
15 KG
14 KG
13 KG
12 KG
11 KG
10 KG
9 KG
8 KG
7 KG
6 KG
5 KG
4 KG
3 KG
2 KG

95%
5%

WEIGHT

4 KG
3 KG
2 KG

body length and increase the size of their head greatly in the first year and then slow down the rate of growth.

Starting at two years of age, the body mass index is the number that represents best the relationship of a child's weight to height. This is a number that can be calculated using pounds and inches or kilograms and centimeters. Use the following equations to calculate the body mass index: weight (pounds)/stature (inches) squared x 703 *or* weight (kilograms)/stature (centimeters) squared x 10,000. You can also put the numbers in at the BMI calculator at www.realage.com.

You want to pay attention to the following:

1. Not just the percentiles of your child's weight and length/stature but the relationship between them to prevent obesity or failure to thrive (underweight).

2. It's important to put your child's growth in the context of both parents' heights. Between one-third and two-thirds of children change growth percentiles over the first two years of life, most frequently related to the height factors of both parents.

3. In general, children should not be losing weight; if they are, there needs to be a search for the cause. Conversely, control of present or pending obesity is usually managed by aiming for slowing the rate of weight gain while continuing the rate of growth of length/stature.

4. Keeping careful records can come in handy when a growth problem develops, as it usually needs to be put in the context of the child's growth history.

Acknowledgments

From the YOU Docs—Mike Roizen and Mehmet Oz

We pulled together another great team of experts, all parents with a total of fourteen kids, to discuss, debate, and deliberate over the golden rules of parenting. What you're reading now is the result of a truly group effort that works because of the diverse and dedicated minds on our team, and we are indebted to all of our co-authors.

Ted Spiker pulled together more diverse opinions than a true congressional leader and crafted an uplifting, enjoyable text that thrills readers with insights spiced with humor. Professor Spiker (he really is one in real life at the University of Florida) keeps his classroom lively as we are pumped with weekly homework assignments. He has crafted an elegant syllabus in this newest creation on parenting.

Gary Hallgren's acclaimed medical cartoons have brought alive every one of our books. We love watching him create magical images that bring alive complex topics so all our readers can enjoy the childlike enthusiasm the YOU docs have for our work.

Craig Wynett has done it again. His brilliant ability to connect seemingly disparate facts keeps us on our toes. His overarching concepts light the pathways to knowledge in our books and he designs and articulates these seamlessly on each call. Craig transforms doctrinal discussions into profoundly insightful meetings on how to change our readers' minds so they act on what we teach.

Superpediatrician Dr. Ellen Rome brought humor and life-changing insights to every chapter in this book. The practical experiences she collects while working at the Cleveland Clinic helped us share the essence of her specialty with our readers.

Developmental-behavioral pediatrician from Rainbow Babies and Children's Hospital Dr. Nancy Roizen joined us full-time for this endeavor and kept us honest as she crafted numerous sophisticated reviews of complicated topics so we get the story right. This is not why Mike married her thirty-seven years ago, but Mehmet is sure glad that he did.

Lisa Oz pushed and shoved behind the scenes to ensure we focused on the needs of the readers and didn't take our academic traditions too far into the practical-minded world of a new mother. Mehmet is thrilled that he was able to lure her into marriage a quarter century ago.

Linda Kahn's meticulous attention to detail improved the quality of the book. She continues to teach the doctors quite a bit about medicine as well as the mother's perspective on life. She provides very profound criticisms of our work and helps us revise the text into the wonderful final result by commenting on both the content and the style.

Joel Harper created a practical YOU: Raising Your Child Workouts for several age groups ranging from age 2 to 5 (even Mike loves these as he searches for nieces, nephews, and grandkids).

Marta Worwag attended every conference call and worked carefully with the authors to fact-check and research many of the questions created whenever scientists are researching a book.

We want to specially thank our many readers: More than two dozen recent mothers commented on each edition and each section or chapter of each edition, bringing clarity to our efforts. Finally, our agent Candice Fuhrman's innovative insights and tough commentary helped redirect our work to truly suit the needs of women having babies.

We also want to thank the group at Free Press (Simon & Schuster) who so enthusiastically supported this material and have dedicated themselves to bringing our ideas to the world. Dominick Anfuso joins Martha Levin (with Carolyn Reidy) as our partners at Free Press (Simon and Schuster). The superb team of Jill Siegel, Carisa Hays, Suzanne Donahue, Mark Speer, Erich Hobbing, Nancy Inglis, Philip Bashe, Leah Miller, and Maura O'Brien are always seeking solutions to our many needs and have committed themselves to making our books the best possible experience for our dedicated readers.

Most of the recipes came from the Lifestyle 180 team of master chef Jim Perko, nutritionist Kristin Kirkpatrick, medical director Elizabeth Ricanati, and full-time doc Mladen Golubic. These Lifestyle 180 recipes are based on guidelines for YOU healthy foods, and were tested for enjoyment and capacity to make by mothers, their children, and their male significant others (who washed the dishes).

We are indebted to our close partners at realage.com, including Val Weaver, Keith Roach, Carl Peck, Axel Goetz, Marty Munson, and Meredith Wade. And we thank the great team at *Good Morning America,* including Patty Neger and all the anchors who made waking up early to discuss health a lot of fun.

Thanks to all of our friends at *The Doctor Oz Show,* especially executive producers Mindy Moore Borman, Amy Chiaro, Lori Rich, and all the great production team members who make our day-to-day lives so much fun. Thanks to the Oprah radio team, including Chris Kelly, Corny Koehl, and Katherine Kelly. The Harpo and www.doctoroz.com web team with Michael Bloom, Samantha Lazarus, and Jenn Horton have kept us digital.

Our books contain so broad a range of topics that we are compelled to ask advice from many world experts who selflessly share their insights in the true academic tradition. We list them all here without details of their contributions in order to save space for the actual book, but we deeply appreciate your dedication to your specialties and willingness to sacrifice your time in helping craft the most scientifically accurate book on parenting possible.

We thank Burton Edelstein, David Albert, Ken Taylor, Thomas Vilt, Emily Smith, Samantha Griffin, Ruth Lemole, Jen Trachtenberg, and all the JCAHO folks who authored *The Smart Parent.* We especially thank Drs. Shari I. Lusskin, Dean Ornish, Mark Hyman, Lise Eliot, Johanna Goldfarb, Paul Offit, Justin Lavin, Rocio Moran, Charis Eng, and Sharon Malon for teaching us and reviewing our work.

We also thank Jennifer Ashton, Mary D'Alton, Sherri Tenpenny, Ivan Kronenfeld, Jon Lapook, Regina Brett, Paul Rosenberg, George Rodgers, Robin Golan, Julide Tok, Evan Johnson, Scott Forman, Bill Levine, Erin Olivo, Rowe Jones, Mary Matsui, Irvin Schorsh, John Ellis, Marsha Lowry, Barbara Gaffield, Michelle Narens, Alan Cichon, Iyaad Hasan, Jodi Hazen, Tiffani Mauldin-Frederick, Sarah Mohr, Suzanne Dixon, Erinne Dyer, Jennifer Hunter, John Mauldin, Dominique Campodonico, Julie Templeton, Meg Zweiback, Louis Z. Cooper, Erica Foreman, Megan Pruce-

Ferington, Susan Parnell, Mitzi Reaugh, Anna Robins, Jennifer Roizen, Rosaleind Wattell, Bethany Yu, Alfonse Gallizia, and Brian Kolonick.

From Mehmet and Lisa Oz:

Dr. Oz thanks his colleagues in surgery for their continued support, including Dr. Craig Smith, Dr. Yoshifuma Naka, Dr. Mike Argenziano, Dr. Henry Spotnitz, Dr. Allan Stewart, and Dr. Mat Williams. The physician assistants, especially Laura Altman and Tom Cosola, and the nurses in the OR and floor, as well as our spectacular ICU team, always care meticulously for my patients. My office staff, including Lidia Nieves and Caroline O'Sullivan, kept me on time and on target as I combined a life of heart surgery with media. Our divisional administrator Diane Amato offered unique insights to books and life and has graced our efforts as my chief of staff at *The Dr. Oz Show*. Thanks to the dedicated staff at New York Presbyterian Hospital, including Herb Pardes, Steve Corwin, Bob Kelly, David Feinberg, Bryan Dotson, Alicia Park, and Myrna Manners for their heartfelt advice. Thanks to the inspired Harpo leadership of Oprah Winfrey, Tim Bennett, Erik Logan, Sheri Salata, Harriet Seitler, and Doug Pattison.

My parents, Mustafa and Suna Oz, taught me how to parent as they struggled to parent their mischievous child. My parents-in-law, Gerald and Emily Jane Lemole, led by example while raising my brothers- and sisters-in-law and raised wonderful human beings who are all great parents themselves. Besides being our co-author, Lisa, the love of my life, has raised four rambunctious kids (Daphne, Arabella, Zoe, and Oliver) who I pray can emulate her magical parenting touch. You have taught us all how to live in relationship.

From Michael and Nancy Roizen:

Dr. Mike wants to thank his administrative associates Qintene Graham and especially Beth Grubb, who made this work possible. And thank you to many of the staff at the Cleveland Clinic and physicians elsewhere, who answered numerous questions. Many of the Clinic's Wellness Institute staff and associates made scientific contributions and constructive criticism, and allowed us the time to complete this work. Cleveland Clinic CEO Toby Cosgrove has said that while the clinic will continue to be one of, if not the best in illness care, wellness is what the clinic will do for every employee and person we touch. I am fortunate to work with such a talented and creative group who helped our thought processes as Nabil Gabriel, Regina Chandler, Dr. Beth Ricanati, Dr. Mladen Golubic, Dr. Martin Harris, Dr. Joe Hahn, Cindy Hundorfean, Chris Vernon, Dennis Kenny, Paul Matsen, Bill Peacock, Cindy Moore and many nutritionists and exercise physiologists, chef Jim Perko, and Drs. Rich Lang, Tanya Edwards, Raul Seballos, Steve Nissen, Jim Young, David Bronson, Anthony Miniaci, and Glen Copeland, as well as clinicians and leaders who run the gamut from inner city school teachers to executive coaches.

Our family was fully engaged—with Jeff as our MD and PhD research associate and Dr. Jennifer as critical reader, and joined full-time by the woman responsible for our kids' developmental successes, Nancy, as well as by the "enlarged family" of the Katzes, Unobskeys, Wattels, and Campodonicos. I also want to thank Sukie Miller, Diane Reverend, Eileen Sheil, Susan Petre, Zack Wasserman, and others for encouraging and critiquing the concepts. Having a great partner to ablate stress daily, and to depend on for her incredible expertise and common sense honed carefully in this area, is clearly a magnificent way to help life be better—thank you, Nancy.

From Ted Spiker:

Above all, I thank my wonderful wife, Liz, whose passion and compassion are just two of the many reasons the three Spiker boys admire and love her. There's no way to thank you for all you do for us to help us, teach us, and make us laugh every day. Every minute we spend with our two crazily awesome kids, Alex and Thad, is one that we'll remember. One day, you two will be able to beat me in H-O-R-S-E, and when you do, I hope you'll still keep playing with me. I also thank my mother Faith, who did a fine job raising three kids on her own (even if she did make us wear winter hats to walk three feet from the car to the school door*), and to my in-laws, John and Karen, for their guidance and support over the years. I also appreciate all the inspiring members of the YOU team for the opportunity to work with such a

---

* In high school!

dynamic group, my students and colleagues at the University of Florida, and a whole slew of folks who have helped me in my career. Finally, to my late father, who died before he got the chance to raise his children: I'm sorry you never got to experience the same parenting joys that I get to now.

From Craig Wynett:

To my family: my wife Denise, sons Ryan and Jim, cat Abbey, and dogs Ned and George. Collectively you have given me plenty of baby-related experience to draw on. A few of these "experiences" we have advised readers to avoid at all cost, many more are truly worthy of emulation.

From Gary Hallgren:

We didn't have this book to work with when my wife Michelle and I were raising our daughter Annabel . . . but I agree totally with its philosophy and its principles of health and common sense, both then and now. Perhaps this is why people congratulate my wife and me on raising such a fine human being and compliment us on our excellent parenting. Aw, shucks, tain't nothin', I say, but it is something. It is caring and thinking and loving and being well informed. It's not being rich and indulgent. It's definitely not letting your offspring play you against each other. Thanks be to Mike Roizen, Mehmet Oz, Ted Spiker, Lisa Oz, and everybody on the team for helping all of us make a better generation. Our children are our future.

From Linda G. Kahn:

Many thanks to Drs. Mehmet Oz and Mike Roizen for the opportunity to engage intellectually with a subject I've been immersed in personally for the past twelve years—raising young children. To Drs. Nancy Roizen and Ellen Rome for providing a weekly tutorial on the latest approaches to caring for children's mental and physical health. To Craig Wynett for stretching my brain and to Ted Spiker for lightening my prose. To Jackie Skeris for her thoughtful insights. And most of all to my husband, Rob, and my three research subjects, Elliot, Eva, and Leda.

From Ellen Rome:

Many people contributed to the shaping of my thoughts that provided content for this book. First and foremost, I thank my father, Dr. Leonard P. Rome, the best pediatrician I've ever known, for his amazing role modeling that impacts daily my approach to the care of all children, and for allowing me to participate as he edited the American Academy of Pediatrics book, *Caring for Your Infant and Young Child*. Second, I thank my mother, Nancy Rome, whose wisdom I use daily in raising our children, and whose support allows me to engage in much of what I enjoy doing today, at work and at home. Thanks to Dr. Barb Kaplan, pediatric gastroenterologist par excellence, for her editing pearls in chapter 6. I thank my general pediatric colleagues, particularly Drs. Elaine Schulte, Allison Brindle, Kim Giuliano, and Laura Gillespie, for their keen intellects, their editing skills when asked, and along with pediatric infectious disease specialist Dr. Johanna Goldfarb, their strength in trying to steer this book closer to an evidence-based approach with respect to content, particularly around the vaccine debate. Our cheers for the AAP and CDC vaccine recommendations continue to ring loudly in my ears! Hopefully those particular vaccine recommendations will resonate with our readers, too, and safely keep more of the world fully immunized and protected.

I would also like to thank Craig Wynett for helping me find Big Ideas in some of the most interesting places, to Ted for training in how best to "Spikerize" text, to Linda Kahn and Nancy Roizen for providing voices of sanity and wisdom when debates got interesting, and especially to Drs. Mike Roizen and Mehmet Oz for allowing me the privilege of working with them and learning from them weekly and often daily.

Last, I thank my husband Fred, as best friend, soul mate, support cast, and wise parent with our own two munchkins. His sense of humor and calm presence bring light to my soul and spring to my step. Andrew and Katherine, thanks for tolerating Mommy's weekly Sunday seven a.m. conference calls and weekend time on the computer. All the work makes each Sunday breakfast and every family dinner all the more precious!

Index

A+D ointment, 147, 314
ABC (Airway, Breathing, Circulation), 278
ABC (Antecedents, Behavior, Consequences), 424
abdomen. *See* stomach
abnormal development, 63–67
absentee parents, 10, 25, 26
abuse, 22, 69, 92, 96, 160, 328
accidents/injuries
    and child-proofing the home, 251–57
    cleaning up after, 149
    family plan about, 243
    risks of, 240–42
    See also type of accident or injury
acellular pertussis, 406, 407, 408, 409
acetaminophen, 174, 177, 188, 189, 208, 211, 272, 274, 275
acid, 161–62, 188
acne, 225
actions
    and abnormal development, 64
    and brain, 48, 78
    consequence of, 38
    imitating, 79
    and parenting styles, 22
    and paying attention to children, 28
    and River of Dreams analogy, 4, 5, 20
    You Tips about, 38
    See also specific action or behavior
activity. *See* exercise
acute lymphocytic leukemia, 437
ADHD (Attention Deficit/ Hyperactivity Disorder), 29, 64, 127, 282, 283, 423–24
adolescent psychiatrists, 282
adoption, 439–41
African Americans, 228, 239, 268
AIDS. *See* HIV-AIDS
airborne allergies, 197–98, 200, 201

Airplane (standing exercise), 383
alcohol, 114, 229, 246, 247, 253
Allegra, 201
allergic salute, 194
allergic shiners, 194
allergies
    airborne, 197–98, 200, 201
    and breast feeding, 204, 211
    and breathing, 200, 203, 212
    and "clean" and "dirty" hypotheses, 194–95, 195*n*
    contact, 209
    diagnosis and treatment of, 199–202, 232, 272
    evolution of, 193–95
    Factoids about, 154, 194, 202
    and firstborn children, 195
    food, 110, 120, 121, 124, 197, 198–99, 200, 201, 203–4, 210, 211, 222
    and formula feeding, 211
    and genetics, 204
    and GI system, 197, 203
    and gluten, 158, 162–63
    and immune system, 192–93, 197, 210
    intolerance distinguished from, 158*n*
    as mimicking cold symptoms, 199
    and obesity, 202
    "outgrowing," 197, 199, 211
    parental assertiveness about, 210
    and pets, 210, 212
    and pregnancy, 204
    prevalence of, 192, 196–97
    and RAST test, 201
    risks of, 210
    and River of Life, 302
    and skin, 219, 220, 224, 226
    symptoms of, 194, 196, 197, 199, 200, 211
    triggers for, 196, 198, 209–10
    types of, 198

    You Tips about, 162–63, 209–12
    See also anaphylaxis; asthma
aluminum acetate, 221
Alzheimer's, 395
American Academy of Pediatrics (AAP)
    brain–screen time study by, 97
    day care recommendations of, 326
    and finding the right pediatrician, 261–62
    as source of information, 270
    and vaccinations, 261–62, 393, 394, 396, 397, 398, 401, 402, 406–7, 415
American Board of Medical Specialties, 260, 281
amygdala, 18, 19
anal fissure, 152, 164
anaphylaxis, 197, 199, 201, 202–4, 231
anemia, 135, 440. *See also* sickle–cell anemia
anger, 39, 104–5
animals. *See* pets/animals
antacids, 154
anti–inflammatories, 207, 250
antibacterial products, 107, 168
antibiotics
    and allergies, 195*n*
    and asthma, 195*n*
    and burns, 246
    and colds, 177
    and cuts, 248
    and ideal medicine cabinet, 272
    for infections, 175, 176, 177, 179, 180–81, 182, 185, 190, 227, 305
    introduction of, 195*n*
    and salmonella, 156
    taking, 275
    and unnecessary medications, 271
    You Tips about, 190

Whole Wheat Brownie Bites
(recipe), 372
Whole Wheat Pizza Dough
(recipe), 330–31
whooping cough, 395, 400, 406,
407, 408, 409, 410
windows: child-proofing, 245,
252
witch hazel, 239
words, 4, 53, 56, 57, 58, 65, 71, 72,
77. *See also* vocabulary
working parents, 288
wounds, 273, 278, 279. *See also*
accidents/injuries; cuts/
scrapes
wrestling, good-natured, 105

X-rays, 244

yards: child-proofing, 255
yeast infections, 116–17, 147,
225, 226
Yellow Spaghetti (recipe), 366

"Yes" points, 290
You: Having a Baby (Roizen and
Oz), 315, 392
YOU: On a Diet (Roizen and
Oz), 131*n*, 144*n*
You Tips
and being the leader, 104
and comforting your child,
104–5
about establishing a healthy
household, 137
and letting your child explore,
38
and letting your child lead, 39
and mental development, 38
and pointing things out, 72
about taking care of yourself,
139
about talking smart, 137
See also specific topic
You Tools
and babysitters/mother's
helpers, 327–28

and choosing a day care center,
325–27
and choosing a nanny, 324–25
and discipline, 417–19
and family fitness, 376–91
and family-friendly recipes,
329–75
and home-based child care,
327
and newborn survival guide,
311–22
and other caregivers, 323–328
on taking child's temperature,
191
and vaccines, 392–416
"Young Living Oils": as
aromatherapy source, 273

Zero to Three, 46*n*
zinc oxide, 238
Zithromax, 180*n*
zoos: visits to, 212
Zyrtec, 201, 272

ABOUT THE AUTHORS

MICHAEL F. ROIZEN, M.D., is a four-time *New York Times* number one best-selling author, and is cofounder and originator of the very popular RealAge.com website. He is chief wellness officer and chair of the Wellness Institute of the Cleveland Clinic and chief medical consultant of *The Doctor Oz Show*.

MEHMET C. OZ, M.D., is also a *New York Times* number one best-selling author and Emmy Award–winning host of *The Dr. Oz Show*. He is professor and vice chairman of surgery at New York Presbyterian Hospital/Columbia University Medical Center and the director of the Heart Institute.